Sex Guides

Garland Reference Library of Social Science
Vol. 312

Sex Guides

Books and Films About Sexuality for Young Adults

Patty Campbell

Garland Publishing, Inc.
New York & London
1986

The first seven chapters of this book were originally published by R. R. Bowker in 1979 as *Sex Education Books for Young Adults, 1892–1979.*

Library of Congress Cataloging-in-Publication Data

Campbell, Patricia J.
Sex guides.

(Garland reference library of social science ; vol. 312)
"The first seven chapters of this book were originally published by R. R. Bowker in 1979 as Sex education books for young adults, 1892–1979"—T.p. verso.
Includes bibliographies.
1. Sex instruction literature—United States.
2. Sex instruction for youth—United States. I. Title.
II. Series: Garland reference library of social science ; v. 312.
[DNLM: 1. Sex Behavior—in adolescence. 2. Sex education.
HQ 35 C189s]
HQ35.C28 1986 016.6139′5′088055 85-45108
ISBN 0-8240-8693-7 (alk. paper)

Cover design by Alison Lew

Printed on acid-free, 250-year-life paper
Manufactured in the United States of America

Acknowledgments

No book is an island. Many people deserve thanks for their share in this one: Gary Kuris, who saved me from split infinitives and the slough of despond with his meticulous and helpful editing and his witty correspondence; Mary K. Chelton, for sharing journals, papers, clippings, and her extensive knowledge of the field of sex education; Joan Atkinson, for extending the geographic coverage of the chapter on religious sex guides; Joni Bodart, for listening and caring and making me laugh when I needed it; and most of all my husband David Shore, for patient counsel and wise comfort.

I wish also to thank the following for permission to reprint illustrations:

Drawings by Ruth Belew from *Facts of Life and Love for Teenagers*, by Evelyn Duvall. Revised edition, New York: Association Press, 1956. Copyright 1950, 1956 by the National Board of the Young Men's Christian Associations. Reprinted by permission of the National Board of the Young Men's Christian Associations.

Drawings by Edward C. Smith from *Love and Sex in Plain Language*, by Eric Johnson. Revised edition, Philadelphia: J. B. Lippincott, 1967. Illustrations copyright 1965, 1967 by Edward C. Smith. Reprinted by permission of Harper and Row Publishers, Inc.

Drawing by Roger Conant from *Ten Heavy Facts About Sex*, by Sol Gordon. Fayetteville, N.Y.: Ed-U, 1971. Copyright Ed-U Press. Also reprinted in *You!* by Sol Gordon with Roger Conant. New York: Quadrangle, 1975. Copyright Sol Gordon. Reprinted by permission of Ed-U Press and Times Books, a division of Random House, Inc.

Drawing by Vivien Cohen from *Facts About Sex for Today's Youth*, by Sol Gordon. Fayetteville, N.Y.: Ed-U, 1985. Copyright Vivien Cohen. Reprinted by permission of Ed-U Press.

Jacket illustration by Janet Halverson from *Forever*, by Judy Blume. New York: Bradbury, 1975. Copyright 1975 by Judy Blume. Reprinted by permission of Bradbury Press, an affiliate of Macmillan, Inc.

Photograph by David Crawford from *Teenage Marriage: Coping with Reality*, by Jeanne Warren Lindsay. Buena Park, Calif.: Morning Glory Press, 1984. Copyright Jeanne Warren Lindsay. Reprinted by permission of Morning Glory Press, Inc.

Photograph by Kim Ecclesine from the film *Condom Sense*. Reprinted by permission of Perennial Education, Inc.

Contents

Preface

We are in the midst of a sex information crisis. Although it is impossible to open a magazine, turn on the radio or TV, or even cross the street without being bombarded by images of sexiness, too many of our teenagers are growing up as practicing sexual illiterates. Studies reveal their ignorance, but so do the statistics on adolescent pregnancy and sexually transmitted disease.

How can this be when there are so many books on the market—115, by my last count—that try to teach young people how to manage their sexuality? Why is it that worried teens and embarrassed parents so seldom seek out these books for answers to their urgent questions? With such a wealth of sex guides for every degree of reading skill and social sophistication and every kind of religious or political orientation, we should long ago have made the right sex information connection for every teen and put all to rights. (Not an impossible goal, as the examples of modern Sweden and Holland show beyond dispute.)

It was to find some of the answers to this puzzle and to offer help in correcting it that I set out to write this book. My goal has been to provide the definitive guide to sex guides, a resource that will give background and understanding and specific title suggestions to librarians, teachers, parents, youth advocates, and young adults themselves.

The history of the teen sex manual is a fascinating revelation of American attitudes toward adolescent sexuality and a vital key to understanding the current problem. The first section of *Sex Guides*, then, traces that development. Since the beginning of the form in 1892 there have been nearly four hundred such books written for young adults. I set myself the task of tracking down and evaluating all of them, and I believe I have come as close as is humanly possible. For the research I visited the Library of Congress and the library of the Kinsey Institute for Research in Sex, Gender, and Reproduction of Indiana University. I also made heavy use of the collections of Los Angeles City Public Library, the University of California at Los Angeles, the University of Southern California, the Los Angeles County Medical Library, and, through interlibrary loan, dozens of other scholarly libraries in the United States.

The second, and larger, section of *Sex Guides* is a detailed analysis of the patterns, content, and usefulness of all the contemporary manifestations of the genre. For this I have expanded my sights to include not only modern versions of the traditional teen sex guide but also other sources of noncurricular sex education information, both print and audiovisual. Young adult fiction is an often-overlooked but extremely effective source of sexual learning, and here I have tried to show what it is and is not teaching. With the swing to conservativism religious sex education books are becoming a necessary part of library collections; I have made an objective effort to explore evangelical, liberal Protestant, Catholic, and Jewish sex guides. The books that have evolved from the sex guides to explore a particular aspect of teen sexuality—venereal disease, contraception, pregnancy, homosexual identity, and so forth—are analyzed. A chapter on audiovisual sex education, by Susan B. Madden, evaluates film, from *Porky's* to *Condom Sense*. The last chapter and appendixes suggest some books for parents and professionals, review sources, an evaluation checklist, core-collection and weeding bibliographies and other tools, and encouragement for adults who care about teenagers and who know that sex guides can never be fully effective unless we become fully effective sex guides.

Patty Campbell

Then—

Introduction

The willingness of the adult world to share with young people whatever accurate and valid information on sexual and reproductive behavior we possess constitutes one of our best gestures of confidence and communication in their direction.
—DR. MARY CALDERONE

The history of the sex guide for adolescents documents the quite unconscious movement of our culture's ideas about sex and youth, revealing the heritage of our own sexual beliefs and codes of behavior. As we shall see, the one characteristic of sex education for young people in America from Victorian to modern times has been the reluctance of sex educators, other professionals and parents to tell teenagers what they really need to know about sex. Indeed, from their first appearance, sex guides for young adults have aimed primarily at preventing them from engaging in any sexual expression whatsoever outside of marriage.

While the theme of sex prevention is most blatant in the earlier manuals, as recently as the 1960s (and now again in the conservative eighties) sex guides have continued to emphasize the dangers of venereal disease and illegitimate pregnancy rather than the cure and prevention of these conditions. Spreading that helpful information was often defined by society in the past as obscene and/or illegal. Generation after generation American teenagers have been taught to fear and deny the impulses of their own bodies. Along with this learning they were indoctrinated with rigid gender roles: girls have been taught to muffle their humanity, to pretend and withdraw and reject, and boys have been indoctrinated with the idea that becoming a man means rigid self-control and muscular effort. The wonder is that so many people have been able to have happy and fulfilling sex lives in spite of these teachings. Nor does harm from this early conditioning pass away from society in twenty or thirty years. Many of the older legislators, judges, and corporate executives now in power absorbed their joyless attitudes toward sexuality and life from Victorian sex education. One source for the just but destructive anger that has hampered the Women's Movement can be found in the dating manuals of the 1950s that preached sexism to young girls now in their forties.

The authors of these books were not conscious villains. They simply reflected the attitudes and apprehension of our fundamentally sex-negative society. Only in the past few years have sex educators begun to acknowledge teenage sexuality to the point of providing young people with the realistic advice and practical information they need to live safely and responsibly. Today a sex education book that is older than ten years is a road map to a country that no longer exists.

Teen sex guides form a true literary genre. They show "a distinct style, form, and content," as the dictionary specifies. Whether the tone is pompous or jazzy, the intent is always to teach teenagers the currently approved sexual behavior for their age group. The content is a combination of anatomical and medical information and ethical exhortation, with the proportions varying according to fashion and each author's expertise. The few books that discuss only ethics or only physiology have usually felt it necessary to justify the one-sidedness of their approach. Despite such variations the genre can be seen as a unique type with its own conventions and even its own jargon (surely the word "petting" was never used in ordinary speech).

The historical development of the sex education book is internally consistent. The authors imitated each other shamelessly, making minor revisions to the established pattern of advice while offering their own works as the first adequate books on the subject. With enthusiastic scorn they often denounced their predecessors' work as worthless and even vicious. The current of social opinion is accurately mirrored in these books, and even minute changes in society's position can be detected in the adjustments made in successive editions of a particular title. Sex guides were the first nonfiction (and perhaps the first fiction) written exclusively for teenagers. Their existence may even have helped form our modern concept of adolescence as a special, dangerous time sectioned off between childhood and adult status.

It is possible to lose sight of a delightful aspect of the old sex guides. These earnest and antiquated pages are quaint, surprising, and often irresistibly funny to modern eyes. Henry Miller is reputed to have summed up sex in America as "Do it in the dark, and for God's sake, don't giggle!" As you read on to find out what every young man should know, it will be quite all right to giggle occasionally.

Chapter 1

What Every Young Man Should Know

"What every young man should know" is a piece of American folklore, a phrase that evokes earnest but irrelevant mini-instruction in sex, a mythical title whose mention evokes snickers and knowing leers. Was there ever actually such a book? Did it deserve the snickers and leers with which it has been remembered? Was this prototype of American sex education a reality?

Not only did it exist, it existed in six editions and eleven translations. It had seven companion volumes that provided sex instruction for both sexes from cradle to grave. It was much admired, widely read, and, although not the first of its genre, set the tone for the sex education of teenagers for fifty years. The many chapters of elementary biology, tracing the reproductive process from the simplest forms of life up to mammals, are remembered as "the birds and the bees"—a phrase that became a common metaphor for embarrassed and clumsy attempts to communicate the facts of life. But most of all the book is characterized by its hortatory tone, its dire warnings and deliberate avoidance of the urgent questions of the young—features of most sex education books for teenagers up until nearly the present day.

The title behind the myth was actually *What a Young Boy Ought to Know*, which the folk memory, with its own aesthetics, has rounded off to the more rhythmic "What every young man should know." It was written by Sylvanus Stall, a retired Lutheran minister with an astute business sense (one of his first books was *How to Pay Church Debts, and How to Keep Churches Out of Debt*). In his career as a sex educator, or "purity advocate," Stall put his clerical background and business savvy to good use. With the success of *Young Boy* Stall almost immediately launched the more ambitious project of producing a series of age-oriented advice manuals based on its format. In the same year in which *Young Boy* was published Stall wrote a sequel for older teens, *What a Young Man Ought to Know*, and a third book, for the newly married male, *What a Young Husband Ought to Know*. Turning to the market for the other half of the human race, he contracted with Dr. Mary Wood-Allen to write companion volumes for girls and women. In 1897 she wrote *What a Young Girl Ought to Know* and the next year turned out *What a Young Woman Ought to Know*. Rounding out the series in the three years, Stall added *What a Man of Forty-five Ought to Know* (1901) and asked another woman doctor, Emma F. Drake, to write *What a Young Wife Ought to Know* (1901) and *What a Woman of Forty-five Ought to Know* (1902).

These eight books were marketed as the Self and Sex series; "Purity and Truth" is embossed on the cover and heads the title page. The portrait of the author in clerical collar that appears on the frontispiece shows a neatly combed man with a modest beard and kindly eyes behind gold-rimmed spectacles. The series was heavily promoted under the slogan "Pure books on avoided subjects." Every volume bears copious advertisements for the others in the series, some even including facsimile pages of translations into French, German, Spanish, Dutch, Swedish, Japanese, Korean, Hindi, Bengali, Telugu, and Persian-Urdu. In 1907 Stall wrote a guidebook for his sales staff, entitled *Successful Selling of the Self and Sex Series*.

Each book opens with a dozen pages of "Commendations from Eminent Men and Women," including citations from officers of the American Purity Alliance, the Society for Moral and Sanitary Prophylaxis, and the Women's Christian Temperance Union, as well as a number of prominent clergymen and evangelists. Accompanying the citations are a series of stiff portraits depicting grim-visaged figures in high collars or muttonchop whiskers. Ironically, early editions included a commendation from Anthony Comstock, solicitor of the U.S. Post Office and sponsor of the prudish obscenity laws that were to hinder American sex education until 1971. Although this impressive gallery warded off any suspicion of lasciviousness or erotic intent on the part of the authors or publisher, the medical authorities were

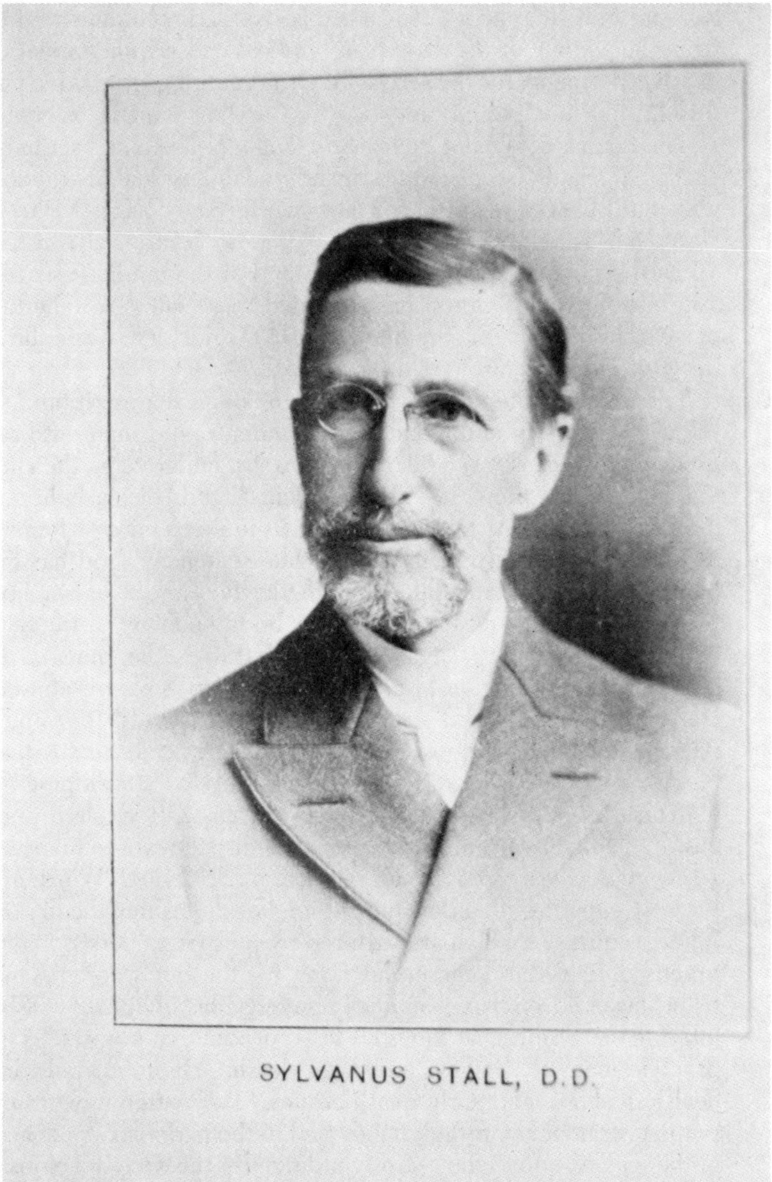

Fig. 1. The Reverend Sylvanus Stall, author of *What a Young Boy Ought to Know*.

cautious in their approval. In 1901 this reserved recommendation from the *Journal of the American Medical Association* appeared in advertisements for the series: "We find nothing from which to dissent, but much to commend."

The format of *What a Young Boy Ought to Know* is a series of chats supposedly recorded on cylinders (audiovisual instruction was modish even in 1897) for a young teenager named Harry. Harry has asked, on the occasion of the birth of a baby sister, "Where do babies come from?" A friend of the family has been asked to instruct him and has recorded these talks "to take the place of his dear mama's nightly visits to the nursery" while she is busy with the new baby.

The first chapters are a heavily theological description of "God's purpose in endowing plants, animals, and man with reproductive organs." We hear about Adam and Eve as the first parents, "father, mother, and baby plants," and "the early life of the baby oyster." At the end of Part I the mechanics of human reproduction are dispensed with in one sentence: "God has ordained that the ovum, while yet in the body of the wife, shall be fertilized by the requisite and proper bodily contact of the husband." Part II warns against masturbation—"the manner in which the reproductive organs are injured in boys by abuse." Harry is told about "God's purpose in giving us hands" (or rather, what is *not* God's purpose in giving us hands). He learns that "some boys weaken and disease their bodies by developing an unnatural appetite for vinegar, salt, cloves, coffee, slate pencils. . . ." Such habits diminish a boy's ability to resist temptation and may lead to the practice of secret and social vice. "Words are scarcely capable," thunders the author, "of describing the dreadful consequences which are suffered by those who persist in this practise." Self-abuse causes suffering for the boy's parents and sister, his children may be born in poverty, his offspring will be inferior because he has "injured his reproductive powers." The practice leads to "idiocy, and even death." His mind fails, his health declines, and early death ensues. "Boys often have to be put in a straitjacket or their hands tied to the bedposts or to rings in the wall." A boy who secretly indulges in this vice develops a shifty glance and "pulls his cap down so as to hide his eyes" when passing people in the street. The closing chapters admonish boys to recover their purity through self-control and to help their comrades do the same. "It is our duty to aid others to avoid pernicious habits and to retain or regain their purity and strength."

As strange as this book may seem to us today, the views it expresses were solidly rooted in the accepted beliefs of the time. In particular Stall's diatribe against masturbation offers significant clues to the Victorian concept of the nature of sexuality and begins to suggest why sex education books for young people began to appear almost explosively at that time in history.

▪ Self-Control in Victorian Sexuality

Lack of restraint in sexual matters was seen throughout much of the nineteenth century as not only morally wrong but also physically and socially harmful. A metaphor that came to be accepted by the late Victorians as scientific fact was the idea that a man's physical, mental, and spiritual health depended upon the retention of semen within the body. Conversely, loss of semen was interpreted as a loss of the essence of vitality. In an unpublished paper titled "The Origins of Sex Education in America 1890–1920: An Inquiry into Victorian Sexuality" Bryan Strong explores how this pseudoscientific theory was used to explain the need to suppress sexuality:

> This theory, which possessed remarkable similarities to Freud's theory of sublimation, was a materialistic explanation of biological and intellectual growth. It stated essentially that the testes, "through some hidden and not yet understood process slowly secreted cells" within the semen which, if the semen were not expended, were absorbed by the blood. The absorption of these cells enabled the young male to develop his body, let his voice become masculine, and grow a full beard. If the physically mature man refrained from sexual excesses and remained continent, then the semen was absorbed by the blood and was carried to the brain where it was "coined into new thoughts—perhaps new inventions—grand conceptions of the true, the beautiful, the useful, or into fresh emotions of joy and impulses of kindness." This explanation, however much disguised as science, in reality reflected Victorian morality since its actual function was to offer positive rewards for sexual repression.

As Strong further explains, the Victorians believed that man's sexual behavior was the model and source for the rest of his character; the habits of restraint developed in that area led to the acquisition of "the Victorian constellation of values which included work, industry, good habits, piety, and noble ideals. Indeed, without sexual repression the Victorians believed that it was impossible for those other values to exist in an ideal character. If a man were pure, he was also frugal, hard-working, temperate, and governed by habit. If, on the other hand, he were impure, he was also a spend-thrift, disposed to speculation, whisky-drinking, and ruled by his impulses."

By expending his seminal power in illicit intercourse, masturbation, lewd thoughts leading to nocturnal emissions, or even excesses in the marriage bed, a man would damage his health drastically. He would waste away, become pale, hollow-cheeked, and silly. He might contract venereal disease, develop "spermatorrhea" (a chronic and involuntary loss of semen), or go insane; his business might fail and he would surely die an early death. Charles Scudder, in *Hand-book for Young Men*, phrased this idea succinctly in 1892: "Bodily vigor and moral integrity depend on personal purity. This great force curbed and restrained, expends itself in the business of life and makes a man useful and successful."

Purity and self-restraint were equally important within the marriage bond. A husband's responsibility to maintain his own health and purity was inextricably bound with his obligation to his family, which resulted in a curious bifurcation of the sexual impulse. Although the restrained expression of sex within marriage was holy and spiritual (the family was the cornerstone of Victorian society and the center of a woman's life as wife and mother), uncontrolled sex between married couples was physical and base. If a man were impure, his wife's health could be ruined by contact with him.

Furthermore, because the Victorians subscribed to Lamarckian theories of heredity, they also believed that the presumed effects of sexual misconduct could be passed on to one's offspring in the form of tendencies toward dissipation.

Thus the vehemence of Stall's argument against masturbation in *What a Young Boy Ought to Know* is typical of Victorian pleas for self-restraint. The purity advocates were most especially concerned that young people should not learn "solitary vice." It was not only the significance they attached to the loss of semen, however, that inspired such strong emotions in addressing the young. The masturbatory act is done solely for pleasure; it can be carried on in secret and is easily hidden from parents; and, most important, it sets a pattern for adult sexual attitudes. A teenager who masturbates is finding out that sex feels good, a very dangerous piece of knowledge by Victorian standards. On the other hand, a boy who can be taught to look on his own genitals and their needs with loathing and fear has been taught to repress sexuality all his life.

Ronald Walters, in *Primers for Prudery*, an excellent survey of mid-Victorian sexual attitudes, carries this explanation even further: "The authorities continually harped on masturbation's supposedly self-destructive nature: it was self-abuse and self-pollution. There could scarcely be a more straightforward way of representing sex as a personal impulse with which each human being (including authors of advice manuals, presumably) must struggle. Concern for masturbation, then, easily became a screen upon which to project one's own unconscious battle with drives that orthodox morality demanded be subjugated." Walters also points out that concern about masturbation increased as changes in nineteenth-century society created new opportunities for privacy and solitary indulgence. Such social factors included "the isolation experienced by new arrivals to urban areas, simultaneous production of larger homes and smaller families, the growth of boarding schools, [and the] increasing removal of middle-class children from the workday world of adults."

The clarion call to parents to face the task of instructing the young in the heretofore unmentionable facts of life was being issued as early as the 1880s, around the same time that anti-masturbation pamphlets for young men had begun to appear. During most of the Victorian era the accepted method of sex education had been deliberate silence, but now parents were becoming increasingly concerned that their children would acquire bad habits from their peers if they were not carefully supervised and provided with the armor of "right knowledge." ("Ignorance is vice," erroneously attributed to Plato, appears on the title page of *What a Young Boy Ought to Know*).

George Franklin Hall, in an 1892 book titled *Plain Points on*

Personal Purity, or Startling Sins of the Sterner Sex, lists signs of self-abuse to alert parents to their sons' possible debauchery. Adults were to watch for any or all of the following: change in character (from cheerful, obedient, energetic to irritable, sullen, stupid, reticent); decline in health; precocious development ("a senile look") or deficiency in development; unnatural lassitude, especially in the morning; love of being alone; shyness or boldness (to hide inability to look a person in the eye); strange appetities for clay, chalk, and slate pencils; use of tobacco; round shoulders; an unnaturally stiff, wriggling gait; twitching; a decided preference for the society of little girls; pain in the back, headache, full veins, bedwetting, palpitations, pimples (especially on the forehead), epilepsy, or wet palms; abnormal development or underdevelopment of the parts; and stains on underclothing or bedding.

Once detected, however, a wayward boy should not be made to feel that all hope is lost, warns Hall. Lest he become discouraged at seeking salvation and sink into a slough of self-gratification, the youth should be reassured that the effects of masturbation are almost entirely reversible for those who learn self-mastery. As we shall see, Hall and his contemporaries provide a variety of techniques for developing the requisite mastery, ranging from hymn singing to sitting in a bowl of ice water.

Published by the White Cross Committee of the Young Men's Christian Association, a group pledged to the promotion of purity, Scudder's *Hand-book for Young Men* also appeared in 1892. Despite the title the book is addressed to parents and other sex educators. The tone of righteousness and missionary purpose is immediately apparent in the opening paragraphs: "The light of knowledge must shed abroad in larger measure, in order to drive away the darkness. This book has been prepared to arm the advocates of purity with arguments wherewith to meet their adversaries." Scudder expounds at length on the necessity for conserving seminal power, the theme that was to appear regularly for the next forty years, and ends on a note of patriotism: "So we conclude our short work with a purely American question addressed to each reader. Does impurity pay? If not, then join your heart, mind, and soul with ours to fight down this hideous vice, and let us all unite in a determined effort to be pure ourselves, to esteem the purity of woman, and to uphold the pure honor of America!"

▪ A New Genre

The years between 1892 and 1920 saw the publication of several dozen sex education tracts addressed to adolescents themselves. Advice manuals for married people and for youth in their twenties had already become plentiful by this time, but the book meant for the teenager's own reading was an innovation. Indeed, the very idea of "teenage" is a Victorian invention, as Walters reminds us: "Nineteenth century writers also fashioned the concept of adolescence, an idea we take for granted although it is actually of comparatively recent origin (previous generations simply expected youth to assume adult duties at a far younger age than at present). Cautionary literature, with its continual fretting about resisting sexual activity in the decade or more between puberty and marriage, encouraged people to regard these years as a special time with special problems (including sexual ones). . . ."

Why was it that sex education books for the young appeared so suddenly and in such quantity at the turn of the century? The ideas they expounded had been generally accepted for most of the nineteenth century, but in the late Victorian era the signs of a disintegration of the old social order, such as those mentioned by Walters in regard to the increased isolation of the individual, aroused an urgency about preserving the sexual attitudes that had been one of its foundations. As the Industrial Revolution grew in America, the work ethic of frugality and self-denial began to give way to an ethic of consumption and self-indulgence. This was inevitably reflected in a loosening of regard for accepted sexual attitudes. New scientific research led to a more realistic understanding of the mechanics of sex—the functioning of the union of the sperm and the ovum, for instance, was discovered in 1875. From the other side of the Atlantic the early works of Freud, Shaw, and Havelock Ellis were challenging accepted sexual ideas. (Although the first title of Ellis's monumental *Studies in the Psychology of Sex* was published in England in 1897, the complete seven-volume work was available in the United States only to the medical profession until 1935.)

These and other advocates of sex as pleasure (the free-lovers of the Oneida Community, for example, who practiced group marriage) panicked the American late Victorians into energetic attempts to indoctrinate the young. The very core of their civilization was challenged. Having long ago eschewed the more relaxed attitudes of the eighteenth and early nineteenth centuries, the late Victorians were convinced that sexual restraint was essential to the development of the individual and the progress of society. Ignoring the lessons of history regarding what Walters has called "cycles of frankness," they now prepared to do battle with the return of that cycle in the twentieth century.

Thus, with the convergence of all these social, psychological, and historical factors, a new literary genre, the sex education book for young adults, emerged. The first true example of the genre that appears in the comprehensive subject catalog of the Kinsey Institute is *Confidential Talks with Young Men* (1892), by Lyman Beecher Sperry, which will be examined in some detail later in this chapter. A second book also published in 1892 is the little volume titled *Almost Fourteen*, by Mortimer A. Warren, which centers its call to purity on the key concept of modesty; one of its chapters relates the harrowing tale of John Onan the masturbator. Other early examples predating the Self and Sex Series are *Almost a Man* (1895), by Mary Wood-Allen, also to be examined in this chapter, and the companion volumes for girls, *Confidential Talks with Young Women* (1893), by Sperry, and *Almost a Woman* (1897), by Wood-Allen, discussed in Chapter 2. The primary purpose of all these early works was to provide just enough anatomical explanation to blunt the curiosity of the young so that they would not seek information from their contemporaries and to warn them away from any sexual thoughts, feelings, or actions.

Stall and Predecessors

Stall's second book for the Self and Sex series, *What a Young Man Ought to Know* (1897), is a predictable product of the foregoing purposes and beliefs. Written for men in their late teens and early twenties, it begins with praise for the value of physical strength, which, of course, results from sexual self-mastery. Stall warns that although lack of personal purity (secret vice) can lead to unmanly weakness, as well as many other horrid conditions, losses of the seminal fluid in sleep are not necessarily abnormal. (Obsessed as they were with sexual control, the Victorians apparently found the prospect of involuntary loss of semen, even in sleep, alarming.) In any case young men should be aware of the

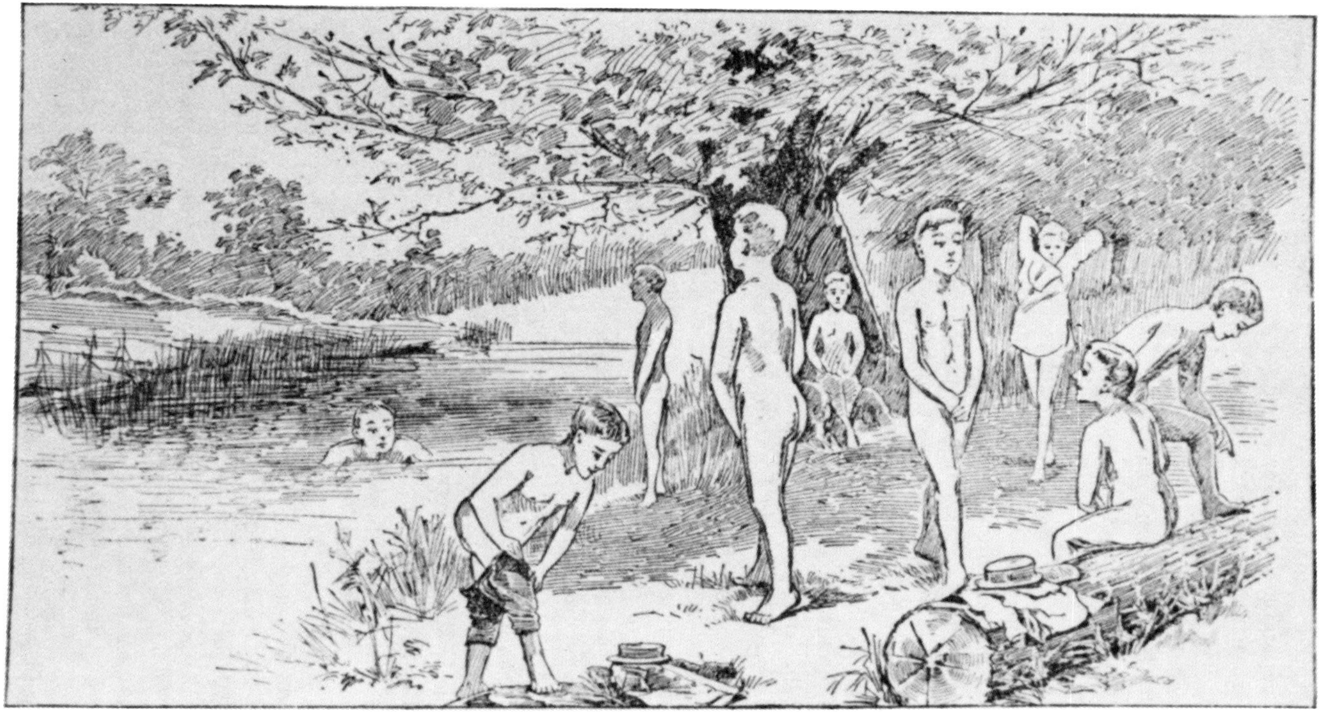

Fig. 2. Modesty. From *Almost Fourteen*, by Mortimer A. Warren.

dangers of consulting quacks and charlatans and seek advice only from reputable physicians.

Alarmed at the ignorance concerning the diseases that accompany vice, Stall presents a lurid picture of the symptoms and complications of gonorrhea and syphilis. He describes how healthy brides become early and permanent invalids and asks (without much hope), "Can it ever be cured?" A chapter on the reproductive organs follows, with some cautionary words on their purpose and their willful debasement. Marriage is a great blessing, he urges, but unbridled sexuality even within that institution can cause great unhappiness. In conclusion, a man should get all the help he can for self-mastery by the right choice of companions, books, pictures, and recreation. He should eschew liquor and tobacco, rise early, and adopt habits of industry. He should rely on the influence of an ennobling affection and, most of all, honor the Sabbath, the church, and the Bible.

Of the other Self and Sex titles for boys and men, *What a Young Husband Ought To Know* (1897) first warns against sexual excesses in marriage and the miseries visited on a marriage by vice in earlier years and then discusses the nature of woman ("God has fitted her for her sphere") and the joys of parenthood and the family. *What a Man of Forty-five Ought to Know* (1901) is that he should at that age enter in a "sexual hush" and prepare himself for some strange behavior from his wife as she goes into menopause. A description of the physical changes and mental manifestations of menopause follows, and the book ends with some cheering words on the "character of hospitals of mental sickness." The four titles for females by Emma Drake and Mary Wood-Allen will be discussed in the next chapter.

Let us look now at Stall's predecessors. Although *What a Young Boy Ought to Know* was the first book of its kind to win wide acceptance, a much more informative work had been published five years earlier in 1892—*Confidential Talks with Young Men,* by Lyman Beecher Sperry (the companion volume, *Confidential Talks with Young Women*, was written by Sperry a year later). A comparison of Stall's and Sperry's books suggests that *Confidential Talks with Young Men* may have provided the pattern for the early chapters of *Young Boy*. Sperry was a "lecturer on Sanitary Science at Carleton College" and a physician. His straightforward and unornamented style and knowledgeable descriptions of anatomy and sexual acts indicate a man of science accustomed to dealing with matters of fact. Sperry also reveals a sense of admiration and wonder for the intricacies of nature that sometimes emerges in un-Victorian metaphors, such as "Flowers are the sex organs of plants." He evidently felt no need for the theological justification and bombast that Stall later employed, although Sperry was no less devoted to the promotion of purity.

Confidential Talks with Young Men opens with an introduction addressed to parents. Explaining the newly felt need for sex education, he urges parents, teachers, and physicians to teach the facts of sex so the young will not get "venomous ideas from corrupt playmates." Although knowledge is not a guarantee of pure living, it is far safer than ignorance or distorted and poisoned notions. There is no hope of raising boys in ignorance of sex; the world has tried it for centuries and failed, says Sperry, adding that since only 5 percent of American youth attend church regularly, there is also little hope for help from that quarter. The problem is serious: "Lust can truthfully claim more victims than tobacco even," and it is " the most common and most serious vice of youth." Explaining the importance to society of training in sexual control, Sperry points to "the far-reaching power of the reproductive system over every other organ and function" and declares that "vigor of body, strength of mind, and integrity of moral character depend largely on personal purity [and] on the proper development and use of the reproductive organs." Youths who indulge in unrestrained sex become defective specimens, passing on to their offspring not only "venereal disease and taints" but feeble bodies, unbalanced minds, and lustful tendencies.

After this introduction the book itself is addressed to boys in their midteens. The early chapters, as imitated by Stall, deal with the reproductive arrangements of various forms of life on an ascending scale of complexity. First he describes reproduction of plants, followed by "the multiplication of oysters and fishes," "the propagation of insects and birds," "the perpetuation of marsupials and mammals," and finally human reproduction. Here Sperry is at great pains to explain the differences between the male urinary and reproductive systems. A most peculiar diagram appears as illustration: all of the major parts of the male genital and urinary anatomy are labeled and described, including the penis and the testicles, but the latter two items do not appear in the drawing. Where they should be are only blank spaces with identifying numerals.

In the next chapter Sperry arrives at a vital subject: puberty and self-abuse. Sperry stresses the contrasts between the gelding and the stallion, the capon and the rooster, to show the benefits of proper masculine development. Since he, like his contemporaries, is convinced that this development depends on the body's reabsorption of sperm, the argument moves quite logically to an indictment of masturbation. He describes this act with surprising accuracy: "an artificial excitement of the penis sufficient to produce an erection and lustful desires terminating in a spasm of the sexual organ which, in those who are sufficiently developed, produces an emission of semen." Noting that "artificial excitement" may be achieved by imagination alone, inflamed by lustful thoughts, lewd reading, or indecent pictures, Sperry cautions that this is as harmful as manual manipulation. For the most part, however, he is cheerfully humanistic in emphasizing the healthy development of the reproductive system, although he mentions the "harvest of horrible conditions" reaped by the masturbator. Unlike Stall, he mercifully refrains from enumerating them.

Sperry then broaches the problem of nocturnal emissions, a source of considerable anxiety to male Victorians. He hastens to reassure the reader that nocturnal emissions are normal and natural. Frequent emissions may sometimes cause debility, but far more often the reverse is true—a weakened condition of the body leads to increased ejaculation. On the whole it would be better if semen were absorbed as produced "to spare the nervous system the shock of emission," but "in some cases . . . emissions really seem to clear up the brain and increase the sensation of bodily vigor."

Unnatural emissions, however, are another matter completely. Sperry advises readers to be alert to signs of spermatorrhea and passes on the widely accepted belief that this condition, "sad to contemplate and terrible to experience," can be caused by physical or mental self-abuse. However, spermatorrhea is not as common as many suppose, comforts Sperry.

For those young men who are worried by too-frequent emissions Sperry provides what was to become staple antimasturbation advice—a list of practical remedies. First, he says, indulge in no lustful thoughts; crowd them out by thinking of your mother's pure love, reading the Sermon on the Mount, praying for help, or singing a soul-stirring hymn. Eat a nonstimulating diet (avoid meat and eggs, pepper, mustard, spices); and avoid tea, coffee, alcohol, and tobacco. Choose physical labor in the open air instead of mental work. Get plenty of sleep and arise immediately on waking. Bathe often (but not every day). Seek the company of sensible women, and quit worrying about sexual matters.

Predictably Sperry uses the chapter on prostitution to demolish the myth of "sexual necessity" (the belief that a sexual outlet is needed for health) and to catalog the horrors of venereal disease. But he also takes the position that a male who visits a lady of the evening is as degraded as she—"a just human judgement will stamp the word prostitute on the one as surely as on the other." He estimates that one third of the population of civilized countries has, or will have, venereal disease and heightens the impact of this alarming statistic by providing vivid descriptions of the primary and secondary symptoms of "venereal ulcers—the Almighty's 'registered stamp' for the act of adultery." He attacks the rationalization, still heard today, that "gonorrhea is no more troublesome than a bad cold." Sperry warns that venereal disease can be transmitted by kissing (a common Victorian warning) but explains that the receiving party must have an open sore on the mouth (an *un*common clarification of that warning). He mentions no cure.

Next Sperry discourses eloquently on the evil of quackery. The intense sexual repressions and anxieties of young men must have made them easy prey for clever advertisements that played on their fears and ignorance. Newspapers were thick with ads by "experienced physicians" or "returned missionaries" promising to cure, for large sums of money, vaguely described sexual ills that might otherwise prove fatal. Lacking basic knowledge of their bodies' sexual functions, young men could easily be persuaded by the unscrupulous that even normal responses like nocturnal emissions were symptoms of disease. In this vacuum of ignorance any explanation was seized upon.

Sperry describes one of the forms of quackery that exploited this hunger for information—the "Museum of Anatomy." These shows (for men only) were free or charged only ten cents. On entering, the boys and men were treated to the sight of a nude reclining female figure in wax, usually copied from a famous painting. Proceeding with passions aroused, they viewed scenes of the horrors of the Inquisition or historical battles (the traditional duo of sex and violence). Next came lurid and exaggerated representations of the dreadful results of venereal disease, self-abuse, and other sexual excesses. As the trembling victim emerged, he was handed a pamphlet advertising a quack whose offices were nearby and who was available right then for consultation.

Sperry ends his book with a section of sensible advice on healthful living. He especially deplores the use of tobacco (an opinion that must have been amusing to readers in the first half of the century, but now, ironically, we find ourselves nodding in agreement). It is interesting to notice what Sperry does *not* include. There is no mention of normal human sexual intercourse, nor is there any talk of courting or marriage or the family. Sperry's only discussion of the relationship between the sexes is in reference to prostitution. Still, *Confidential Talks with Young Men* is extraordinarily candid for its time and deserved better than the oblivion it received.

Another forerunner of the Self and Sex series was *Almost a Man*, by Mary Wood-Allen, M.D., first published in 1895. Evidently it was this volume and its counterpart, *Almost a Woman* (1897), that brought Wood-Allen to the attention of Sylvanus Stall when he was casting about for someone with prestige and experience to write the volumes for women of his series. Wood-Allen was not shy about sex education; in 1892 she had written a booklet on the subject titled *Teaching Truth* ("Its sweet truth is like the breath of a May morning," claimed an advertisement), which was later expanded to become the flagship of the Teaching Truth series. And in 1895 she had written a treatise for laypeople on human physiology, a daring project for a woman, even if she was a doctor. This work had the cumbersome title *The Marvels of Our Bodily Dwelling: Physiology Made Interesting; Suitable as a Text-book or Reference Book in Schools, or for Pleasant Home Reading*. Some, but not all, of the editions of 1895 cautiously added a sixteen-page supplementary chapter, "The Birthchamber," which was also published separately as a pamphlet.

But it was the pseudo-fiction *Almost a Man* that most clearly showed Wood-Allen's devotion to the cause of purity. With its skeletal plot and didactic tone this book could be called the first young adult novel. Certainly it has all the earmarks of the genre that was developed in the 1950s by such writers as Jeannette Eyerly and Betty Cavanna, including the awkward attempt to use current teenage speech patterns, the depiction of an all-wise adult who advises the young person, and the transparent manipulation of plot to make a moral point.

As the book opens, four young boys—Guy, Frank, Carl, and Rob—are lolling about by a stream in a field, discussing how boring life is at home and how much fun it would be to run away. The author hints that one or two of the boys may have a more serious reason than boredom for wanting a change of scene—Guy, for instance, has a tendency to pull his cap down over his eyes. Along the road comes Dr. Lynn with her satchel, and seeing the boys up to no good, she crosses the field and sits down with them on a log. After a bit of conversation she senses the problems on their minds and invites them to come to her house the next week, with their parents' permission, to be told the facts of life. The boys are delighted and rush off to get the requisite parental consent.

A few days later Guy, cap in hand, appears on the doctor's doorstep. He has not been able to wait until the meeting to talk about his problem, and besides, he doesn't want the other fellows to know about it. Guy, as the reader has been led to suspect, is a self-abuser. He confesses his vice to Dr. Lynn, but she is not a bit shocked. Instead she gives him a pat on the back and some practical advice. Overcoming this evil practice takes willpower and he must train like an athlete to succeed, the doctor begins. Guy must give up tea and coffee, keep his bowels open, sleep on a hard bed, and get up the minute he wakes. And before retiring he must take a cold bath and then sit in a bowl of cold water. Dr. Lynn's encouraging words hearten Guy, and he goes away confident in his ability to conquer himself.

On the agreed-upon day the boys assemble at Dr. Lynn's house. She begins by assuring them that sex is beautiful and the basis of human life. Then comes a short version of the birds and the bees—explanations of plant and animal reproduction, stopping short of human beings. Dr. Lynn passes around a generous supply of a temperance and antimasturbation tract entitled "A Gateway and a Gift, Written for the Land of Teens" and impresses the boys with the Victorian misconception that behavior influences heredity: "You can change yourself by education so that the inheritance of your children may be quite changed."

After a few more discreet words on solitary vice the doctor hands around copies of the "White Cross Pledge" (sponsored by the same organization of the Young Men's Christian Association that had published Charles Scudder's *Hand-book for Young Men*) for the boys to sign. This pledge, headed by the motto "Blessed are the pure in heart: for they shall see God," provides an interesting summary of the guiding laws of purity:

I PROMISE, BY THE HELP OF GOD:

1. To treat all women with respect, and endeavor to protect them from wrong and degradation;
2. To endeavor to put down all indecent language and coarse jests;
3. To maintain the law of purity as equally binding upon men and women;
4. To endeavor to spread these principles among my companions, and to try to help my younger brothers;
5. To use all possible means to fulfill the command "Keep thyself pure."

A few days later the doctor again has a visitor. This time it is Frank who has the problem. In a panic over something strange that had happened to him (we gather that he means nocturnal emissions) he noticed an advertisement that promised help for his "ailment." Hopeful, he sent for advice and medicine, which didn't help. Now he has received a bill for $20—a huge sum in an age when $10 a week was a living wage. Dr. Lynn assures him of his normalcy (but doesn't tell him what to do about the bill).

When the boys again visit Dr. Lynn, she has had time to suspect that their problems are caused by idle hands. Suddenly she has an idea. Her attic is not being used, and there are some carpenter's tools up there; they will form a manual-arts workshop club. Her enthusiasm carries the project through, and she also helps to set up a manual-arts program in the schools. The clubroom is also outfitted with Indian clubs and other exercise equipment and a library (which gives an excuse to end the book with a list of good reading for boys).

Despite its obvious contrivances *Almost a Man* tried to meet young people on their own level instead of thundering at them from the pulpit. There is almost no factual content, of course, and a boy who was ignorant about masturbation or nocturnal emissions would learn nothing here except that the former was forbidden and the latter was normal. Coitus, as might be expected, is never mentioned. Still, Wood-Allen's warmth and kindness must have been some comfort to Victorian boys, who were faced with sexual warnings and horrors in every direction.

■ BIBLIOGRAPHY

Drake, Emma Frances. *What a Woman of Forty-five Ought to Know*. Self and Sex Series. Philadelphia: Vir, 1902.

———. *What a Young Wife Ought to Know*. Self and Sex Series. Philadelphia: Vir, 1901.

Hall, George F. *Plain Points on Personal Purity*, or *Startling Sins of the Sterner Sex*. Chicago: Columbian, 1892.

Scudder, Charles D. *Hand-book for Young Men*. New York: White Cross Committee. Young Men's Christian Association of the City of New York, 1892.

Sperry, Lyman Beecher. *Confidential Talks with Young Men*. Chicago: Revell, 1892.

———. *Confidential Talks with Young Women*. Chicago: Revell, 1893.

Stall, Sylvanus. *Successful Selling of the Self and Sex Series*. Philadelphia: Vir, 1907.

———. *What a Man of Forty-five Ought to Know*. Self and Sex Series. Philadelphia: Vir, 1901.

———. *What a Young Boy Ought to Know*. Self and Sex Series. Philadelphia: Vir, 1897; rev. eds., 1905, 1909.

———. *What a Young Husband Ought to Know*. Self and Sex Series. Philadelphia: Vir, 1897; rev. ed., 1907.

———. *What a Young Man Ought to Know*. Self and Sex Series. Philadelphia: Vir, 1897; rev. ed., 1904.

Strong, Bryan. "The Origins of Sex Education in America 1890–1920: An Inquiry into Victorian Sexuality." Located in library of the Kinsey Institute for Research in Sex, Gender, and Reproduction, Indiana University, n.d.

Walters, Ronald G. *Primers for Prudery: Sexual Advice to Victorian America*. Englewood Cliffs, N.J.: Prentice-Hall, 1974.

Warren, Mortimer A. *Almost Fourteen*. New York: Dodd, Mead, 1892.

Wood-Allen, Mary. *Almost a Man*. Ann Arbor, Mich.: Wood-Allen, 1895.

———. *Almost a Woman*. Ann Arbor, Mich.: Wood-Allen, 1897.

———. *The Marvels of Our Bodily Dwelling: Physiology Made Interesting; Suitable as a Text-book or Reference Book in Schools, or for Pleasant Home Reading.* With supplementary chapter "The Birthchamber." Ann Arbor, Mich.: Wood-Allen, 1895.

———. *Teaching Truth.* Ann Arbor, Mich.: Wood-Allen, 1892.

———. *Teaching Truth.* Teaching Truth Series. Ann Arbor, Mich.: Wood-Allen, 1903.

———. *What a Young Girl Ought to Know.* Self and Sex Series. Philadelphia: Vir, 1897.

———. *What a Young Woman Ought to Know.* Self and Sex Series. Philadelphia: Vir, 1898.

Chapter 2

What Every Young Girl Should Know

In 1887 Dr. J.W. Howe, an eminent physician, wrote *Excessive Venery, Masturbation, and Continence.* His subject was the curing of the "disease" of masturbation. In Chapter 6 he mentions in passing that the appropriate medical treatment for young girls who show excessive sexual interest is amputation of the clitoris. An appalling theory, but even more appalling is the fact that Howe was professor of clinical surgery at Bellevue Hospital Medical College in New York City and very likely had many opportunities to put his theories into practice.

Howe's ideals were not universally accepted, but they are symptomatic of the Victorian attitude toward feminine sexuality. A woman who showed erotic feelings was perceived as demented, diseased, or evil, and sometimes all three. The ideal Victorian lady was delicate, refined, and pure. Her nature was defined in terms of her role as "the angel in the house" who ministered to the spiritual and physical needs of the family. Her sexuality was acknowledged only in connection with the exalted function of childbearing and thus, in a way, transcended sex. The purpose of sex education for a girl, then, was to prepare her for the demands of motherhood and impress her with the grave moral and spiritual responsibilities of the role. She was given just enough information about her own body so that she could stay healthy, care for herself during menstruation, and preserve her virtue from evils that were never really explained to her. The books of this period constantly return to the refrain of the sacred joys of motherhood—the ultimate purpose of a girl's existence.

There were a number of changes afoot in the woman's sphere at the turn of the century that made the late Victorians feel the need to reinforce this rigidly defined feminine role. The first women's-rights convention had been held in 1848 in Seneca Falls, and from it emerged a vocal feminist leadership. Agitation for women's suffrage had begun and in England would soon lead to demonstrations and arrests. Higher education for women was becoming accepted—Vassar, Smith, Wellesley, and Barnard were building fine academic reputations.

Male writers rose to these challenges with ridicule and condemnation for the "new woman," often disguised as praise for the fair sex in general. In 1895 Charles H. Parkhurst wrote a volume of essays, *Talks to Young Women*, that refers to women who demand equal rights as "andromaniacs" and stresses woman's mission of motherhood: "Nature has so wrought its opinions into the tissue of woman's physical constitution and function that any feminine attempt to mutiny against wifehood, motherhood, and domestic 'limitations' is a hopeless and rather imbecile attempt to escape the inevitable. . . . A true mother lives for her children, and knows no other ambition but to live in her children." He approves the idea of college for women ("It is one of the pleasant features of our generation that increased attention is being given to the discipline of the female mind") but only if that education is used for motherhood ("'There is no 'strong-mindedness' and no completeness of college training that will unsex her, provided only such possessions and acquisitions are dominated by the feminine instinct and mortgaged to maternal ends and purposes"). Suffrage for women will get his reluctant sanction only when women have exhausted the opportunities for excelling in their own sphere: "I have not even uttered a word against so serious an innovation as that of woman's going to the polls. I have only tried to show the infinite stretch of opportunity that opens before her in the line of service which the general instinct and the revealed word of God show to be primarily pertinent to her. When the sex has succeeded in doing perfectly what God and nature evidently intended to have her do, it will be ample time for her to think about doing some things upon which God and nature have expressed themselves less definitely."

In *Steps up Life's Ladder* (1905), a book of inspirational essays for teenage boys, Charles A. Ingraham took Parkhurst's idea of andromania to its logical conclusion—women who broke through the accepted boundaries of feminine behavior had ceased to be women and had defined themselves as male: "The girls of masculine proclivities can hardly be admitted into the decorous circle of elect maidens. They may succeed in stunning the corner loungers with the exhibition of their horsemanship and the mannish cut of their coats; they may be able to converse intelligently and fluently on political topics; they may have the capacity to buy and sell and make money; but, after all, what the world wants of a girl is to be a girl, not a tom-boy."

This was the social setting, then, in which Mary Wood-Allen was asked to write *What a Young Girl Ought to Know* in 1897. Who was Mary Wood-Allen? What kind of a woman did Sylvanus Stall select to join in his profitable sex education enterprise? The frontispiece photograph in *Young Girl* and *Young Woman* shows her as sweet-faced and a bit plump, in a lacy collar and brooch, and with wavy hair pulled back into a bun from a high, rounded forehead. From all the evidence she was a person with considerable strength and independence of thought. She was a medical doctor at a time when obtaining that degree was a difficult accomplishment for a woman; she wrote prolifically on subjects that were previously taboo for women writers; and she published her early works herself under the imprint "Wood-Allen Publishing Company." Her maiden name was Wood and her married name Allen; the hyphenated Wood-Allen must have been a statement of identity for her. (The Library of Congress and most other U.S. libraries have robbed her of that statement, however, by entering her books in the files under "Allen, Mary [Wood]" in strict adherence to *Anglo-American Cataloging Rules*.) After her reputation as a sex educator was established by the Self and Sex series, she was offered, and accepted, the post of World Superintendent of the Purity Department of the Women's Christian Temperance Union.

Wood-Allen's first books were the Teaching Truth series ("Treats of the instruction to be given the young regarding sex and parenthood"), which she at first published herself, beginning with *Teaching Truth* in 1892. *Almost a Man* and *Almost a Woman* were early titles in this series; later titles included *Child-Confidence Rewarded* and *Caring for the Baby*. Another series launched by Wood-Allen was the American Motherhood leaflets. These dealt with family relations and had such titles as *Keep Mother and Me Intimate*, *Adolescence*, and *A Noble Father*. Her physiology text, *The Marvels of Our Bodily Dwelling* (first published in 1895), was popular for years and was published in five editions, the last appearing in 1915. In 1901, after the success of

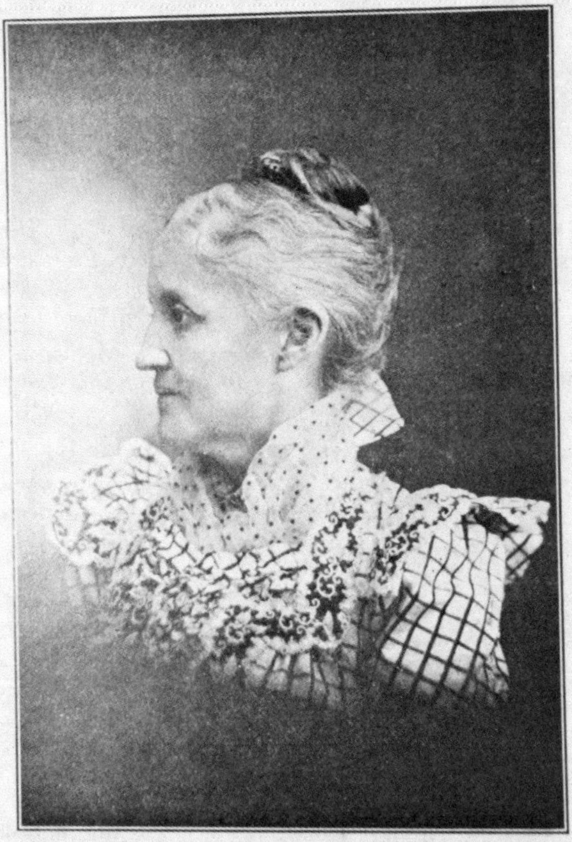

MARY WOOD-ALLEN, M.D.

Fig. 3. Dr. Mary Wood-Allen, author of *What a Young Girl Ought to Know.*

What a Young Girl Ought to Know, she tried her hand at marital advice with *Ideal Married Life: A Book for All Husbands and Wives* (could it be that she felt slighted by Stall's choice of Emma Drake to write the Self and Sex volumes for adult women?). Wood-Allen continued to write on family living and sex education until her death in 1908. A posthumous collection of her works, *Making the Best of Our Children* (1909), was edited by her daughter, Rose Woodallen Chapman, who was herself a well-known sex educator and columnist for the *Ladies' Home Journal*.

▪ Preparing for Motherhood

Like all the books in the Self and Sex series, *What a Young Girl Ought to Know* opens with a formidable battery of "Commendations from Eminent Men and Women." Wood-Allen's choice of members in these galleries is revealing not only of Victorian standards of prestige but also of the author's changing patterns of friendships and alliances. For *Young Girl* the eminent women are representative of causes and professions closely connected to the purity movement. Included are the national and international presidents of the Women's Christian Temperance Union, the president of the National Christian League for the Promotion of Social Purity, and one or two minor authors of works on domestic arrangements ("The Model Nursery," "House and Domestic Decorations"). Among the eminent men cited are the physical director of the Young Men's Christian Association, a few academics (the president of Berea College and a professor from the University of Michigan), and the "famous gospel singer and hymn writer" Ira Sankey.

The book opens with a preface for parents and other adults that justifies the need for limited instruction of the young girl in certain delicate matters. Like all early sex educators, Wood-Allen acted on the belief that knowledge of sex is dangerous to young people unless it is meted out in small quantities. Her preface reassures parents that her approach will be cautious: "It is thought wise to put the information suited to different ages in different volumes so that the girl will find what meets her present need and not be led into fields of investigation wider than the immediate case demands."

The dramatis personae of *Young Girl* are Nina and her mother, Mrs. Grant, who, like the characters in Stall's book, are having a series of talks after the birth of a baby brother. The instruction begins with the usual descriptions of plant reproduction, pollen and the role of bees, and fish fertilization (favored, perhaps, by Victorian sex educators because it requires no embarrassing description of physical contact between the participants). Mrs. Grant proceeds to mammals' care of their offspring and gingerly describes human birth. Sexual intercourse is only hinted at in delicate terms: "The germ of life . . . would never wake up unless it were touched by the power that only the father could give." Nina is warned that a good girl will not listen to her playmates' versions of these facts and is forearmed with a sample rebuff: "'I would rather you would not tell me about it. I will ask my mother and she will tell me. Mother tells me everything that I ought to know and she tells it to me in such a way that makes it very sweet to me, and so I have my little secrets with mother, and not with other girls.'"

A chapter on moral heredity reveals Wood-Allen's predictable Lamarckian ideas. Mrs. Grant explains that her early lack of effort to control her bad temper has resulted in Nina's difficulties with the same trait. On the other hand, languages are easy for Nina to learn because her mother studied them diligently as a child. The point, of course, is that Nina must be made aware of the far-reaching consequences of her own behavior, which, presumably, she will pass on to her own children.

The next chapter is on masturbation. Girls are warned against this practice, but gently, as was appropriate for their presumed lesser temptation. As in the manuals for boys, constipation is discussed at length in connection with masturbation. (Sex educators reasoned that constipation produced pinworms, which led to local itching, which led to local scratching, handling of the genitals, and solitary vice.) The lack of fresh fruits and vegetables and whole grains in the American diet probably made constipation a universal condition, and dietary advice to relieve the problem became obligatory in sex education books. Tea and coffee were routinely forbidden, as were alcohol and tobacco (for men, that is; there was no question of a woman smoking). In *Young Girl* Wood-Allen recommends "milk, eggs, oatmeal, entire wheat flour, and fruits."

After physical hygiene the doctor turns to mental hygiene:

"Evil thoughts create actual poisons in the blood, good thoughts create life-giving forces." Posture (or "carriage") affects the mental state, and so it is important to stand upright in correct alignment. The value of work is extolled (surprisingly, she has "no objection to a girl learning to use nails, saw and hammer") along with the complementary value of wholesome play, such as gymnastics. Wood-Allen illustrates the evils of wrong recreation through an anecdote about a young man who died of delirium tremens after two weeks of "visiting saloons."

Wood-Allen emphasizes that girls should choose good reading (defined as "the books that make you desire to be better") from the categories of history and biography, science and art, travel and exploration, morals and religion. On no account are girls to read "silly stories" of robbers and pirates and bandits in scenes of murder and robbery and intrigue. Education is of value to a woman because it can be morally uplifting and is useful in running a household. Also it ensures that her children will not be ashamed of their mother. Anticipating that girl readers will begin to feel the burden of society's expectations a bit heavy on their sex at this point, Wood-Allen digresses here to explain that boys should be as pure and good as girls.

Young Girl mentions menstruation only obliquely: "some physical changes which take place at puberty of which I will more fully tell you as the time approaches." Without specifying why, Wood-Allen recommends plenty of sleep and exercise at puberty. Exercise is to be had most conveniently in the form of housework: "Dish-washing is especially beneficial as the hot water calls the blood to the hands and so helps to relieve the headache or backache," and "it is far better to the young girl at puberty to be gently active in household duties than to be lying around reading love stories."

In the concluding section Wood-Allen sums up *What a Young Girl Ought to Know:* women's work is to make a home for men and to train future men and women. Perhaps feeling the need to modify the harsh truth of this arrangement, she adds that this allows women the leisure to entertain: "If the mother, as well as the father, went away in the morning to business, and both came home tired at night, there would be little of the social life which we all find so enjoyable." She also notes encouragingly that women can use their free time to advance social causes, such as temperance and social purity. (Like most Victorian writers,

Wood-Allen assumed that her readership was of the privileged upper classes.) Thus, with this amount of information and advice, the young girl was considered appropriately equipped to face the storms of puberty.

■ "Your Body Is Your Dwelling"

Wood-Allen's next book, *What a Young Woman Ought to Know* (1898), is intended for girls in their mid- to late teens and is equally reticent in tone. However, this time the eminent persons cited on the opening pages are strong women who in some way had transcended the role limitations imposed on their sex and were leaders in the feminist movement: May Wright-Sewall, president of the International Council of Women and nominee of the International Congress of Women; Mary Lowe Dickinson, president of the National Council of Women and professor of literature at Denver University; Matilda B. Carse, founder of the Woman's Temple, Chicago; Helen Campbell, dean of home economics at Kansas State University and author of *Prisoners of Poverty* and *Wage Earners*; Elisabeth Robinson Scovil, associate editor of the *Ladies' Home Journal*; and Elizabeth Cady Stanton, "noted woman suffragist." The roster is impressive, but if Wood-Allen selected these women because she admired their achievements she did not permit their ideas to infiltrate her book for young women, nor did she allow her own success as a doctor and author to alter her stance on the importance of a woman's place in the home.

Sparing older readers another recitation of the birds and the bees, Wood-Allen launches immediately into practical matters, with a minimum of rhetoric and theology. The emphasis in *What a Young Woman Ought to Know* is on health: "Your body is your dwelling." After a discussion of diet and the need for plenty of sleep she takes up a topic troublesome to the corseted Victorian woman—breathing. For many women of this era, when the eighteen-inch waist was the ideal of beauty, a deep breath was impossible. Wood-Allen considered the topic important enough to devote three chapters to it. After explaining the function of oxygen in the blood and the action of the diaphragm, she describes the damage done by tight lacing. Not only is breathing hindered, but the stomach and the liver are squeezed up under the diaphragm or down into the pelvis, with consequent malfunctions. The circulation is hampered and the heart overloaded. Sometimes a condition called "corset liver" results, in which the organ is pinched into two parts connected only by a thin strip of tissue. Wood-Allen pronounces judgment on these fashionable tortures by declaring that a tiny waist is a deformity and a mutilation.*

Exercise, therefore, should always be taken in loose clothing. Wood-Allen's first recommendation, of course, is the "home gymnasium," that is, housework. But skating, lawn tennis, and swimming are also approved, as is bicycle riding (*if* the girl does not sit on her perineum). Dancing is excellent exercise in itself but cannot be recommended because it involves late hours, immodest dress, and heavy late suppers and may lead to promiscuous associations.

After some words on bathing and care of the complexion she moves on to a detailed explanation of the function and hygiene of menstruation. The female organs of reproduction are briefly described, although there is no diagram and no mention of the external genitalia. Then Wood-Allen pictures the internal events of the menses, betraying the fact that she, like her medical contemporaries, believed that ovulation and menstruation were simultaneous:

> The uterus is lined by a mucous membrane similar to that which lines the mouth, and at this time of ovulation this membrane becomes swollen and soft, and little hemorrhages, or bleedings occur for three or four days, the blood passing away through the vagina. This is called menstruation.

It is not necessary that a woman be a periodical semi-invalid, says the doctor; menstruation should be painless, but the majority of civilized women suffer more or less. She blames this on tight, unhealthful clothing, lack of exercise, constipation, twisted postures, standing on one foot, and disturbed nerves from reading novels (the latter because it causes an abnormal excitement of the sexual organs and can also cause premature sexual physical development).

*Clothing reform was a constant plank in the feminist platform. The loose Turkish trousers and tunic designed by Amelia Bloomer were worn for a time by a few leading suffragist women as a protest.

Precautions should be taken during the menstrual period, since the girl's energy is being used to "establish a new function." She should guard herself from cold, overexertion, social dissipation, and mental excitement, especially the aforesaid novel reading. An abdominal support bandage can be used for taking pressure off the bowels. Contrary to old wives' tales, it is all right to change underwear and to wash, although full tub baths are not advisable. Wet feet and clothes can be dangerous at this time because the girl is weaker and more susceptible to infection.

If she has severe pain, a girl should assume the "recumbent position," drink warm liquids, and apply warm cloths (but she should never make use of alcohol, either internally or externally). It is a bad practice to consult traveling doctors or take hot douches. Remedies for extremely heavy flow are bed rest, cold cloths over the abdomen and between the thighs, and two or three enemas a day. Wood-Allen cautions that nervous strain, such as the pressures of school, may stop the menses but assures readers that this is not a symptom of tuberculosis. Rather the reverse is true; tuberculosis can lead to cessation of menstruation.

Wood-Allen's description of Victorian sanitary arrangements for menstrual "protection" in *Young Woman* gives us some insight into the difficulties of menstruation in the days before tampons:

> I would suggest that the napkins be fastened to straps that go over the shoulder and are then joined together in front and back to an end piece, on each of which a button is sewn. Buttonholes in the napkins at the corners, diagonal from each other, will make them easily attached or removed.

Directions for sewing napkins follow.

While she is on the subject of vaginal discharges, Wood-Allen takes up the matter of leukorrhea. This is not a disease, she maintains, but results from congestion of the blood vessels due to improper dress, taking cold, or "a debilitated condition of the stomach" (providing another example of the curious but common assumption of the times that the reproductive and digestive systems were somehow closely linked).

After such a long discourse on menstruation Wood-Allen mercifully gets to the point on masturbation:

> It destroys mental power and memory, it blotches the complexion, dulls the eye, takes away the strength, and may cause insanity. It is

> a habit most difficult to overcome, and may not only last for years, but in its tendency be transmitted to one's children.

In an echo of the doctrine of seminal power she states that the release of sexual energy through masturbation represents a "waste of vital force" and implies that the expenditure of this force is acceptable only in marital intercourse for the purpose of procreation: "One can feel justified to lose a part of her own life if she is conferring life upon others, but to indulge in such a waste of vital force merely for pleasure is certainly never excusable." Self-abuse may be accomplished by fantasies of love making, without manual stimulation. Reading romances can lead to this mental masturbation. To overcome the habit girls should remember that sex is holy and intended for reproduction. They should avoid pelvic congestion from constipation or tight clothes and keep the mind healthfully occupied with other thoughts.

Next the doctor talks about flirting. Later sex educators were to call it "petting" and devote many fevered pages to exploring its evils. Wood-Allen's arguments foreshadow the writings of Ann Landers and Evelyn Duvall. Many girls feel, she says, that they have to allow intimacies to get young men to notice them. They may think a few stolen kisses and unobserved hand pressures don't matter, but they are "playing with the fire of physical passion." Moreover, young men talk about flirts. A girl who arouses a boy may cause him to lose his honor and purity by going to prostitutes; it is a girl's responsibility to discourage intimacies and keep matters within the bounds of propriety even during her engagement. As for friendships between girls, they, too, should be kept at a physical distance. The attitude of "gushy" girls who fondle and kiss "if probed thoroughly might be found to be a sort of perversion, a sex mania." As a matter of fact, young girls should keep everybody at a physical distance and kiss only their mothers. This doctrine of distance is reinforced in the next chapter on venereal disease. Millions die annually from these diseases, which can be transmitted by a kiss. For further facts girls are referred to *What a Young Man Ought to Know*.

Wood-Allen's interest in eugenics is reflected in several chapters on heredity, which caution girls to choose a husband carefully on the basis of his behavior and genetic inheritance. The concluding chapters deal with the engagement and the wedding, bringing the reader to the next book in the series.

Predictably, Emma Drake's two books match the advice Sylvanus Stall had provided in his companion volumes for men. *What a Young Wife Ought to Know* (1901) glorifies home and family, and *What a Woman at Forty-five Ought to Know* (1902) is a less-than-comforting guide through menopause. Like the other volumes of the Self and Sex series, these books for women were very popular and ran to several editions—*Young Woman* was reprinted as late as 1936.

▪ Earlier Titles for Girls and Young Women

In Chapter 1 we saw how Lyman Beecher Sperry's *Confidential Talks with Young Men* and Wood-Allen's *Almost a Man* preceded the publication of the Self and Sex volumes for boys and young men. In the same way ground had been broken for the sex instruction of girls and young women by Sperry's *Confidential Talks with Young Women* and Wood-Allen's own *Almost a Woman*. Both predated the more popular Self and Sex books, and both set themes that sex educators were to reiterate and elaborate for many years to come.

Published in 1893, Sperry's *Confidential Talks with Young Women* was the very first sex-advice manual addressed to teenaged girls. It established many of the themes that were later orchestrated by Wood-Allen and her followers, including the benefits of fresh air, moderate exercise, and healthful diet and the dangers of late parties, masturbation, sentimental novels, indiscriminate kissing, and wet feet and fatigue during menstruation. We can be sure that Wood-Allen was influenced by, or at least was aware of, *Confidential Talks with Young Women* because she wrote the introduction (Wood-Allen had already gained some recognition with the publication of her first Teaching Truth booklet the previous year).

Although Sperry was as obsessed as his contemporaries with preserving virginity and preventing masturbation, his primary concern in *Confidential Talks with Young Women* is the unhealthful practices and social expectations that made early invalids of many women—the lack of fresh air and exercise and the stifling, choking burden of fashionable dress: "The expected physical condition of the modern American woman over thirty years of age is a sofa, a shawl, and the neuralgia." Modern society (of 1893) puts obstacles to healthful development in women's way, says Sperry: malnutrition, the practice of keeping girls indoors—and, worst of all, fashionable dress. Corseting and tight lacing can be blamed for prolapsed or tipped uteruses; characteristically, Sperry provides a careful anatomical description of how this can happen. Crowding and injury of the rectum and the bladder can also take place in corset-squeezed abdomens. The development of the sexual organs can be affected and, consequently, all maturing. Western man is horrified at the Chinese practice of foot binding, yet corseting and lacing are every bit as cruelly wrong. Tight shoes and garters and the weight of heavy skirts also hamper circulation and development. Sperry quotes from *The Relation of Dress to Vice*, by Frances E. Willard, as he maintains that hampering dress is a remnant of primitive society: "Every punctured ear, bandaged waist, and high heeled shoe is a reminder that manhood and womanhood are yet under the curse transmitted by their ignorant and semi-barbarous ancestry."

How, then, could the young girl who wanted to be healthy modify her clothes to make them comfortable but still not be an object of ridicule on the street? Like many "radical" thinkers of the day, Sperry admired Amelia Bloomer's costume in principle but did not seriously advocate wearing it in broad daylight. He proposed instead a three-point program of moderate dress reform. To paraphrase:

1. Leave off corsets and loosen the dress.
2. Reduce the weight of clothing and shorten skirts so they do not drag on the floor.
3. Clothe each limb, legs as well as arms, individually and evenly (presumably, he means under the skirts).

Many women are reluctant to adopt dress reform because they fear men may be hostile to it. Nonsense, says Sperry: "If the women will but make convenient, comfortable, healthful, modest dress *fashionable*, the men will admire it and praise it far more than they ever approved the grotesque upholstery, drapery, flummery and murderous toggery in which women have so long and so submissively masqueraded." As support Sperry quotes at length a corset manufacturer who has found it profitable to switch over to producing loose "waists" with buttons for attaching skirts. The standard corset measurements, he explains, are bust fourteen inches larger than the waist and hips sixteen inches larger (36–22–38, for instance). His new product, the "waists," have a difference of only ten inches between waist and hip. True, they do have steel reinforcement up the front and sides, but this can easily be slipped out if the wearer wishes to be completely unfettered. The manufacturer describes this new healthful Victorian version of le minimum: "At the foundation is the union undergarment, covering the arms, legs and body in one piece. Then there will be the stockings and the waist, the stockings being supported by hose supporters attached to the waist. Over this cotton drawers can be fashioned directly to the waist; or, the cotton drawers and waist-cover can be combined in one garment, to be used in place of the old fashioned chemise. Over this again is a single skirt; better still, the divided skirt. This with a dress in which the waist and skirt are made in one piece, completes the costume."

Sperry's depiction of the physical and mental changes of puberty may seem exaggerated to a modern reader, but it was probably based on the doctor's clinical observation of the Victorian teenage girl, who was expected to be occasionally neurasthenic and hysterical and who referred to her menstrual period as being "unwell." The mental manifestations of puberty, Sperry says, are a new weariness and indifference to passing events, bashfulness, a fondness for love stories, giggling and gossiping with one close friend, and a tendency to be absentminded, nervous, and notional. A girl may often "feel like having a good cry about it." Although the physical changes of puberty result in a glow of attractiveness, the subjective symptoms are not so pleasant, he adds: "Quite likely you experienced wandering pains and shifting aches, heaviness in the small of the back, a sort of pressure in the spine, and a great many little 'bad feelings.'" These and other discomforts of painful menstruation are the habit of civilized, sedentary women, explains Sperry, and are not at all the normal state in nature.

Sperry is quite comfortable in describing the anatomy of menstruation, including the function of the ovum and the sperm, although he, like Wood-Allen, is convinced that ovulation occurs during the menses. He is not so comfortable, though, in advising girls on the hygiene of their periods and suggests that a girl ask her mother or a trusted teacher about this or go to a woman doctor: "Fortunately, there are now many educated and trustworthy physicians of your own sex to whom you may properly and safely apply for counsel in such matters. You may thereby avoid the strain which, very naturally (although unnecessarily) you might experience in calling upon a physician of the opposite sex."

Now Sperry turns to a subject he finds less congenial: masturbation. He turns over the chapter to Mrs. E. P. Miller, author of "A Mother's Advice," explaining that "it seems most fitting that the needed words of admonition should come direct from one who is a mother as well as a physician." Mrs. Miller takes over with gusto: "When I see a little girl or a young lady wasted and weak and listless, with great hollow eyes and a sort of sallow tint on the haggard face, with the red hue of the lips faded, the ears white like marble and the face covered with pimples, I dread lest they have committed the sin which, if not abandoned, will lead them down to death." Many women "die of consumption and liver disease and brain disease and many other diseases just because they have wasted their best blood and weakened the system by this vile habit. Some become idiots . . . some become crazy; in the insane asylums all over the land are very many who have practiced self-abuse. Many of those who commit suicide do it because they practiced this habit when they were young."

Confidential Talks with Young Women concludes with a promising picture of the future of feminism, which is, unfortunately, short on specifics: "Woman may, if she will, secure perfect development of all her powers, perfect freedom of action in all spheres of activity possible for her, and perfect equality with man, socially, politically and commercially."

Mary Wood-Allen's *Almost a Woman* was published in 1897 as a companion volume to *Almost a Man* (1895), and, although it appeared in the same year as *What a Young Girl Ought to Know*, it almost certainly is an earlier work. It clearly shows the author's lack of commitment to female emancipation and, like the moralistic tale of Guy, Frank, Carl, and Rob, uses fiction to make its point.

The prelude finds Mr. and Mrs. Wayne discussing their thirteen-year-old daughter, Helen. "Have you explained her approaching womanhood to her?" asks Mr. Wayne. His wife responds that she has been waiting for the right moment: "I have thought that perhaps she would indicate by some question that her mind was becoming ready for the disclosure. It always seems to me that to force information before the mind is ready to receive it, is to jeopardize its reception."

"Don't wait, Mary," says her husband sternly. They agree to seize the first opportunity.

In the next chapter that opportunity presents itself. Helen and her father are alone in the house, and he uses the occasion for a chat on the dangers of being free with young men. Helen is troubled by the double standard: "But, Father, tell me why it's so much more important for girls to be particular about what they do than for boys?"

"Well, it's not," he says, but adds that everybody thinks it is. He explains the high ideals society holds up for women and reads her several pieces of literature to illustrate, among them this passage from John Ruskin's *Sesame and Lillies:*

> Woman's power is for rule, not for battle, and her intellect is not for invention or creation, but for sweet ordering, arrangement and decision. Her great function is Praise. There is not a war in the world, no, nor an injustice, but you women are answerable for it, not in that you have provoked, but in that you have not hindered. Men, by their nature, are prone to fight. They will fight for any cause or none. It is for you to choose their cause for them, and to forbid when there is no cause. There is no suffering, no injustice, no misery in the earth, but the guilt of it lies with you.

Helen is polite but not impressed. She chafes at the limitations imposed on her by her sex. Her father's answers are unconvincing, and our sympathy is all with Helen. "It seems so much grander to be a man than a woman. A man's life is so much freer, and he can do so much greater things, you know. Of course, I shall try to be a good woman, but I wish women could do big things, the way men can . . . women just sit in the house and look on. I'd like to *do* something."

"It only seems like men do bigger things," her father responds; "it is *mind* that does the real work and women have minds, you know."

"Yes, I know, but they must devote their minds to cooking and dishwashing," she says. But Mr. Wayne persists and eventually convinces her to be content with her lot, because, after all, while "man makes *things*; woman makes *men*."

Mrs. Wayne soon has her turn. As she and Helen are sitting by the front window, a flirtatious young woman of Helen's acquaintance passes by. This leads to talk about the impropriety of accepting expensive presents from young men and allowing them to take liberties.

"Mother," says Helen after a pause, as two girls pass the house with their arms about each other's waists, "Don't you think it silly for girls to be so 'spooney?' Lucy is always having such lover-like friends and then quarreling with them. Now, she and Nellie are going to have a mock wedding next week. They call themselves husband and wife even now—isn't that silly?" Mrs. Wayne thinks it is worse than silly—"morbid unnatural sentimentality" she calls it.

(The subject of quasi-sexual relationships between girls occurs frequently in these books, demonstrating the Victorian abhorrence of any hint of homosexuality. Although affectionate friendships between young women have never been uncommon, the hugging and kissing of Victorian girlfriends was probably a response to the absence of physical affection in the home. Forbidden any other expression, the sexuality of young women emerged in such fevered and sentimental attractions. While a few of these romances may have been lesbian love affairs, the great majority of them were probably not.)

The next time Mrs. Wayne is alone with Helen, she delicately brings up the subject of how girls become women. It soon becomes clear that while Helen has absorbed a detailed knowledge of human physiology at school, the reproductive system has never been mentioned in those lessons. The words "womb," "uterus," and "vagina" are new to her, and she is surprised to hear about "the little room where the baby grows." She shows an apprehensive interest in her mother's explanation of menstruation but is on more familiar ground when the talk shifts to the internal damage done by the corset. (Mrs. Wayne shows her a drawing comparing the ideal shape of the Venus de Milo with the corseted figure of a popular actress.) Helen asks for an explanation of the plight of a girlfriend who has had an illegitimate child, which gives her mother a chance to expound on the evils of permitting "even the slightest unwarranted familiarity." With married people, on the other hand, "it is perfectly proper for them to do what before would not have been proper." That proper action needs some clarification, so Mrs. Wayne explains, but not very directly: "You can understand that, for the spermatozoa to be placed where they can find their way into the uterus, means a very close and familiar relationship of the man and woman."

No Wood-Allen book would be complete without some mention of the obligation to improve heredity by right action and the related importance of temperance. Alcohol and tobacco are evil, and she illustrates that fact with two stories: the first about a little boy who attempted to murder his baby brother with scissors because his father was an alcoholic and had passed on the mental degeneration to him, and the second about a tobacco-addicted baby born to a woman who was an inveterate smoker and who found that the only way to quiet her child's cries was to put the pipe between its lips.

At the end of this model of parental instruction the reader finds Helen resigned to her fate. She says, a bit sadly, "I think after this I'll try to feel that even I am of importance to the world, instead of regretting that I am not a man."

Sperry's and Wood-Allen's books are typical of the flavor and content of most sex education books for girls from the turn of the century through its first and second decades. The late Victorian social hygienists were prolific, and many other titles exist, among them *The Doctor's Plain Talk to Young Women* (1902), by Virgil Primrose English, *Personal Information for Girls* (1909), by Ernest Edwards, and *Confidences* (1910), by Edith Belle Lowry. While sex educators continued to caution girls against coquettish behavior and too much exercise, however, the literature for boys began to urge them to strive toward a redefined—and impossibly rigorous—masculine ideal.

■ BIBLIOGRAPHY

Drake, Emma Frances. *What a Woman of Forty-five Ought to Know*. Self and Sex Series. Philadelphia: Vir, 1902.

———. *What a Young Wife Ought to Know*. Self and Sex Series. Philadelphia: Vir, 1901; rev. ed., 1908.

Edwards, Ernest. *Personal Information for Girls*. New York: Fenno, 1909.

English, Virgil Primrose. *The Doctor's Plain Talk to Young Women*. Cleveland: Ohio State Publishing, 1902.

Howe, Joseph William. *Excessive Venery, Masturbation, and Continence*. New York: Treat, 1887; reprint, New York: Arno, 1974.

Ingraham, Charles A. *Steps up Life's Ladder: An Old Doctor's Letters to a Young Friend*. Poughkeepsie, N.Y.: Haught, 1905.

Lowry, Edith Belle. *Confidences: Talks with a Young Girl Concerning Herself*. Chicago: Forbes, 1910.

Parkhurst, Charles H. *Talks to Young Women*. New York: Century, 1895; rev. ed., 1897.

Sperry, Lyman Beecher. *Confidential Talks with Young Women*. Chicago: Revell, 1893.

Wood-Allen, Mary. *Adolescence*. American Motherhood Leaflets no. 32. Cooperstown, N.Y.: Crist, Scott and Parshall, 1907.

———. *Almost a Man*. Ann Arbor, Mich.: Wood-Allen, 1895, 1897.

———. *Almost a Man*. Teaching Truth Series. Cooperstown, N.Y.: Crist, Scott and Parshall, 1907.

———. *Almost a Woman*. Ann Arbor, Mich.: Wood-Allen, 1897.

———. *Almost a Woman*. Teaching Truth Series. Cooperstown, N.Y.: Crist, Scott and Parshall, 1907.

———. *Caring for the Baby*. Teaching Truth Series. Cooperstown, N.Y.: Crist, Scott and Parshall, 1907.

———. *Child-Confidence Rewarded*. Teaching Truth Series. Ann Arbor, Mich.: Wood-Allen, 1903; Cooperstown, N.Y.: Crist, Scott and Parshall, 1903.

———. *Ideal Married Life: A Book for All Husbands and Wives*. New York: Revell, 1901.

———. *Keep Mother and Me Intimate*. American Motherhood Leaflets no. 31. Cooperstown, N.Y.: Crist, Scott and Parshall, 1907.

———. *Making the Best of Our Children*, ed. by Rose Woodallen Chapman. Chicago: A. C. McClurg, 1909.

———. *The Marvels of Our Bodily Dwelling: Physiology Made Interesting; Suitable as a Text-book or Reference Book in Schools, or for Pleasant Home Reading*. Ann Arbor, Mich.: Wood-Allen, 1895, 1896; Philadelphia: Vir Publishing Co., 1915.

———. *A Noble Father*. American Motherhood Leaflets no. 10. Cooperstown, N.Y.: Crist, Scott and Parshall, 1907.

———. *Teaching Truth*. Ann Arbor, Mich.: Wood-Allen, 1892.

———. *Teaching Truth*. Teaching Truth Series. Ann Arbor,

Mich.: Wood-Allen, 1903; Cooperstown, N.Y.: Crist, Scott and Parshall, 1907.
———. *What a Young Girl Ought to Know*. Self and Sex Series. Philadelphia: Vir, 1897; rev. ed., 1905.
———. *What a Young Woman Ought to Know*. Self and Sex Series. Philadelphia: Vir, 1898; rev. eds., 1905, 1913.

Chapter 3

The Bully Boys and the Rosy Girls

Theodore Roosevelt, like Queen Victoria, was one of those leaders who came to represent the ideals and aspirations of an age, who symbolized the unfocused yearnings of their people. A complex and fascinating character with enormous charm but many inner contradictions, Roosevelt was perceived by the popular imagination as the champion of American capitalism and a man who had used his fierce competitive instincts to create his own manhood. Roosevelt was wracked with asthma as a child; his illness kept him at home and isolated him from his peers. Although he disciplined his mind, he grew up with a feeble body. As a teenager he was so shamed at being easily overpowered by a group of young toughs that he determined to build himself a strong body. Using great resources of willpower and energy, he did just that and became a man whose skill and endurance in the outdoor life won him the loyalty and companionship of seasoned cowboys, grizzled soldiers in the Spanish-American War, and big-game hunters in Africa.

This aspect of Roosevelt's colorful life became an example for young boys in America: the idea that virile manhood must be created by strenuous self-discipline, vigorous effort, and self-denial. Along with this muscular ideal went a denial of the feminine quality: although women were to be treated with almost reverent respect, the ultimate insult to a man was to be called a "sissy"—a word derived from "sister." Men were not allowed to express their more sensitive, aesthetic, and emotional nature for fear of discrediting their hard-won masculinity. American men are straitjacketed by this syndrome even today and have only recently begun to struggle against it.

The sex educators seized on this pervasive and popular ideal of manhood. They encouraged the enthusiasm for bodybuilding, outdoor sports, and self-discipline as a method of diverting sexual energies and squelching masturbatory temptations. In a book of instruction to parents, *Sex Education*, author Ira Solomon Wile said in 1912: "Activity diverts energy into channels free from sexual suggestion. Idleness and laziness involve a sluggish circulation and a will flabby from disuse. There is little manliness to withstand the assaults of the degenerate sex lore of the gang, the train of horrors like dance-halls, saloons, and boat excursions."

Like the Victorians, sex educators in the early years of this century were primarily interested in sex education as a form of sex prevention. Their methods differed from those of their predecessors in that instead of terrifying their young readers, they emphasized the joys of building manliness through exercise and self-discipline. In 1914 William Trufant Foster edited a collection of essays, *The Social Emergency*, that distilled the ideas of the time on the aims of sex education. The essays had been adapted from a series of lectures delivered at Reed College by authorities in the field to an audience of teachers and social workers. They reveal an almost unanimous agreement on the proper content of education in sex. (The "emergency" in the title refers not to an epidemic of venereal disease, as might be suspected, but to the breaking of silence on the subject of sex and the lack of competent teachers.) Although the contributors to this book were still firmly convinced that conservation of semen was essential to manhood, they were beginning to rebel against the earlier hysterical fear of self-abuse. "To warn boys against horrible effects of masturbation and to tell them things not to do is a poor method. It is far better to explain that by keeping clean a boy may acquire virility," wrote Harry Hascall Moore, whose invocation of the usefulness of sports in helping boys to keep pure here became the theme of his own book, *Keeping in Condition*, published in 1916:

> Athletics are to be recommended as possessing a positive prophylactic value against the indulgence of sensual propensities. Physical exercise serves as an outlet for the superabundant energy which might otherwise be directed toward the sexual sphere . . .

The Teddy Roosevelt ideal emerges clearly in this passage by another contributor to Foster's book, Edward O. Sisson:

> The lad who plays vigorously, even violently; who can "get his second wind," turn a handspring, do a good cross-country run, swim the river, possesses a great bulwark of defense against sexual vice, especially in its secret forms.

Andrew C. Smith's essay summarizes the content of sex education for a boy, which, according to Smith, should begin "when more thrilling sensations command his attention." The boy should be taught that this new function is for reproduction only, that sexual activity is not necessary for health, and that involuntary emissions are normal and not harmful. Moore, in his own essay, adds that boys should also be disabused of belief in the double standard and the idea that gonorrhea is no worse than a bad cold. A girl, however, needs only to be instructed on menstruation and to be impressed with the idea that the purpose of her sex mechanism is maternity. She should be taught to guard her purity against both sexes, and "it will only fortify her maidenliness to tell her that much of the world is deceitful and degrading in sex matters."

One of the first books for young men to advocate the muscular path to sexual abstinence was Elisha Alonzo King's *Helps to Health and Purity*, a tiny pocket-sized handbook that appeared in 1903 (although it had been published in 1897 under the title *A Talk to Men*). King also later wrote *Clean and Strong* (1909, 1917), a book with similar content, for the United Society of Christian Endeavor. After providing reassurances about the normalcy of nocturnal emissions, King discourses on the evils of masturbation. He recommends cold baths as a remedy to temptation and advises at length on techniques for overcoming constipation. The second half of the book describes health-building exercises, each one beginning with the command "Attention!" A photograph of King's exercise class—rows of leotard-clad figures with folded arms—adorns this section.

The organization that most clearly grew out of this American ideal of manhood is the Boy Scouts, which was founded in 1910. It is no accident that Teddy Roosevelt is listed in the first handbook as honorary vice-president, right after the obligatory first choice of then-President William Taft. An advertisement for shredded wheat on the inside cover of that first handbook gives the flavor of the 1911 Boy Scout philosophy: "Building buster boys is bully business!" That basic philosophy has not changed much over the years—Scouting is still characterized by an enthusiasm for strenuous outdoor exercise and clean living. Taking cold baths and avoiding constipation remained a ubiquitous refrain in Boy Scout literature and scoutmasters' lectures for the majority of those years.

The sexual attitudes reflected in the 1911 Boy Scout *Official Handbook for Boys* were equally predictable and long-lived. Chapter 5, "Health and Endurance," was written by George J. Fisher, a doctor with the physical department of the Young Men's Christian Association. The last paragraph, headed "Conservation," explains in careful euphemisms the need to avoid wrong habits and retain the sex fluid for manliness. Readers are referred to Winfield Scott Hall's *From Youth into Manhood* (1909) for further information. Thirty-four years later, in the 1945 edition of the handbook, the passage remained substantially unchanged, although a few words about nocturnal emissions had been added and Fisher had become national Scout commissioner. Only after a protest in that year by sexologist Alfred Kinsey was the sexual advice modernized. (Recent editions of the handbook only advise boys who have questions about sexual matters to talk them over with parents and spiritual or medical advisers.)

▪ The Bully Boys

The most full-blown example of the "bully boys" school of thought is Harry Hascall Moore's *Keeping in Condition: A Handbook on Training for Older Boys* (1916). The book's contents and its bluff and hearty tone are so representative of its type that it is worth examining in some detail. In the preface the author makes it clear that he is attempting "to set up an ideal of vigorous manhood, a program of training now used by many expert leaders of boys to relieve them of the sex excitation and temptations so clearly part of the dangers to our present-day social life." He proposes to lay out "all the essentials of training for manhood—

exercise, fresh air, diet, rest, and 'the control of inner force.' " The book is illustrated with photographs of groups of boys engaged in various manly outdoor activities: climbing a snow-covered mountain peak, finishing a race, diving into a lake, shooting rapids in a canoe, and "roasting 'hot-dogs' over fires built in the rain after a morning hike." The frontispiece adds a reference to Spartan life with a photograph of a Greek statue, "the relay runner."

Moore begins with a pep talk about the six qualities of virility—strong muscles, endurance, energy, courage, self-control, and willpower. Young readers are exhorted to get right to work on building their manhood now before it is too late: "It is the function of the boy to develop the powers that will be used in adult activities, such as vital and nervous energy, skill, willpower, and courage. This development cannot be secured after maturity." Self-development aimed at the attainment of the racial and national ideal is a boy's responsibility.

So to work. A boy should start the year by visiting the doctor and getting a clean bill of health and by having taken two or three photographs of the body in various positions. This is for comparison as bodybuilding progresses, so that the boy can have a plan for competing with himself. The best exercises are baseball, rowing, canoeing, skating, and especially hiking. Boxing, wrestling, and gymnastics are good, too, if they can be done in the open air. A set of calisthenics is also given for posture and muscle building. Exercise should be followed by a short warm bath, a cold plunge, and a rubdown.

The diet Moore recommends seems to our sensibilities to be deficient in bulk—no salads, fresh vegetables, or raw fruit—and very heavy in starch and fats. "Bread and milk," he says, "provide all the important elements in food." Each mouthful of this diet is to be chewed thoroughly to a paste, and coffee, tea, alcohol, and tobacco are absolutely forbidden. Fresh air is an important element in training for manhood; the candidate should exercise in it at least two hours a day and sleep out-of-doors if at all possible.

This hard-won virility can be lost by yielding to the temptation of self-abuse. A boy who would be a real man must be mentally clean and keep dangerous thoughts and suggestions away by willpower or with physical exertion: "By *immediately* turning to vigorous exercise, or hard mental or physical work, this impulse may be converted in a wonderful yet mysterious manner into a great constructive force in his life." In summary, "He who would possess virility must work for it."

Virility can also be endangered by tuberculosis, colds, typhoid fever, venereal disease, constipation, and worry about nocturnal emissions. This last should be no cause for alarm, says Moore. The manly essence of the fluids is not lost in natural emissions; only when a boy allows himself to become sexually excited does the discharge involve the whole system. Therefore manhood candidates should keep away from suggestive pictures and stories, "certain vaudeville acts," and all impure thinking. Moore illustrates with an anecdote: "A short time ago a football player on one of the big university teams began to play poorly. His coach investigated the trouble and found that the man had a suggestive picture hanging in his bedroom. The coach at once tore it down . . ." and the player's game improved very soon afterward.

Moore briefly touches on the mechanics of plant and animal reproduction, ending with the union of the sperm and the ovum. When it comes to human beings, however, he says only: "In a true man, the beauty and wonder of it all awakens tenderness and a protective sense toward all women and girls." Moore returns to the issue of feminine delicacy repeatedly in *Keeping in Condition*: "A youth should regard all girls as the future mothers of the race" and "should treat every girl as he expects other fellows to treat his own sister." Girls are to be given special consideration during those times when they are sensitive to exercise because of their "monthly sickness."

For these and other reasons the sex drive, which can be compared to fire or rushing water, must be controlled for good use. Indeed, "it is not enough to repress the sex instinct; it must be directed into constructive activities." There is a temptation to gratify desire, "the race instinct," with prostitutes or immoral girls. This must be resisted by keeping in mind the dangers of venereal disease. Remember, sex is not necessary for health. Controlling his instincts is "the biggest fight ever waged by man—a fight in secret—without applause."

Introducing another major theme, the implications of manhood training for race progress, Moore explains that it is important to consider heredity when choosing a mate. He adds, however, that it is not true that acquired characteristics are transmitted to one's children. National progress also calls for virile men. There are certain political and social problems on which a real man must take a firm stand: child labor, trade unionism, unemployment, and alcohol abuse. The nation needs virile men in the professions and the sciences, in business and trade, labor, public office, and social reform. In short, national purity equals national power.

Many similar books for boys were published during the two decades before World War I. The title recommended in the Boy Scout handbook of 1911—Hall's *From Youth into Manhood*—was published by the Young Men's Christian Association, which took up the promotion of muscular manhood with zeal. A prolific pamphleteer for sex education, Hall was a professor of physiology at Northwestern University Medical School. His pamphlets were not limited to a male audience and included *Margaret, the Doctor's Daughter*, published by the American Medical Association in 1911. Hall wrote a second book for boys in 1913 with the triple title *Father and Son; John's Vacation; What John Saw in the Country*. Since the vacation was at a farm with the usual component of copulating livestock, what John saw was sufficiently surprising to prompt him to ask his father a number of interesting questions. In response, however, John's father limits himself to the standard advice about seminal conservation and good health habits.

Another prolific producer of pamphlets was Edward Bok, whose Books of Self-Knowledge for Young People and Parents grew out of articles on sexual subjects previously published in the *Ladies' Home Journal*. These thin volumes of advice on intimate matters sold for twenty-five cents and had various authors. Volume 2 of the series is typical—*When a Boy Becomes A Man* (1912), by H. Bisseker, an English schoolmaster, who addresses boys from ages thirteen to fifteen on the dual themes of the perils of masturbation and the benefits of health.

The Misanthropes

Despite the emphasis that the virility advocates placed on the positive rewards of physical development in these books, the theory itself is in many ways grounded in disgust with the human body and represents an effort to control, and thereby overcome, the fact of man's animal nature. Thus it is not surprising that alongside the health and conditioning books there appeared a number of works that border on misanthropy in the stern relish with which they hold forth on the horrors of the body and of sexuality in particular. This attitude is most clearly evident in books written for girls (which emphasized the weaknesses of the female body), although it is not limited to them. A good example is *Confidential Chats with Girls* (1911), by William Lee Howard, which makes the "bully boys" books seem benevolent by contrast.

Reflecting the social changes of the Industrial Revolution that were beginning to result in the employment of large numbers of women in the factories, Howard addresses himself, with considerable condescension, to working girls. He defines his ground right from the beginning: "I do not intend to talk to you about the process of procreation or the physiology of conception." That can be read in other books. Rather he intends to convey the warning that a girl who does not "protect her growth may ruin herself that, when she marries, she is unable to be a mother." A worthy message, although it "may seem a little indelicate," he cautions.

Launching into instruction on the care of the female sex organs, Howard explains that the ovaries are sensitive to emotion and movement. (The belief that the developing female sex organs required a girl to be extraordinarily careful of her body appeared regularly in early sex education books. It was felt that jumping, running, and standing would tangle and twist the uterus and ovaries, or even jar them loose from their moorings entirely.) At puberty a girl should cease all rough play, sports, late dancing, and standing for long periods, says Howard. For the first two years after the onset of menstruation she should have no exercise except walking, swimming, and "bending of the body." Sledding is especially dangerous in that it may cause a rupture or strain of the ovaries or womb. Girls who disregard this advice may later regret it: "The ovaries may be so twisted and put out of order that nothing can be done for them in later life but to cut them out with a knife." Exercise during a menstrual period may displace the womb and cause difficulties in pregnancy: "the child is smothered while trying to grow, and then must come a horrible operation."

A girl should stay at home and rest during this period, Howard declares. To emphasize the point he tells a tale about a young girl with menstrual pain who asked to go home from school. Her unfeeling teacher sent her to the principal, who asked embarassing questions. A few days later, when the girl returned to school, the boys laughed at her. According to Howard, her mortification was so great that she attempted (by some unexplained means) to stop her menstrual flow, which resulted in permanent internal damage. Furthermore, school is also harmful because of the physical stress of gymnastics classes. Girls who are too shy to ask permission to go to the bathroom may develop menstrual irregularity from retention of urine.

Beware of mumps; they can destroy the ovaries, Howard warns. But the worst fate of all is reserved for the girl who goes to dances lightly clothed, in short sleeves and low neck. She will surely end up in the doctor's hands or become a drug fiend.

Next comes a peculiar passage in which Howard unwittingly reveals a deep revulsion for the feminine body. Girls have bad odors, he says, but saturating the system with many glasses of water dilutes them so that "scarcely any of them will make their presence known to those around you." The effect of this accusation on an adolescent girl's self-confidence must have been devastating.

In a section on health and hygiene even pimples are made a source of guilt: "Muddy and contaminating thoughts will cause a muddy skin." In a set piece of advice that holds the rudiments of the standard pimple talk for teens he admonishes: (1) don't squeeze; (2) use your own brush; (3) ignore ads for remedies; (4) avoid constipation; and (5) go to a reputable doctor. And don't kiss other girls, he adds.

Howard's dietary advice in *Confidential Chats with Girls* is also eccentric. Cereal and stewed fruit should be eaten for breakfast. The author agrees with "most girls" that eggs, fish, and milk are repulsive. In any case one should never drink milk with meat. Eating before bed is perfectly all right, as are candy, pickles, and almost anything else one wants to eat—as long as the bowels are kept open.

Like most of his contemporaries, Howard puts great faith in the healthfulness of cold baths. He also advises girls to perform "waist exercises" regularly and to take sodium phosphate once a week (as a laxative). He vehemently attacks the rats and falls with which young women elaborate their coiffures because, he says, "dead" hair smells and such hairstyles may lead to baldness.

Another Edwardian favorite, the high collar, also reaps his scorn: tight collars with points up under the ears cause headaches and bad complexions.

Howard also assumes that women are especially subject to nervous disease. The nerves are destroyed by exercising or working when not inclined, he says, but (in an unconscious paradox) adds that developing willpower depends on healthy nerves. And willpower, of course, is "the rudder of life." Therefore Howard provides some advice about maintaining healthy nerves: "Sleep always alone. Sleeping with another person is unsanitary. Don't use coffee to overcome fatigue. Shouting and yelling exhaust the nervous powers. Never drink nerve tonics such as 'Dopie' or 'Bromo Tonic.'" We are inclined to agree when he says "Most of the bottled drinks sold at five cents should be thrown into the sewers, and how many diseased lips do you think have touched the glasses passed around at the circus and similar shows?" A final word of advice on this topic suggests that Freud's ideas were beginning to have a wide impact by 1911 (even on working-class girls): "You have heard much about psychotherapy, suggestion and a lot about certain Movements in church circles" as a cure for nerves. A better practice for healthy nerves would be to examine the inner self daily at home.

Uncongenial as it may be to present-day readers, *Confidential Chats with Girls* probably reflects better the daily realities of life at the turn of the century than the more polite and restrained books written for the middle class. Howard's closing chapter of miscellaneous health advice is particularly revealing: Don't giggle—it distorts the face. Don't hold hat pins or theater tickets in the mouth, or use the teeth to pull off glove fingers—there is a danger of contracting consumption from such unsanitary habits. Using arsenic to plump up the face is not recommended. And it probably is not very healthy to eat candies with cocaine in them.

A similar attitude of distaste toward feminine and masculine sexuality is evident in Irving David Steinhardt's *Ten Sex Talks to Girls* and *Ten Sex Talks to Boys* (both 1914), which were based on a lecture series the author had delivered to the Hebrew Educational Society of Brooklyn and the Emanu-El Brotherhood of New York. A respected member of society, Steinhardt was on the faculty of Cornell University Medical School and had worked with a clinic for delinquent girls. Like most contemporary sex educators, he was a member of the American Society of Sanitary and Moral Prophylaxis. Yet Steinhardt's finickiness seems old-fashioned even for 1914. The ways of female masturbation, he declaims are "too disgusting for utterance." A girl who indulges in excessive self-abuse will end her days in an insane asylum or in an early grave. Even excessive sexual indulgence in marriage can lead to such unhappy endings. In a passage extraordinary for the time in its veiled references to lesbian seduction he warns against overaffectionate girlfriends. A young girl should avoid a friend who admires her breasts and invites her to stay overnight or sleep in the same bed. If a girl does accept an invitation from such a sinister person, she should keep her gown and robe close around her, beware of snuggling, and ask to sleep in a separate bed because it is more sanitary. On no account are girls to lie in each others arms all night and talk about sex.

Steinhardt shows an extreme respect for the physical evidence of virginity. Douching is not advisable, he maintains, because it might interfere with the hymen by accident. If a doctor must violate the hymen he should give the patient a signed statement for her "future protection against unfounded suspicions." He ends with a warning against those girls who take pay to bring about the moral ruin of other girls. "Beware of strange women!" he intones biblically.

In *Ten Sex Talks to Boys* Steinhardt demonstrates that his misanthropy is not restricted to the female half of the human race. He begins by justifying sex education in negative terms:

> A criminal silence has been maintained which permitted innumerable girls to be morally ruined by the male sex. These girls, as they became more and more degraded, likewise became diseased, yet were allowed without question or restraints, to ruin the health of their male companions. . . .

Steinhardt fills his chapter on male reproductive anatomy with enough technical detail to discourage anyone but the serious medical student (one illustration, for example, is labeled "Cast of ampullae and seminal vesticles, showing winding and sacculation of lumen"). To further impress the reader with the seriousness of the book Steinhardt includes exercises at the end of each chapter ("Describe fully the interior of the testicles." "What might produce feeble-mindedness or insanity in children at birth?").

In contrast to the abundant details he supplies in the anatomy section Steinhardt is utterly uninformative on the physiology of coitus:

> All of you should know, and probably do, that children are the result of the proper union of the male and female elements of generation. Also all of you should know, and probably do, that these elements are brought into contact with each other by a certain act or relation which unites the male and the female. This relation is designated as sexual intercourse or the marriage relation, and should never be indulged in before marriage.

This is followed by the declaration, in capital letters, that "THE SEXUAL RELATION IS ABSOLUTELY UNNECESSARY TO YOU OR TO ANY OTHER MAN."

Steinhardt next launches into a recitation of the horrors of venereal disease that is remarkable not only for its lurid detail but also for its persistence even into the 1940 edition: "Seventy to eighty percent of the men who indulge their animal desires are infected with gonorrhea by the fallen woman with whom they consort sexually," he begins. The full extent of damage caused by gonorrhea and syphilis is of comparatively recent discovery. In a case of gonorrhea the primary symptoms cause intense suffering and may lead to abscesses of the bladder, kidney, and prostate and testicles, or even to gonorrheal rheumatism, causing "the most excruciating continuous pain that can be imagined." The end result may be sterilization, blindness, or the deaths of innocent loved ones. Steinhardt invites readers to imagine a tiny grave and tombstone with this pathetic inscription: "Here lies a little blind baby, so afflicted from birth, offered up by its father as a sacrifice to his pre-marriage sacrilege of the sexual relation."

Steinhardt refuses to discuss methods of treatment: "It would only harm you were I to recommend specific modes of treatment. There are many kinds of treatment, and none of them has any place in my talks." Far better to guard against contracting the disease in the first place through sexual abstinence. Never sit on a toilet seat without cleaning it and covering it with paper; never wear other people's clothing, especially rented bathing suits; never swim nude in indoor pools; don't drink alcohol, read licentious matter, or dance. In other words, says Steinhardt. "Just be a real man!"

Having finished with gonorrhea, Steinhardt gives equal attention to the ravages of syphilis. He describes the five types of syphilitic chancres in full detail, while affecting an inability to convey the full horror of the disease:

> To tell you what follows during the acute and chronic stages of this most horrible of diseases is to commence with the hair on the top of the head, to go down to the soles of the feet, and to include every part of the head, body and extremities lying between. . . .

Nevertheless, he steels himself for the challenge ("It will do no harm to touch upon these sequels") and commences the parade of horrors from head to toe, emphasizing again that not only the transgressor is affected: "The sowing of wild oats in the springtime of youth can make a man later on the murderer of his own child." Steinhardt punctuates his argument by including a photograph of a hideously deformed syphilitic baby, probably a corpse.

By this time the shaken reader is in a frame of mind to pay strict attention to the author's instructions on disease prevention. Most important, lead a moral life, says Steinhardt. Avoid common drinking cups and towels, shaving brushes and mugs, and all unnecessary physical contact with other people. If one should contract syphilis and have to submit to two years of cure, he should not consider himself clean until he has had negative Wasserman tests from three different doctors. There should be laws, Steinhardt says (and there soon were), requiring Wasserman tests before marriage and the application of silver nitrate to the eyes of newborn babies to be sure they are not afflicted with gonorrhea (which can be passed from mother to child during birth).

Having expended most of this thunder in the chapters on venereal disease, Steinhardt is relatively mild on the subject of masturbation. He suggests that the harm of this practice is psychological rather than physical. It is unhealthy, he says. Being a solitary activity, it can be done to excess, because some masturbators lose the desire for sex with a partner and because deception about it leads to dishonesty in other areas, too. But after this restrained and modern-sounding passage he ends the chapter with a reference to masturbatory insanity.

Steinhardt concludes *Ten Sex Talks to Boys* by offering the young male some encouragement and instruction on appropriate attitudes and action toward womankind. He deplores the "freak-

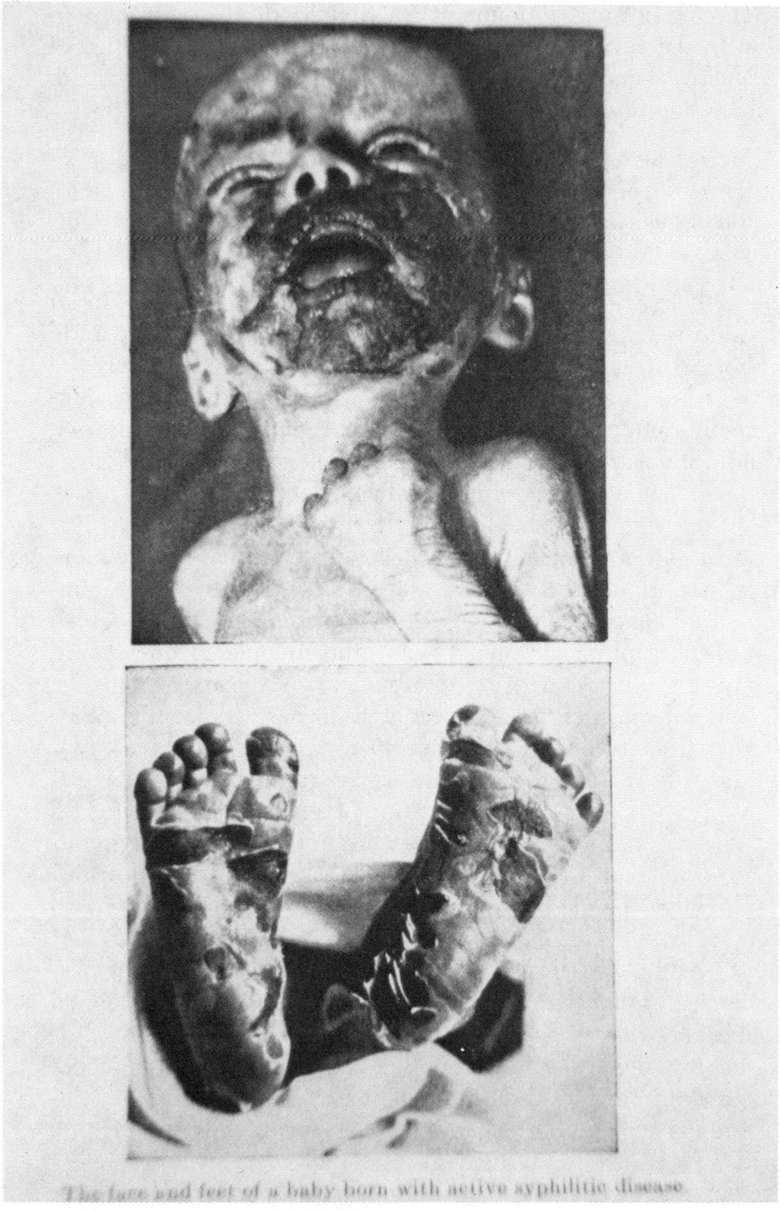

The face and feet of a baby born with active syphilitic disease

Fig. 4. Syphilitic baby. From *Ten Sex Talks to Boys*, by Irving Steinhardt.

ishness and immodesty" of fashionable female dress and suggests a remedy:

> We want them [women] to understand that, while not posing as their masters or "bosses," we still have ideas to what is right and wrong; and, being convinced of the justness of our ideas, we expect them to conform to these. Certainly our wishes should have as much weight with our women as the dictates of a so-called style.

The young man should keep a tight eye on his female sibling: "Take enough interest in your sister to ascertain where and for whom she works, if she is so unfortunate as to be compelled to go outside of her home to make a livelihood." In that event he should check his sister's wardrobe frequently to make sure it contains no items suspiciously beyond the reach of her salary. Even toward his fiancée he should be cautious about physical contact, because "kissing in couples is always dangerous" and spreads tuberculosis, syphilis, and other diseases.

Just before World War I, in stark contrast to works like Howard's and Steinhardt's a few books began to appear that attempted a less didactic and more scientific (though not necessarily more successful) approach to sex education. A particularly unsavory example of this type of book is *My Birth: The Autobiography of an Unborn Infant* (1916), by Armenouhie T. Lamson. In sentimental and breathless prose the fetus tells the story of its development from conception to the moment before it "appears on the stage of life." Not only is the fetus given a voice but also every cell and organ it encounters speaks and has its own personality and point of view. The overall effect is reminiscent of an utterly humorless cartoon script. Here, for instance, is the ovum describing her meeting with the sperm (how he got there in the first place is carefully ignored). The scene is the fallopian tube:

> As it was very dark and very close about me, I was sure my end was at hand. But then I suddenly felt myself forcefully held and lovingly embraced by a friendly little stranger known as the male germ cell or "Spermatozoon"—during which act the male element disappeared within my body.

A more successful attempt at scientific objectivity is found in Bertha Louise Cady's *The Way Life Begins: An Introduction to Sex Education*. First published in 1917, it was reissued with few changes in 1939. Cady's stated intent is to teach "the deeper meaning of nature study" by examining the reproductive biology of plants and animals in successive chapters on the lily, the moth, the fish, the frog, the chick, the rabbit, and the child. Only the final chapter attempts to address "the personal problems of life." The illustrations are handsome; color plates (hand-colored and pasted in the 1917 edition) depict "sphinx moths gathering nectar from the lily flower," "the life story of the frog," "a nest of newly-born cottontails under cabbage leaves," and, later, the human embryo and the reproductive organs of the male and the female (these last color pictures often have been torn out of extant copies of the work). The information is presented simply and with scientific accuracy, although Cady makes no attempt to move past biological description or to deal with coitus in any terms—physical, psychological, or social. In the last chapter she asserts that knowledge is the key to right living and self-control, and ignorance creates disharmony, disillusionment, pain, and misery (meaning vice, as Sylvanus Stall had maintained twenty years earlier). Cady's inclusion of this last section is clearly obligatory, however, and incidental to the main purpose of her work. Apart from their relative flaws and their differences in style and content both Cady's and Lamson's books foreshadow later attempts to separate the presentation of biological information from moralizing discussions of character and sexual contact.

▪ The Rosy Girls

Even as the post-Victorian era of sexual repression began to wane, many books written for girls continued to follow the model that had been set by Mary Wood-Allen almost twenty years earlier. There were marginal differences in emphasis, as in Nellie M. Smith's book *The Three Gifts of Life: A Girl's Responsibility for Race Progress* (1913), which stressed the ability of girls to contribute to the betterment of humanity by selecting husbands with superior genetic and behavioral characteristics. Rose Woodallen Chapman, the daughter of Mary Wood-Allen, also followed her mother's model. She succeeded Wood-Allen as National Superintendent of the Purity Department of the Women's Christian Temperance Union, taking office in 1908, the year of her mother's death. From 1910 to 1913 Chapman wrote a popular sex education column for the *Ladies' Home Journal* called "What Shall We Tell the Children?" and in her later years she held office as field secretary of women's work for the American Social Hygiene Association.

Although, like her mother, Chapman enjoyed a wide and responsive readership, her advice tended to be cautious and prudish in contrast to Wood-Allen's relatively forthright and definite approach. Chapman's *In Her Teens* (1914) warns that the first step on the road of danger can be such "innocent" pleasures as holding hands or allowing an arm about the waist or a good-night kiss. She quotes from her fan mail: "Some girls write to me that they are so afraid of young men, since hearing of the dangers that exist for girls, that they can hardly speak to them." Goodness, no, says Chapman, she didn't mean to give that impression. A girl need not fear men if she is master of herself. But remember, "No one ever touched another's soul by becoming the plaything of his senses." Yet despite her exaggerated conservatism, Chapman shared the warmth, dedication, and real concern for her young readers that had distinguished her mother's work.

Gradually, however, the works of many sex educators began to show signs of changing times, even as they remained within the Wood-Allen tradition. *The Changing Girl: A Little Book for the Girl of Ten to Fifteen* (1913), by Caroline Wormeley Latimer, is unusual in its acknowledgment of female sexuality. Latimer was an instructor in biology at Goucher College and was ahead of her time in conjecturing that "the apparent absence of sex instinct in girls is largely a matter of training extending over many generations." Other writers seemed to alter the pattern almost unconsciously. Mary Gould Hood's *For Girls and the Mothers of Girls* (1914), for example, is a fulsome tract on the pleasures of self-sacrifice and the joys of motherhood and probably was written in reaction to feminist calls for new freedoms. However, Hood's book stands apart from its predecessors in that it contains the first clinically accurate (if strangely disembodied) description of coitus ever offered in print to girls: "This muscular tube [the penis] deposits the semen in the upper part of the vagina, where the sperm can readily reach the ovum. Such union of the sexes is commonly called intercourse."

As the war years approached, there were frequent references to proper feminine conduct at the office, reflecting the new acceptance of the working woman. Dating, too, began to be mentioned, although with disapproval. *Preparing for Woman-*

hood (1918), by Edith Belle Lowry, illustrates contemporary attempts to reconcile these emerging social patterns with inherited attitudes.

Lowry, a physician, had previously written several sex education books, including *Truths: Talks with a Boy Concerning Himself* (1911) and *Confidences: Talks with a Young Girl Concerning Herself* (1910), which her publisher had promoted as "the only series of books on sex hygiene which has received the endorsement of the leading medical, educational and religious authorities." Addressed to girls aged fifteen to twenty-one, *Preparing for Womanhood* consists mostly of the usual advice on health, recreation, and personal appearance, with an emphasis on the need for girls to learn homemaking skills. Lowry includes an unusual feature, however—an entire chapter on the special problems of women in business: "Times have changed greatly, and the girl of today, besides being independent, is a dominant factor in the life of this country and most notably in the cities, where the women not only sway the business world but even the sacred world of politics."

Evidently feeling the need to justify this new role, Lowry explains that a knowledge of business methods enables a girl to run a home better. Furthermore, it is wise for women to prepare for a career in case their husbands die or they encounter "sudden financial misfortune." She then makes the paradoxical accusation that many girls do not succeed in the business world because they do not take their work seriously and are only waiting to get married. The girl who wants to do well, says Lowry, should not be afraid to start at the bottom and to do menial chores like dusting the office in addition to her regular duties. She should also be careful to dress modestly and inconspicuously.

Lowry was well aware of the demanding conditions under which most working women labored. A twelve- to sixteen-hour day was not unusual (although New York State had passed "an enlightened law" in 1912 limiting women to a nine-hour workday). Average wages were six dollars a week, but a diligent girl might hope for eventual raises to ten dollars. Lowry deplores the fact that after paying rent and laundry, many working girls have little left for food, but her advice is less than helpful: "The only solution of this problem that I can see is for each girl to pause and plan her future course carefully."

In a number of other less obvious ways *Preparing for Womanhood* incorporates and yet departs from the common repertoire of advice to young women. Lowry, for instance, feels that the corset is not so bad after all: "I believe that a large percentage of the objections to the corset originated from women wearing improperly fitted corsets which pushed the organs out of place. A corset fitted to the wearer is not injurious and often serves as a support."

She describes the female reproductive organs in terms of their use by a fetus, not the owner; the uterus is the baby's nest and the vagina is its birth channel. Although she gives the usual cautions against cold, bathing, and exercise during the menstrual period, Lowry excuses girls living away from home from the onerous task of washing out pads made of old rags. (Disposable commercial napkins were not yet available.) She recommends "absorbent cotton enclosed in a thickness of gauze" as an alternative, because these "may be burned instead of laundered."

However conventional, Lowry's discussion of correct behavior for women while in the company of men reflects the emergence of the new pattern of courtship called dating. In particular, she warns against meeting young men at "the corner drugstore"; properly a girl should be called for at her home. Furthermore, girls should dress modestly and bear in mind always that "a man who seeks to destroy your chastity under the guise of love only is cloaking selfish passion under the raiment of affection."

While other writers also attempted to address the practical problems of contemporary girls, Lowry's warning to girls to ignore evident changes in sexual morality and conduct is more representative of the current literature. Indeed, similar cautions in other books for girls from this period constitute the primary evidence that a trend toward sexual freedom in the coming decade was underway. A particularly reactionary example is a pamphlet titled *Why the Roses Bloom: A Message to Girls*, written about 1919 and attributed to Sina Stratton, superintendent of moral education for the Women's Christian Temperance Union. A labored metaphor of the young girl as a newly opened rose runs throughout its twenty-three pages ("Your individual rose is finished, the perfect bloom of womanhood has come . . ."). The explanation of "why the roses bloom" is, of course, those vital bodily fluids, which are held in reserve in

> two little store rooms called ovaries. From their very substance a fluid is thrown into your blood, which recreates you, physically, mentally, spiritually and causes you to grow rounded and have color in your cheeks. God wants to use this fluid which is being

> poured into your bloodstream, to recreate you into the perfect woman, before there can be any surplus, to create through you, that second individual, your child, your rose. It is this creative force in you, that if rightly used, will enable you to go through your school and college work with credit, and after you leave, to make a success of whatever line of work you may select.

Every girl should be alert to protect her bloom from the hazards of loose behavior. Girls must not tempt men, Stratton says in a passage foreshadowing the image of the "flaming youth" of the twenties, by meeting them for "dates" or at the "movies," or by dressing indecently, bleaching their hair, painting or powdering, or taking part in promiscuous fondling and kissing. "Indulgence in these liberties, and thus catering to, and arousing this sex instinct, outside the marriage vows, leads to many a clandestine mating, and many an unwelcome child is born to a life of sin." Such behavior, or even solitary vice in the form of prurient thoughts, can interfere with development. The sad result can be colorless cheeks where no roses bloom and that must be painted to simulate the real blossoming of God's purpose.

As we shall see in the next chapter, from the same generation of sex educators who continued to reassert the function of motherhood as "God's purpose" for women rose a few impassioned activists who challenged the very core of this argument.

■ BIBLIOGRAPHY

Bisseker, H. *When a Boy Becomes a Man: A Little Book for Boys*. Edward Bok Books of Self-Knowledge for Young People and Parents. No. 2. New York: Revell, 1912.

Boy Scouts of America. *Official Handbook for Boys*. New York: Doubleday, Page, 1911; Irving, Texas: Boy Scouts of America, 1976.

Cady, Bertha Louise (Chapman). *The Way Life Begins: An Introduction to Sex Education*. New York: American Social Hygiene Association, 1917; rev. ed., 1939.

Chapman, Rose Woodallen. *In Her Teens*. New York: Revell, 1914.

Foster, William Trufant, ed. *The Social Emergency: Studies in Sex Hygiene and Morals*. Boston: Houghton Mifflin, 1914.

Hall, Winfield Scott, *Father and Son; John's Vacation; What John Saw in the Country*. Chicago: American Medical Association Press, 1913.

———. *From Youth into Manhood*. New York: Young Men's Christian Association Press, 1909.

———. *Margaret, The Doctor's Daughter*. Sex Education Pamphlets. Chicago: American Medical Association, 1911.

Hood, Mary Gould. *For Girls and the Mothers of Girls: A Book for the Home and the School Concerning the Beginnings of Life*. Indianapolis: Bobbs-Merrill, 1914.

Howard, William Lee. *Confidential Chats with Girls*. New York: Clode, 1911.

King, Elisha Alonzo. *Helps to Health and Purity*. Des Moines, Iowa: Personal Help, 1903.

———. *A Talk to Men*. Des Moines, Iowa: Personal Help, 1897.

———, and F. B. Meyer. *Clean and Strong*. Boston: United Society of Christian Endeavor, 1909; rev. ed., 1917.

Lamson, Armenouhie T. (Tashjian). *My Birth: The Autobiography of an Unborn Infant*. New York: Macmillan, 1916.

Latimer, Caroline Wormeley. *The Changing Girl: A Little Book for the Girl of Ten to Fifteen*. Edward Bok Books of Self-Knowledge for Young People and Parents, No. 5. New York: Revell, 1913.

Lowry, Edith Belle. *Confidences: Talks with a Young Girl Concerning Herself*. Chicago: Forbes, 1910.

———. *Preparing for Womanhood*. Chicago: Forbes, 1918.

———. *Truths: Talks with a Boy Concerning Himself*. Chicago: Forbes, 1911.

Moore, Harry Hascall. *Keeping in Condition: A Handbook on Training for Older Boys*. New York: Macmillan, 1916.

Smith, Nellie May. *The Three Gifts of Life: A Girl's Responsibility for Race Progress*. New York: Dodd, Mead, 1913.

Steinhardt, Irving David. *Ten Sex Talks to Boys*. Philadelphia: Lippincott, 1914.

———. *Ten Sex Talks to Girls*. Philadelphia: Lippincott, 1914.

Stratton, Sina. *Why the Roses Bloom: A Message to Girls*. Philadelphia: Women's Christian Temperance Union, ca. 1919.

Wile, Ira Solomon. *Sex Education*. New York: Duffield, 1912.

Chapter 4

Two Trials

From the appearance of the earliest examples of the genre in the 1890s until almost the present day most sex guides enjoyed warm approval from mainstream thinkers of their era. This is probably because the books accurately reflected, or even lagged a bit behind, accepted sexual ideas. Only with the onset of conservatism in the early 1980s did this previously inviolable form begin to be attacked by would-be censors. In the first eight decades of the history of sex guides there were only two major obscenity trials involving an adolescent sex education book. In both these cases the obscenity charges were merely an excuse for a political vendetta against the authors. The real issue was the legality of birth control, and the targets of official wrath were Margaret Sanger in 1916 and Mary Ware Dennett in 1929. Both were prosecuted under the notorious Comstock Law, which prohibited the distribution of contraception information and any other "obscene" material through the United States mails.

▪ "What Every Girl Should Know"

Margaret Higgins Sanger first became aware of the legal restraints on the distribution of contraception information as an outgrowth of her work as a nurse in the slums of New York City in the early 1900s. Having "asked doctors what one could do" to circumvent the bans, she learned (as she relates in *My Fight for Birth Control*) that "I'd better keep off that subject or Anthony Comstock would get me." Later, after she had indeed been "got" by Comstock, she was to refer to him as "that flamboyant and pathological zealot." Comstock's life merited both adjectives. He brought a wild-eyed energy and enthusiasm to the abolishment of obscenity, which he defined in terms of his personal aversions and which he saw everywhere. In his book *Traps for the Young*, written in 1883, he revealed a vision of contemporary America in which vice spread and ensnared the young through newspapers, books, advertisements, classic literature, and almost every other form of human communication.

Comstock had been a powerful figure for forty years before he clashed with Sanger. In 1872, when he was twenty-eight years old and a private citizen living in Brooklyn, New York, Comstock became an officer of an antivice committee of the Young Men's Christian Association (the committee that in 1875 became the New York Society for the Suppression of Vice, which supported Comstock's censorship activities throughout his career). With this official backing he went to Washington and lobbied vigorously for the passage of an antiobscenity bill he had written and succeeded in ramming it through an inattentive Congress at the closing session of March 1873.

Amended and slightly reworded in 1876, the Comstock Law forbade the dissemination through the U.S. Post Office of "every obscene, lewd, lascivious, indecent, filthy or vile" object or publication, as well as any object or publication "intended for preventing conception or producing abortion, or for any indecent or immoral use." This law, which was subsequently reclassified from the Post Office Code (Section 211) to the criminal section of the U.S. Code (Title 18, Sections 1461–1462), declared such materials "non-mailable" and allowed for the punishment of offenders through fine, imprisonment, or both.

Shortly after the bill was passed, Comstock was commissioned a special agent (solicitor) of the Post Office to see that the law was enforced. Supported by the law and the authority of his position, Comstock quickly assumed the role of public censor. Working at both national and local levels (the Comstock Law opened the way for the passage of numerous state laws prohibiting the publication, sale, and distribution of obscene matter and information about abortion and contraception), Comstock was unimpeded in effecting the suppression of any material he considered "unmailable." By the time of his death in 1915 he had made 1,792 arrests and seized forty-five tons of obscene matter.

Margaret Sanger was equally zealous in devotion to her own cause—birth control, a term she claimed to have coined herself.

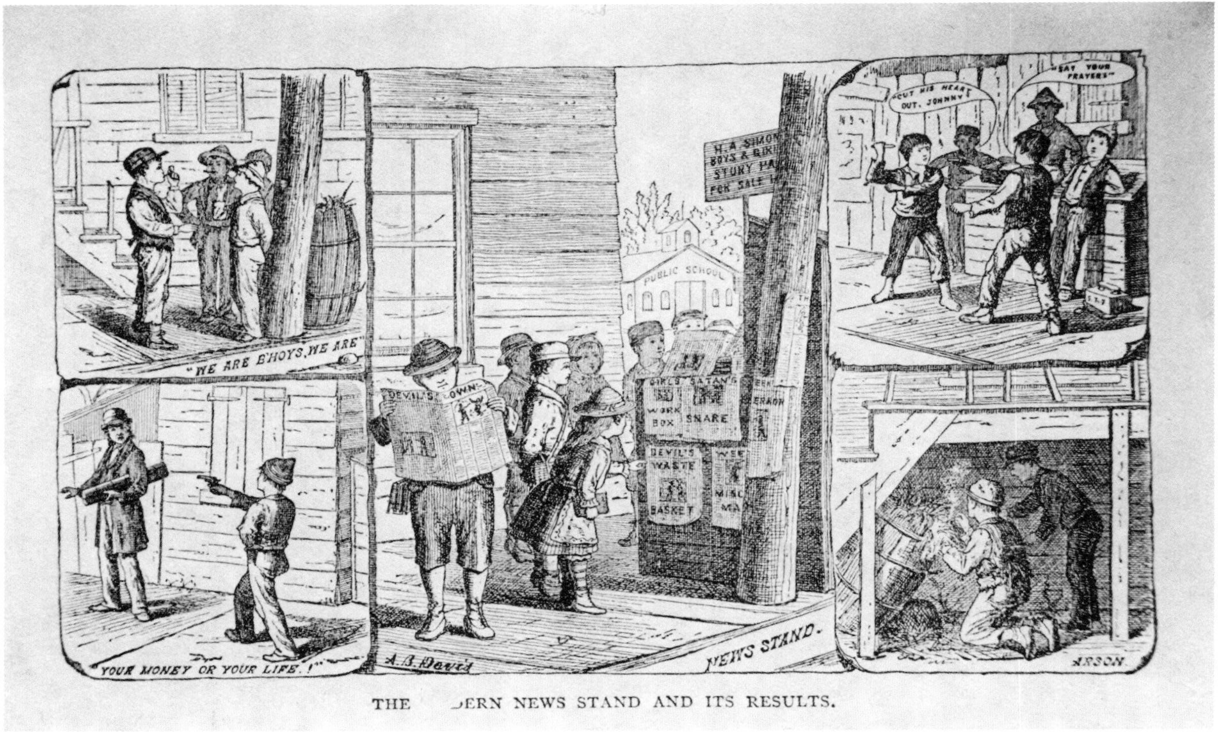

Fig. 5. "The Modern News Stand and Its Results." From *Traps for the Young*, by Anthony Comstock.

In her *Autobiography* (1938) and in *My Fight for Birth Control* (1931) she tells of her harsh childhood as one of eleven children and of her mother's premature death at age forty-eight. Born in 1883 in Corning, New York, she was married in 1900 to architect William Sanger. In 1912 the couple moved to Manhattan, where their home soon became a gathering place for intellectuals and activists of the left—socialists, anarchists, and wobblies—and where Margaret's work in the Lower East Side further exposed her to the suffering caused by unlimited breeding in poverty.

One night that year she was asked by a socialist friend to fill in for a speaker at a meeting for working women. Out of that speech Sanger developed a series of articles called *What Every Girl Should Know* for a radical newspaper, the *Call.* When the paper announced that one of the final installments in the series would discuss venereal disease, it was informed by the Post Office Department, led by Comstock, that the paper's mailing permit would be revoked if it attempted to include the article. Faced with this ultimatum, the *Call* printed the ironic caption "What Every Girl Should Know—Nothing!" in place of the suppressed article. Undeterred by the brush with censorship, Sanger had the full series printed and distributed as a pamphlet in 1914.

Dedicated to "the working girls of the world," *What Every Girl Should Know* is characterized by a straightforward style and a burning concern for women's rights. After detailed descriptions of the male and female sexual anatomy, conception, and birth (with a diagram of the female internal genitalia) Sanger discusses the delicate mental state of the pubescent girl and proposes that the nervous strain of menstruation would be relieved if working women banded together and demanded one day's rest a month during their periods. Even more radical, Sanger dares to hint that unmarried motherhood may be an enriching experience and that "women should know that creative energy does not need to be expended entirely on the propagation of the race." She defines the difference between the young male and female sexual impulse in these terms: girls desire to touch, caress, and speak to the opposite sex; boys desire to discharge the accumulation of sex cells and relieve nervous tension. Masturbation is a habit that is easily acquired by girls as well as boys, and girls who do it may (in a ground-breaking but oblique first reference to female orgasm) "find themselves incapable of any relief in the natural act, tossing about nervously for hours after."

Convinced that "in Anglo-Saxon women the sex desire is latent until the age of thirty," Sanger refers to this as an advantage in that it allows women to sublimate their energies into "the bigger and broader movements and activities in which they are active today." In a section on pregnancy she enumerates the dangers of abortion and induced miscarriages and gives the symptoms and duration of gestation. She expresses conventional views on the theory of seminal power and denies the myth that sex is necessary for health, but the double standard reaps her scorn: "Every girl should look upon the man who indulges freely in sexual relations without social responsibility, as a prostitute far more degraded than the unfortunate girl compelled to sell her body to sustain life."

Sanger is indignant at the number of wives who are infected with venereal diseases by their libertine husbands: "Three out of every five married women in New York have gonorrhea." Further, "if women voluntarily exposed themselves to diseases which sapped the husband's vitality, making him a dependent invalid or exposed him to the shock of a mutilating operation, or death—would men continue to suffer?" In the section objected to by the postal authorities Sanger gives the symptomatology and means of transmission of syphilis and deplores the difficulties for working people in obtaining treatment. Only in the later editions (the pamphlet was reissued in 1927 under the title *What Every Boy and Girl Should Know*) did Sanger conclude this work with a veiled reference to birth control: "Stop bringing to birth children whose inheritance cannot be one of health or intelligence. Stop bringing into the world children whose parents cannot provide for them. Herein lies the key of civilization." An advertisement on the last page announced that "Socialist Party Locals, Branches, and dealers can obtain this book at the following prices . . . "

Also in 1914 Sanger began to edit a periodical, the *Woman Rebel*, in which she published articles advocating sexual freedom for women and closely skirting the birth-control issue. This, too, was declared unmailable, but Sanger continued to publish it in spite of repeated warnings from the Post Office Department. She was soon in serious trouble with the law and in late 1914 was forced to flee to Europe to gain time to prepare a legal defense against charges of obscenity. It was during this period of exile that she met the British birth-control advocate Dr. Marie Stopes and became the friend and admirer of Havelock Ellis, whose theories on the spiritual and emotional aspects of sex left a deep impression on her. (Stopes was then writing *Married Love*, which was vigorously banned in the United States following its publication in 1918.)

Meanwhile, Comstock sent a decoy to William Sanger's home to buy a copy of Margaret's pamphlet *Family Limitation* (1915), a practical guide to birth-control methods that Margaret had arranged to have distributed in her absence. Comstock personally arrested William Sanger the next day. The game was for high stakes: Comstock offered William acquittal in exchange for information about Margaret's whereabouts. Indignantly refusing, Sanger asked Comstock what he would consider appropriate punishment for the author of the pamplet. "Five years hard labor for every copy printed!" he snapped. Within the year William was tried and found guilty of distributing obscene literature and subsequently served thirty days in jail.

Soon after William's trial in September 1915 Margaret returned voluntarily for her own trial. She found that in her absence a National Birth Control League had been formed and had been given her files and mailing lists. Meeting with this group, she was astounded to be told by its president, Mary Ware Dennett, that the league could not support her illegal methods because it was committed to changing the laws in an orderly and proper manner rather than to defying them. But public opinion had grown in favor of Sanger during her year's absence, and the league reversed its opinion just before the trial. Furthermore, Margaret was no longer faced with the personal opposition of Anthony Comstock, who had died (after catching a chill at William Sanger's trial), and when Margaret's case came to trial in February 1916, it was immediately dismissed. The postal authorities were not appeased, however, and bided their time.

Turning to more concrete action later that year, Margaret opened a birth-control clinic in a working-class neighborhood of the Brownsville section of Brooklyn. Assisted by her sister, Ethel Byrne, and a young friend, Fania Mindell, she worked from morning until night fitting diaphragms and giving birth-control information to the women who flocked to the clinic for help. Margaret's venture was in direct opposition to New York State laws, which said that only doctors could prescribe contraceptive devices and only for the cure or prevention of disease. It was not long before the police arrived. All three women were arrested.

Margaret was charged with conducting a birth-control clinic; Ethel, with disseminating birth-control information; and Fania Mindell, with selling an indecent publication—*What Every Girl Should Know.*

Amid lurid press coverage and deafening public outcry Ethel was convicted and nearly died in prison on a hunger strike. Fania Mindell was convicted and fined fifty dollars, later reversed on appeal. Sanger, also found guilty, was sent to prison for thirty days and although she, too, appealed her case, her conviction was upheld. However, the judge who heard Sanger's appeal significantly altered the interpretation of the state statute regarding the prescription of contraceptives for the cure or prevention of disease (previously understood to mean venereal disease only); he allowed that a doctor could give contraceptive advice to any married woman who required it for the maintenance of her health. On the strength of this decision Margaret reopened her birth-control clinic in Manhattan in 1923, paving the way for the establishment of numerous other clinics across the country.

In succeeding years Sanger wrote and lectured widely on birth control. At one point she noted ironically that "the section on venereal disease in *What Every Girl Should Know*, which had once been banned in the New York *Call* and for which Fania had been fined, was now, officially but without credit, reprinted and distributed among the soldiers going into cantonments and abroad." Before her death in 1966 Sanger saw the fulfillment of many of her dreams for liberalized access to birth-control information. However, it was not until 1971 that the Comstock Law was modified to allow the mailing of contraceptives and birth-control information to the general public.

▪ "THE SEX SIDE OF LIFE"

In one of history's minor ironies Mary Ware Dennett, the president of the National Birth Control League, who had self-righteously refused support for Sanger's illegal methods, in 1929 found herself the defendant in the second obscenity trial of an adolescent sex education book. The testimony and evidence in the case are recorded in detail and with considerable emotion by Dennett in her book *Who's Obscene*? (1930), written immediately after the trial. Although it is clear that the real matter at issue was her political activities on behalf of birth control, the nature of the testimony is an interesting commentary on the state of sex education literature in 1929.

The title accused of obscenity was a slight pamphlet of only twenty-one pages—*The Sex Side of Life* (1918). Dennett wrote the pamphlet for her own two boys, aged eleven and fourteen, "after examining about sixty publications on the subject and forming the opinion that they were inadequate and unsatisfactory." "I found none," she explains, "that I was willing to put into their hands without first guarding them against what I considered very misleading and harmful impressions." And so she set out to write her own book.

In Dennett's opinion her work differed from that which had gone before in several important respects. First, she used "proper terminology" in calling things by their right scientific names. She emphasized the *un*likeness of human reproduction to that of plants and animals, and she was honest in saying that venereal disease was becoming curable.

But the most significant difference in her mind, and in the minds of the hostile witnesses at the trial, was the fact that she dealt with what she called "the emotional side of life." As she explained, "In not a single one of all the books for young people that I have thus far read has there been the frank and unashamed declaration that the climax of sex emotion is an unsurpassed joy." And so Dennett said the unsayable—she told young people that sex was pleasurable. The passage in question, while it probably would not have provoked a censorship attempt had it not been for the political issue, is a more explicit description of coitus than anything that had ever before been offered to adolescents:

> When a man and a woman fall in love so that they really belong to each other, the physical side of the relation is this: both of them feel at intervals a peculiar thrill or glow, particularly in the sexual organs, and it naturally culminates after they have gone to bed at night. The man's special sex organ or penis, becomes enlarged and stiffened, instead of soft and limp as ordinarily, and thus it easily enters the passage in the woman's body called the vagina or birth-canal, which leads to the uterus or womb, which as perhaps you already know is the sac in which the egg or embyro grows into a baby. The penis and the vagina are about the same size, as Nature intended them to fit each other. By a rhythmic movement of the

> penis in and out, the sex act reaches an exciting climax or orgasm, when there is for the woman a peculiarly satisfying contraction of the muscles of the passage and for the man, the expulsion of the semen, the liquid which contains the germs of life. This is followed by a sensation of peaceful happiness and sleepy relaxation. It is the very greatest physical pleasure to be had in all human experience, and it helps very much to increase all other kinds of pleasure also. It is at this time that married people not only are closest to each other physically, but they feel closer to each other in every other way, too.

The large part of the pamphlet is taken up with physiological descriptions related to the two very clear drawings by Dr. Robert L. Dickinson showing the male and female internal reproductive systems. Dennett briefly explains the mechanics of conception and birth and laments that "at present, unfortunately, it is against the law to give people information as to how to manage their sex relations so that no baby will be created unless the father and mother are ready and glad to have it happen." About masturbation she says, "Recently many of the best scientists have concluded that the chief harm has come from the worry caused by doing it. There is no occasion for worry unless the habit is carried to excess," but the young person should not yield to the impulse unless the pressure is overwhelming. Dennett concludes with a warning against venereal disease and prostitution, and praise for sex relations between people who love each other.

Dennett's essay was first printed privately, then in the *Medical Review of Reviews* for February 1918, and finally as a pamphlet sold for twenty-five cents through the mails to meet a growing demand. The venture was distinctly secondary for Dennett, however; the main part of her attention and energies was taken up with her activities as director of the Voluntary Parenthood League. In the years 1919 and 1920 those activities took the form of a survey of Congress to find a sponsor for a bill to remove the words "preventing conception" from the Comstock Law. In 1921 the league was given new hope by the appointment of William Hays as Postmaster General. Hays was vociferous in repudiating the role of censor in his new job but, unfortunately, soon resigned to work with the censorship problems of the movie industry. His successor, Hubert Work, vigorously supported the obscenity laws and lost no time in issuing bulletins to that effect to local post offices. Sorely disappointed, Dennett wrote a steamy editorial for the *Birth Control Herald* in July 1922, attacking Work's stand. Two months later she was informed by the solicitor of the Post Office (the position held for so many years by Comstock) that *The Sex Side of Life* had been declared unmailable. Dennett ignored this decree and continued to meet the demand for copies through the mails.

By 1925 public acclaim for the pamphlet had grown to such proportions that Dennett asked some of the most prestigious users for a statement of support. This was submitted to the solicitor with a request that the ban be removed. The Post Office refused. Dennett pressed on, demanding to know which passages were considered obscene and, in a lengthy correspondence, pushed to know how the Post Office could be aware of the contents of sealed first-class mail. It was a surprise to no one when, in January 1929, she was indicted on charges of mailing obscene matter. The penalty was a maximum fine of $5,000 or five years in jail.

After many postponements the case was heard in April of that year. The judge, Warren Burrows, charged the jury to determine whether the pamphlet's "language has a tendency to deprave and corrupt the morals of those whose minds are open to such things, arousing and implanting in such minds lewd and obscene thoughts or desires." Defense attorney Morris L. Ernst presented an imposing array of endorsements from twenty scientific, educational, and religious authorities, including John Dewey, representatives from Union Theological Seminary, the YMCA, the YWCA, and the Child Study Association of America. At the judge's request twelve of these witnesses for the prosecution were invited to submit statements to the court. These letters Dennett later included in *Who's Obscene?* Those for the defense praised *The Sex Side of Life* as "healthy," "sane," and "wholesome," and many compared it favorably with other pamphlets distributed by educational, religious, or government organizations. Statistical and medical testimony to support Dennett's attitudes about masturbation were provided by several of the medical authorities.

The prosecution, on the other hand, evidently had a hard time rounding up expert witnesses. Only eleven relatively obscure clergymen, doctors, and civil servants could be found who were willing to go on record. Their contributions were not distinguished by moderation. Reverend John Roach Straton, pastor of

Calvary Baptist Church of New York, labeled the pamphlet "utterly ruinous in its effect on the young" and "a positive and deadly menace." Dr. Howard Kelly, professor of gynecology at Johns Hopkins University, was even more emphatic: "With one exception the most prurient statement that has come to my notice. . . . Language could not be used more calculated to excite illegitimate, unrestrainable passions than the nasty minutiae upon which Mary Dennett lingers with such obvious unction." Kelly declared that Dennett's "contention is absolutely false that women discover any such extreme gratification in their sex relations; many women are and remain utterly indifferent, and their participation is but a matter of complaisance."

The other witnesses for the prosecution were equally disapproving. Their criticism centered on what they considered a "brazen defense" of masturbation, a lack of emphasis on self-control, and the danger of the pamphlet being read by younger children. They felt that Dennett was advocating birth control and that her emphasis on love in sex relations was a negation of marriage and akin to approval of free love. They found the pictures vile, or at least unnecessary. And most of all they objected to the vivid description of intercourse, called it titillating, alluring, and an "unnecessary glorification of the sexual act." They worried that young people reading the passage might be tempted to act it out (an argument that was to resurface in the fifites during the controversy over sex education in the schools). John Sumner, the secretary of the New York Society for the Suppression of Vice, deplored Dennett's revelation of a cure for venereal disease because it minimized the "punishment following sex iniquity." One of the witnesses even stooped to personal attack; New York State Senator William Lathrop Love wrote: "There is also a recital of intimate experiences that give the impression that they were anticipated for a great many years and when finally realized made such an impression on her that she doesn't hesitate in telling the world."

During the trial prosecutor James E. Wilkinson, who referred to Dennett's pamphlet as "perverted sex instruction," repeatedly blocked evidence showing that the pamphlet had been used in large quantity for ten years by many respectable organizations. A jury of middle-aged and elderly family men found Mary Ware Dennett guilty of mailing an obscene publication. In spite of vociferous objection in the press and many letters asking Judge

Burrows to override the verdict, Dennett was sentenced to pay a fine of $300.

The verdict was reversed on appeal by Judge Augustus N. Hand, who wrote: "The old theory that information about sex matters should be left to chance has greatly changed. . . . We have been referred to no decision where a truthful exposition of the sex side of life evidently calculated for instruction and for the explanation of relevant facts has been held to be obscene." In a precedent-making decision he ruled that any tendency to arouse sex impulses was incidental to the main purpose of this sex education pamphlet.

Mary Ware Dennett combated censorship all the rest of her life through the New York Civil Liberties League and the National Council for Freedom from Censorship. At this writing the Comstock Law still remains a part of the American legal code.

■ BIBLIOGRAPHY

Comstock, Anthony. *Traps for the Young*. New York: Funk and Wagnalls, 1883.

Dennett, Mary Ware. *The Sex Side of Life: An Explanation for Young People*. Astoria, N.Y.: Published by the author, 1918.

———. *Who's Obscene?* New York: Vanguard, 1930.

Sanger, Margaret. *Family Limitation*. New York: Published by the author, 1915.

———. *Margaret Sanger: An Autobiography*. New York: Norton, 1938.

———. *My Fight for Birth Control*. New York: Farrar and Rinehart, 1931.

———. *What Every Boy and Girl Should Know*. New York: Brentano's, 1927.

———. *What Every Girl Should Know*. Reading, Pa: Sentinel Printing, 1914; New York: Maisel, 1915.

Chapter 5

Between the Wars

The years between the two world wars saw a dearth of new sex education books in America. The flood of literature for the young that had been written to assuage Victorian fears dwindled to a trickle as new liberal attitudes toward sex emerged in the twenties. With less urgency to indoctrinate teenagers in sex prevention fewer books were written. For the conservative minority many older titles continued in print or were reissued in new editions; the new titles that did appear in this decade and the next tended either to ignore changing patterns of behavior or to warn against them. The purpose of sex education for the young continued to be the prevention, not the encouragement, of sexual behavior.

At the beginning of the decade Louise Frances Spaller offered *Personal Help for Boys* (1921), which was in the tradition of the "bully boys" books. Spaller had written *Personal Help for Girls* in 1918 but felt, as she explained in her preface, that she had a special rapport with boys: "Hundreds of them have said that I seemed to know how it is with a feller." Typically, Spaller holds up Teddy Roosevelt as an ideal ("He had the grit and willpower to keep up his daily training, and, the result was, he built a weakling of a boy into a giant of a man"). With heavy jocularity and labored spriteliness she lays out "the fun trail" of pep and bully things to do, extols Scouting as a way to become "a dandy scrapper," and emphasizes camping, outdoor activities, and hobbies ("Betcha life! Gee, it's jake!"). Two of her stories are heavily racist even for that bigoted decade: a description of some "chinks" at a Chinese New Year's celebration and a tale about an "old darky" who was scared by some boys' ghost tricks, proving, as Spaller explains, that "fear is especially deep-rooted in the ignorant and the negro."

Perhaps feeling some limits to her vaunted rapport with boys, Spaller delegates the actual sex instruction to Professor Thomas W. Shannon, who subsequently wrote a complementary "Personal Help" volume for men. In eight short supplementary chapters Shannon tells "The Story of Life." A look at the chapter headings indicates a predictable and derivative approach: "Boys make men," "The story of life among the plants," "The story of life among oysters and fish," "The story of life among insects and birds," "The story of animal and human life," "Strong boys make strong men," "Weak boys make weak men," and "What kind of a boy will you be?" The expected diatribe against masturbation points out that prisons and insane-asylum inmates are masturbators and that a boy who wastes his sex fluids is liable to end up either there or in an early grave. Shannon's only original words are a broadside against tobacco. He describes a scientific experiment in which leeches were applied to the arms of both smokers and nonsmokers. Those that were sucking the blood of smokers soon began to tremble and jerk and presently fell to the floor dead.

It was such books as Spaller's that prompted Marie Stopes, the influential sex education pioneer, to deplore the whole genre in *Sex and the Young* (1926):

> Almost without exception I must warn teachers against the books at present existing, rather than encourage them to place them in young people's hands. . . . There are now many works professing to give full details which so overload the horrors and dangers of sex experience, prostitution and other evils as really almost to terrify young people about the future awaiting them in their adult life. . . . Lurid warnings and pronouncements about masturbation are best kept away from healthy young people.

Stopes felt that rather than being singled out for special instruction, sex education should be incorporated throughout school curriculums.

A book that has more of the look of the twenties is *Letters to My Daughter*, by Leslie J. Swabacker (1926). Modishly printed in art deco style and with a format reminiscent of that of Kahlil Gibran's *The Prophet* (which had been published in 1923), the book consists of letters of advice from a father to his four-year-old daughter in anticipation of her teen years. Swabacker attempts to take a modern, enlightened stance. His writing is sprinkled with Freudian terms—"inhibitions," "repressions," "Electra complex," "the subconscious"—but demonstrates little comprehension of their meanings. He professes to welcome the new sexual attitudes, but it soon becomes apparent that his real purpose is to keep his daughter a virgin at all costs.

Like *The Prophet*, Swabacker's advice is packaged in sections labeled Religion, Duty, Conduct, Love, Marriage, and so on. In the section on religion he discourages his daughter from attending church and points out the historical shortcomings of both the Jewish and the Christian traditions; the Golden Rule should be quite enough. As for duty, she should dress well and be loyal to her employer but be unconcerned about duty to her parents. Smoking, drinking, and dancing are all right since everyone does it, but petting is another matter—"a dangerous game," "a dingy ante-room to passion," and "an open gateway to hell." Honesty is a useful virtue, and lies should be limited to ten a week. Swabacker praises monogamy and, to ensure its preservation, suggests that the art of love and the Kama Sutra be taught in school (although he offers no specifics).

Regarding men, Swabacker warns his daughter that most of them "never miss an opportunity to enjoy any woman they can secure. . . . The game of flirtation is played by different rules by the two sexes." For men a visit to a prostitute is like a visit to the barber or the chiropodist, while women bring a quality of "emotional longing" to sexual experience. In short, "Preserve your chastity for your husband." She should pick a man no more than three to seven years older than she, to make sure there is no Electra complex involved. He should be her mental equal or superior, physically attractive, with a sense of humor, and should provide her with a doctor's certificate attesting to his being untainted with venereal disease or hereditary insanity and certifying the fact that his "virility is unimpaired."

The engagement should last no more than three months because it is a "time of sweet danger." Due to the unsettling effects of the war and of women's suffrage and liberation, it is "the custom in this year, A.D. 1926, for a great many girls to give themselves completely to their husbands-to-be during this period." However, Swabacker is sure that the pendulum will soon swing back from this extreme. On marriage he is unenlightening except for the ominous observation that the average bride goes to the marriage bed "with the same feeling that we approach a precipice in the dark." A new husband should be considerate of his bride, and "if he behaves like a beast hit him with a suitcase." And they should both study the art of love to keep enjoyment fresh.

Although they were not sex education books, two titles that much interested young people in these years were *The Revolt of Modern Youth* (1925) and *Companionate Marriage* (1929), by Judge Benjamin Lindsey of the Juvenile and Family Court of Denver. Impressed by the honesty and forthrightness of young people in sexual matters, Judge Lindsey proposed in his books to recodify existing sexual patterns according to his concept of "companionate marriage." As he explained it, "Companionate marriage is legal marriage, with legalized birth control, and with the right to divorce by mutual consent for childless couples, usually without payment of alimony." To bring this about, three bills were needed: to repeal the laws against birth control, to legalize birth-control clinics, and to allow divorce by mutual consent. This proposition caused a great stir in Judge Lindsey's time, and it is only now that his ideas are becoming reality.

The sex education book that was undoubtably the most widely read in these years was *Growing Up*, by Karl De Schweinitz (1928). Although it is very simply written and was probably intended for third- and fourth-grade children, it appeared frequently in recommended bibliographies for teenagers. The first edition was reprinted fifteen times in the first three years of publication. Its biological approach won great favor in an era that equated "scientific" with "modern" and had the added advantage of making it possible to sidestep psychological and ethical problems.

Although De Schweinitz sticks to the biological facts of conception, fetal development, and birth, without digressing into the topic of correct sexual behavior, he interlaces his clinical descriptions with sentimental prose and coy illustrations. The frontispiece of *Growing Up*, captioned "Out of the everywhere," depicts a chubby and surprised-looking naked baby sitting incongruously on a cliff somewhere in what appears to be the Swiss Alps. A few pages later there are drawings of a calf in the uterus, showing the cow in silhouette, and a human fetus in the uterus (but without a corresponding outline of the woman). Photographs of eggs in the nest, an Easter lily, a butterfly and a phlox, and a drawing of the sperm and egg of a minnow illustrate

Fig. 6. "Out of the Everywhere." From *Growing Up*, by Karl De Schweinitz (1928 edition).

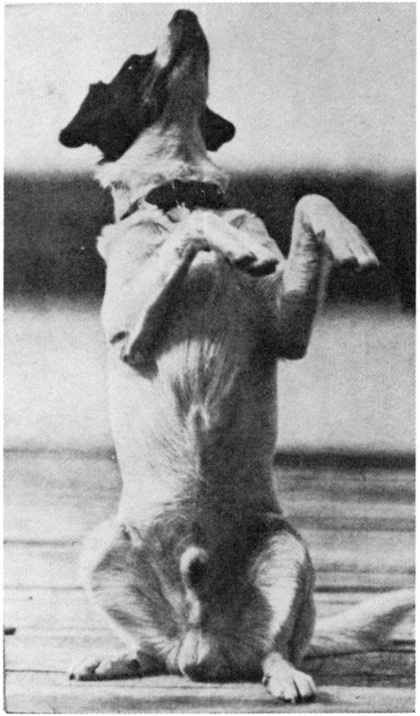

Fig. 7. "Dog Sitting for His Picture." From *Growing Up*, by Karl De Schweinitz (1928 edition).

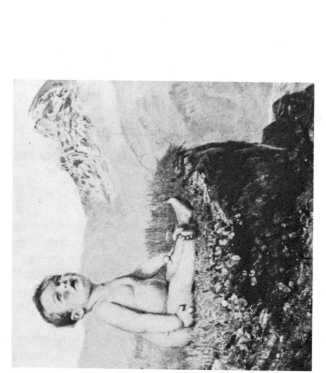

the chapter on fertilization. A small drawing of a human sperm is tucked in at the bottom of a page. A picture of a lactating sow appears near an Italianate painting of a mother nursing an infant. The structure of the penis and testicles is discreetly illustrated through a snapshot of a male dog sitting up on his haunches. Other examples from the animal kingdom—a German shepherd feeding pups, a buffalo calf nursing, a lion cub—lead up to a statue of a nude boy by Alexander Calder appropriately titled "Man Cub." Female nudity is also shown in statuary—a slim, teenage "Bathing Girl." The last chapter, on mating, depicts a bull moose and his mate and reproduces a painting of *Sleeping Beauty* in which round-faced children play at being sweethearts.

The "birds and bees" format of *Growing Up* derives directly from the opening chapters of Sylvanus Stall's *What a Young Boy Ought to Know*. The question is "Where do babies come from?" and the answer is a description of the fertilization arrangements of plants, fish, birds, mammals, and—at last—humans. In its own time *Growing Up* was most similar to Bertha Cady's *The Way Life Begins* (described in Chapter 3), which was first published in 1917 and reached new popularity in the 1939 edition.

De Schweinitz tackles the facts of conception by generalizing that "everything starts as eggs." To the egg is added the male contribution—pollen, milt, sperm—to add up to the seed or the embryo. The dog, the elephant, the mouse, and other mammals differ from lesser creatures in that the mother has a "nest" for the eggs inside her body and the father has a "tube" through which to pass the sperm safely into the female. In animal mating the penis fits inside the vagina, and the sperm stays in the testicles until it is needed.

This is the way it is for humans beings, too, De Schweinitz explains cautiously: "The father places the sperms in the body of the mother in very much the same way that the four-legged animals do, only the mother and father can lie together facing each other. The penis then fits into the vagina of the mother which has its own opening underneath the opening for the urine or waste water." This passage is typical of a number of oversimplifications in *Growing Up* that could have led to some serious misinterpretation by young readers. (The author can attest to the confusing effect of this particular description of coitus, having been given De Schweinitz to read at age ten. The book's joyless and clinical tone led to the impression that sexual intercourse was a medical procedure.)

In another passage De Schweinitz suggests that conception is an inevitable result of every sexual encounter. At the same time he fails to take advantage of the opportunity to describe menstruation: "If no sperms have been sent to meet it, the egg stays in the uterus for a little while and then passes out through the vagina." De Schweinitz's oversimplified approach blithely ignores the whole problem of sexual ethics: "Like the animals a man and a woman may feel like sending the sperm to join the egg but they do not do this unless they love each other."

The final chapter lapses into rhapsodic praise of mating throughout nature. The flowers in spring are "dressed as if to welcome the tiny visitors who carry the pollen from flower to flower." From this lowly example to the mystery of human love, attraction between male and female is the source of beauty in the world.

Many of the shortcomings of *Growing Up* probably result from the fact that it was intended for much younger children than its eventual readership. Although the lack of moralizing in De Schweinitz's book is refreshing in comparison with its predecessors, it is difficult to imagine that its bare biological facts and sentimentalities offered much help to a teenager trying to manage a nascent sexuality.*

Some old favorites appeared during the decade in new editions that showed only token attempts at modernization. Margaret Sanger rewrote *What Every Girl Should Know* in 1927 to reach a broader audience with a new title *What Every Boy and Girl Should Know*. In 1926 Armenouhie Lamson updated *How I Came to Be* by removing some of the sillier personifications (the fetus is no longer "embarrassed" by its tail) and by adding a chapter on evolution as recreated in the growth of the embryo. In 1924 Harry Hascall Moore's *Keeping in Condition* reappeared almost unchanged. *What a Young Boy Ought to Know* was tentatively reissued in 1926. (Although Stall had died in 1915, no new name appears on the title page as author of the revision. However, the copyright is attributed to Fannie C. Cash.) Evidently well received, the book was reprinted two years later when the other seven volumes of the Self and Sex series were also issued in new editions.

*The British edition of *Growing Up*, published in 1931 by Routledge and Sons, has some notable omissions. It leaves out the dog sitting up on its haunches, the nude female statue (but not the male), and the two sentences describing coitus.

Young Boy remained almost unchanged, with all of its Victorian prose on the horrid effects of masturbation nearly intact. *Young Man*, on the other hand, was rewritten in "bully boy" style, although the message remained the same. The revised version puts heavy emphasis on business success as proof (or result) of manhood, using such inspirational slogans as "Be a human flashlight!" and "Avoid a heavy stomach and a cloudy brain!" In an economic metaphor Cash points out the high cost of low living—"this world should be run for the decent and decency; this world must not be run for the nasty." She extols exercise, continence, and clean living and deplores venereal disease, whose symptoms she describes vividly but ungrammatically as "the abscesses that fill the liver, turns the kidneys into gristle and rottens the bones." The book, nevertheless, is still very much Stall's own, as evidenced in the last chapters that discuss such topics as "The appalling penalties exacted by vice" and "Lost manhood and how to regain it."

▪ The Reaction Against "Modern Liberties"

While sex instruction in the twenties largely ignored the upheavals in sexual behavior patterns that characterized the decade, the books of the thirties began to show a reaction to the new freedoms. Although sex educators of that decade were careful to disassociate themselves from the Victorian horror stories about masturbation, they focused sharply on the dangers of teenage sex play, which they called "petting." Such modern liberties, they feared, could lead to premarital intercourse and all its unhappy consequences, from pregnancy to permanent disgrace. Realistic measures, such as new scientific advances in birth control and the prevention and cure of venereal disease, were never mentioned—due only in part to the Comstock Law. It remained socially unacceptable to teach adolescents to deal with their sexuality in this practical way.

So Youth May Know: New Viewpoints on Sex and Love, by Roy Ernest Dickerson, written in 1930, heralded this return to repression. The book opens with descriptions of growth freaks and the results of castration—hardly a comforting subject for adolescent sensibilities. The long and dreary first chapter takes up hormones, heredity, chromosomes, conception, and detailed embryology, with some obscure and technical illustrations. This scientific veneer disappears in the second chapter, when Dickerson poses the question "Abstinence or promiscuity?" In case a youth should opt for the latter, he reminds readers that "drugstore" methods of birth control are only 60 percent effective and that abortion is murder.

Dickerson's book is tedious and overwritten and becomes even more labored when he takes up the subject of petting.

> At the very outset it must be said that it would be indeed ultra-puritanical and ill-advised to denounce altogether all the ordinary minor, more or less incidental, and chiefly matter-of-fact physical contacts between the sexes. . . . The first girl a boy thinks of for a "petting party" is not often the first one he thinks of for a wife. She may be all right for his "good times," but ordinarily he does not want "second-hand goods," or a woman who has been freely "pawed over" for sweetheart, wife, and mother of his children! . . . The boy who . . . thinks it is smart to "mess around" with girls, who—to be plain-spoken—has intercourse with first one and then another girl may very seriously affect his thinking and feeling about girls. He may never become able to be genuinely and permanently interested in any one girl.

To develop self-mastery over these unwelcome sexual temptations Dickerson offers a collection of preventative techniques that come directly from Victorian antimasturbatory literature: keep busy, don't drink, pray, keep your bowels open, walk about rapidly, shadowbox, go through calisthenic exercises—and remember that kissing transmits syphilis.

Dickerson also broaches the forbidden subject of homosexuality: "A man who differs in this way is very unfortunate to say the least. . . . He is usually very uncomfortable and unhappy about it. . . . The medical specialists known as psychiatrists are often able to help a homosexual become quite normal." Women, on the other hand, do not have nearly as many sexual problems as men, according to Dickerson: "A woman's sexual energies are apt to be largely diverted into the maternal channel." Men should respect women's heroism in this, though, because "childbirth may involve suffering unequalled in masculine experience." This denial of feminine sexual enjoyment is reflected in the omission of the clitoris from the diagram of the female sex organs that appears as an appendix. Other subjects that are relegated to the appendixes are venereal disease, the male sexual anatomy, and masturbation (occasional incidents are acceptable, but habitual indulgence is not). Dickerson wrote another book in 1933, *Growing into Manhood*, which was more popularly written but expressed essentially the same ideas.

A widely respected title, and the last of the "bully boys" texts, was *In Training* (1933), by Thurman Brooks Rice, professor of bacteriology and pathology at the University of Indiana School of Medicine. The author's prestige and his hearty, outdoorsy approach made *In Training* the only sex education book to be recommended in the Boy Scout handbook for many years. The text is liberally decorated with photos of boys at sports, and the style is bluff and manly. "There isn't any doubt that the fellow who is strong and healthy has a big lead in these times when every one has to be on his toes," Rice begins. "The real man is a fighter," he points out and holds up Teddy Roosevelt as a prime example of manliness. With this preamble he launches into the familiar tale of sperm and ova and birth (which he terms "a considerable ordeal"). As to the father's role in fertilization, well, it resembles the relationship of the bee and the pollen, but "the details are, of course, different." When intercourse is imminent (between married people), "the male penis becomes much larger and stiff." It is then moved in and out of the vagina; there is a pleasurable sensation; the muscles contract and inject sperm cells into the vagina. Rice explains that the purpose of intercourse is (1) children and (2) pleasure, and although methods of preventing conception do exist, it is not fitting for a doctor to pass this knowledge on to inexperienced boys. Among the hazards of premature intercourse Rice emphasizes venereal disease, which causes death, blindness, and terrible deformity. There is a treatment for venereal disease, but it is long, painful, expensive, and uncertain. Nevertheless, "I don't want you to be good because you are afraid to be otherwise," he reassures.

Further reassurance is offered about masturbation. The old stories are certainly untrue, but a boy who does it "too much" will be tired and weak, and "the fellow who sneaks off to a dark corner to practice masturbation is going to feel pretty badly about it." Athletics, Scouting, and hiking will help a boy keep his thoughts off sex. It also helps to use light bed covers, to go to bed tired, and to eschew "sissy" love stories.

Rice never mentions homosexuality by name, but he refers obliquely to "several other methods of sexual abuse, which are even more disgusting" than masturbation. "Persons who practice these methods are looked on with greatest contempt by all normal persons" and are "utterly ruined for all normal" sex. Nocturnal emissions and morning erections, however, are entirely normal. One should pay no attention to the scare literature of quacks or believe in the "wild oats" fallacy, which leads to venereal disease. Home and family are the cornerstone of society, and a boy should never do anything that would injure his future children.

In the same year (1933) Thurman Rice also wrote a companion volume for girls called *How Life Goes On and On: A Story for Girls of High School Age*. Here he is as enthusiastic in encouraging female passivity (in preparation for motherhood) as he had been in urging male aggressiveness through sports: "Domestic arts are of vast importance to the welfare of the human race." Teachers, as career women themselves, are prone to hold up before girls the ideal of a brilliant career, he observes. This is all right, but girls should remember that the family is most important and motherhood is the best career. Rice describes the function of the female reproductive organs (pregnancy) and the physiology of the male organs, although he omits the specific description of intercourse that he offered to boys. Sex "is perfectly proper when the man and woman are husband and wife," he assures his readers. Menstruation is not a sickness, although girls should avoid chilling and excess exercise during their periods. "Excess" exercise he defines as basketball, hockey, or swimming, adding that "girls should not indulge in athletics that require long periods of training or excessive effort; they should go in for individual rather than for competitive effort." Vigorous sports train "blood vessels to favor the muscles rather than the organs of reproduction." Girls "must not permit improper relations" under penalty of venereal disease or pregnancy, and they are prettier if they don't drink or smoke. Rice deplores modern morality—"There are coming to be a number of people who think that marriage and the vows made in the wedding ceremony are old-fashioned and that they need not be observed"—and reiterates his theme: intelligent women should use their energies to bear children for the good of the race and not leave this important function to less-bright housewives.

Sex Education Books in the Library

How readily available were these books to teenagers? Until the 1930s the dissemination of sex information—whether by book, pamphlet, or word of mouth—had been seen as primarily the parents' job. Sex education books addressed to teenagers often added prefaces for parents assuring them that it was safe to "put this volume into the hands of your son or daughter." But in the course of this decade there were signs that many librarians were beginning to feel a responsibility for stocking and distributing sex information. This new idea caused considerable discomfort to older librarians, who had, after all, learned their own sexual attitudes from Stall and his peers. A controversy developed that still occasionally arises when two generations confront each other in the library profession.

During the thirties the *Wilson Library Bulletin* ran a monthly column in which readers were invited to contribute their solutions to a specified library problem. Cash prizes were awarded for the best answers. The problem posed in the January 1934 issue came from an anxious librarian from a midwestern town who wrote:

> What should one do when a small boy, about fourteen years old, whose family I am not acquainted with but who seems of a quiet and rather studious temperament, comes into our public library and shyly asks for a book that will tell him "all about boys and girls and things like that"? There is no school library here, and we do not have any "sex books" in our library of less than 11,000 volumes. I wonder if I did wrong in telling the boy that he would have to go to his parents for instruction in such matters. I do not know of any books of this nature that it would be safe to put into the hands of an adolescent, though I believe there are some especially written for the purpose. And, furthermore, it seems to me that many conservative parents would object to having the librarian interfere in this delicate phase of education. Just what are the librarian's duties in such a case, and what should be her course of procedure? I should very much appreciate hearing the opinion of others in your valuable publication.

There were twenty-six responses. The consensus was that the librarian was remiss in not providing the information, although many felt that it was advisable to stall for time in which to contact discreetly the parents for permission. A goodly number were of the opinion that supplying sex information was none of the library's business. Others suggested keeping the books locked up, circulating them only to young people who presented written permission from their parents. The more liberal letters indignantly stated that a library of 11,000 volumes definitely ought to have a few books on sex; some of these letters also pointed out that any boy who got up the courage to ask for such information at the library probably did so because he had been failed at home by tongue-tied parents.

The *Bulletin* itself, in an editorial comment, came out staunchly on the liberal side: "The librarian who interposes a barrier between the child and an essential part of his education is failing her duty to society, is weaving another strand into the net of taboos and inhibitions and circumlocutions that enmesh the adolescent and from which modern psychologists and educators would set him free." These brave stands were not backed with sound bibliographic knowledge, however, as is shown by the very few titles that were actually recommended in the letters. Several mentioned encyclopedias, adult physiology or genetics textbooks, or nature books for children. A few referred vaguely to pamphlets from the government or the American Social Hygiene Association. The two titles that were most frequently named were *Growing Up*, by Karl De Schweinitz, and *The Way Life Begins*, by Bertha Cady. Four other titles rated one mention each: *The Sex Side of Life*, by Mary Ware Dennett; *What Every Boy and Girl Should Know*, by Margaret Sanger; *So Youth May Know*, by Roy Dickerson; and Marie Stopes's much-banned *The Human Body*. The Self and Sex series, too, received its share of praise.

The Late Thirties

A book that closely resembled those of De Schweinitz and Cady in its biological approach was *Being Born* (1936), by Frances Strain. The title is still in use with younger children, the third edition having been issued in 1970. The chapter headings show an organization that follows the pattern set by the two earlier authors: "Where the egg is made," "Where the sperm is made," "Two uniting cells," "From embryo to baby," "Coming into the world," "Like father, like son," "Mating and marrying." Strain adds a new dimension to her presentation of biological facts by including several questions from young people at the end of each topic, a method that allows her to raise psychological and ethical problems and to discuss teenagers' apprehensions without making these issues the focus of her book. As a literary technique the question-and-answer format soon became a common feature of sex education books.

Strain's description of intercourse, while somewhat hushed and unearthly, is a bit more informative than De Schweinitz's:

> Outwardly the father and mother lie close together, arms about each other, while the sperm-bearing fluid enters into the mother by way of the perfectly fitting passages. . . . The sperm should be able to find the egg cell and fertilize it. It doesn't always, and if it doesn't, another mating must take place. . . . Because mating is also a way of expressing their love, husbands and wives unite when no baby is to be started. . . . Mating takes place in quiet and seclusion . . . the presence of another person would spoil the deep inner feelings.

The controversial subject of birth control is touched upon briefly and cautiously: "If a husband and wife decide they should not have children, then the sperm cell must not be allowed to enter the uterus and find the egg cell." For further clarification she explains that "one may have a baby though one is not married," but unwed mothers "lead a sorry life."

A chapter on conception and embryology elicits the question "Does the mother have to tell the father when she is pregnant?" Strain describes birth from the baby's point of view. Labor pains, she asserts, are natural, but anesthetics can be given if the mother "becomes tired." The use of forceps is often helpful and is not harmful to the baby. A mother stays two weeks in the hospital afterward. The questions on birth reveal young readers' anxiety: Does birth hurt a lot? What is a Caesarian?

The new science of genetics is the basis for a chapter on heredity, chromosomes, genetic defects, and birthmarks. Strain takes a stand against miscegenation: "Mixed marriages between races so widely different as Negroes and whites or as Chinese and whites are not thought to be desirable. The children suffer. They feel that they do not belong." On mating and marriage she avoids the sentimental pitfalls of *Growing Up* but copies that title in using statuary to illustrate the nude human body. She urges caution in choosing a marriage partner because "we must save the love acts and the mating acts for the chosen one." The book ends with a glossary of scientific terms, another innovation that was soon to become standard practice.

The pervading fear of sex outside of marriage was summed up in an extremely influential and widely reprinted article published by the *Reader's Digest* in August 1937—"The Case for Chastity," by Margaret Culkin Banning. Addressed only to young girls, the article was in preparation over a year. The author claimed to have spent that time interviewing doctors and psychologists about "the widespread whispering campaign that is now condoning unchastity and even advocating premarital relations." In her research she discovered that five percent of Americans had syphilis and ten percent gonorrhea. Banning also came to the conclusion that contraceptives are only partially effective, and she quotes Hannah Stone, the director of the birth-control clinic founded by Margaret Sanger, to this effect: vaginal jelly is only sixty percent safe, suppositories forty to fifty percent safe, and douches only ten percent. (She does not include any statistics on the condom and diaphragm, long known to be the most effective forms of birth control.) The dangers of abortion are also well known, Banning reminds readers. In spite of all this modern talk, she says, men still prefer virgins for wives. Clandestine sex is uncomfortable, and the girl is usually abandoned afterward and may become promiscuous. Banning points out that girls naturally have a sense of guilt about illicit sex even if they are not religious. If the couple eventually marry, their earlier experience may give them cause not to trust each other later. Nor is petting a safe substitute—it may unfit a woman for satisfaction in "normal sex relations." Banning recommends early marriage as a solution, with financial help from the parents if necessary. The article exactly summed up popular attitudes, if not practices, and continued to be recommended in bibliographies. As late as 1962 it was reprinted in the *Reader's Digest*, substantially cut, but with its message essentially unchanged.

Two books that were far above the rest of the genre at this time in presenting humane and sensible sex advice were *Attaining Manhood: A Doctor Talks to Boys About Sex* (1938) and *Attaining Womanhood: A Doctor Talks to Girls About Sex* (1939), by George Washington Corner. The author, a professor of anatomy at the University of Rochester,* writes in a simple, direct, and friendly style and conveys more information in sixty-seven pages than most of the far wordier books that appeared in the next two decades. He presents the anatomical facts with spare precision, and, within the context of the sex attitudes of the thirties, he is calmly matter-of-fact about sex behaviors. The anatomical drawings, although not done by Corner himself, are remarkable for their clarity.

Attaining Manhood is addressed to "the intelligent boy of high school age." Corner catches that reader's attention immediately by admitting in his first sentence that "everybody is interested in sex." But why has nature arranged things in this way? So that every living creature has more than one single line of ancestry, he explains. A clear description of the function of the sperm and ova in fish, birds, and mammals follows. In the next chapter, on the human reproductive system, Corner the anatomist is at his best. With the sureness of the man who knows his subject he describes the structure and function of the male and female reproductive systems, using correct technical terms and illustrating the text with crystal-clear drawings. "Some practical matters" are dealt with in an aside printed in a different typeface—worries about undescended testicles, varicoceles, and penis size.

When it comes to describing the central event of sex, however, Corner shies away: "In the act of mating the sperm cells are deposited in the vagina." He justifies his approach by explaining that "sex attraction in the human race is not a subject which can be dealt with on a purely scientific basis." Furthermore, "About human sex desire the important thing to remember is that it depends upon attraction of the mind as well as the body." The physical changes in puberty can, however, be described scientifically, and Corner does so, using a simple nude drawing to illustrate. He points out that in primitive societies manhood was acknowledged at an early age through puberty rites, whereas in

*Dr. Corner was evidently an extraordinary teacher. At least three of his students credit his classes with being instrumental in inspiring their outstanding careers in sex education: William Howell Masters, author of *Human Sexual Response*; Alan Guttmacher, past president of the Planned Parenthood Federation; and Dr. Mary Calderone, founder of the Sex Information and Education Council of the U.S. Corner also was important in the early development of the Kinsey Institute.

modern society physical maturity precedes marriage by several years.

Corner now offers comfort on the two traditionally worrisome topics of nocturnal emissions and masturbation. The former is "thought by some scientists to have a useful purpose, being perhaps a method by which old stale sperm cells are cleared out in order to make room for a fresh supply from the testes." No sensible boy should pay any attention to the "wicked nonsense" of quacks on the subject. Masturbation is something that "all boys discover for themselves," and it "happens at one time or another to practically every boy and man." Although it is admittedly unnatural and secretive, masturbation is not the terrible thing it has been made out to be. People who offer advice with "an air of horror" have often caused "tragic mental suffering." Corner himself would explain the practice as a kind of substitute for intercourse, because, as he has explained, marriage is ordinarily postponed in our society. However, he is quick to add a counterargument: "People who expect to do well in study and on the playing field cannot permit themselves to yield to every mood of self-indulgence. . . . Sensible boys and men will avoid as far as possible unnecessary sexual stimulations, especially those which tend to cheapen and degrade one's ideas of sex."

"In girls the sex feelings are not expressed in quite the same way as in boys," Corner continues. "Girls," he says, "tend to have much vaguer sex thoughts and feelings. Whether a girl knows much or little about the facts of sex and reproduction, her own emotions are not at first directed toward actual physical sex actions. In fact the thought of sexual relations is often distasteful. Usually it is only when completely under the sway of love that frank sexual desires are developed." Introducing male readers to menstruation, Corner emphasizes the mystery of the process rather than its known purposes: "For reasons which are still very puzzling to science, females of the human race (and also some of the higher animals) are subject to periodic bleeding from the uterus." He gives no further explanation of the function of the menses but does caution boys that girls' cycles are responsible for changes of mood and disposition.

As presented in *Attaining Manhood*, the problem of human sex conduct is how to behave as an animal with a mind. Corner sees some rules as just good biology—the incest taboo, for instance. Other rules are universal throughout humanity: "The human race has decided . . . that the ideal expression of sex is the life-long union of marriage." Any other sexual relationship can be considered immoral, he states flatly. There are many temptations to break this rule, but boys should remember that prostitutes transmit venereal disease and satisfy the animal nature only. Petting or necking is "playing with dynamite" and may result in pregnancy and "grave embarrassment and difficulty." The only safe course is to say "no to all physical intimacies" outside of marriage.

The final chapter of *Attaining Manhood*, on sex disorders, provides a brief and factual description of the symptoms of syphilis and gonorrhea and warns boys that not only prostitutes may be carriers but also "any persons who may be willing to take part in illicit sexual relations." Protection is "dangerously uncertain," and while Corner freely admits that venereal disease is curable, he adds that the treatment is long and painful. A second class of sex disorder is homosexuality, which Corner discusses much more freely than earlier writers, most of whom found the subject too distasteful to mention. He says, "Strange as it may seem, there are a few men who develop sexual attraction toward members of their own sex; a man so disturbed is interested only in sexual contacts with other men and boys. This quirk of the mind is called 'homosexuality.' . . . To normal men it is a very disgusting thing, but the person involved is not to be considered wicked but rather as the victim of a disease. Skillful treatment by a physician experienced in mental guidance may in fact cure the aberration." Corner confuses homosexuals with child molesters, a misunderstanding that was to be nearly universal among sex educators for the next twenty years. A boy who is approached by one of these unfortunate men, he counsels, should seek out the advice of an older man he trusts.

In *Attaining Womanhood* (1939) girls are given almost the same anatomical instruction as the boys, with one interesting difference—Corner seems to have become aware of the function of the sex hormones estrogen and progesterone sometime between the writing of the two books. He mentions them several times, and in the description of menstruation, a phenomenon that in the earlier book he found "still puzzling to science," he gives a full account of their function as triggering mechanisms. Another ground-breaking inclusion in this title is a complete drawing of the female *external* genitalia with all the parts labeled, including the clitoris.

As might be expected, *Attaining Womanhood* has far more detailed information about pregnancy and birth than the boy's book. There are diagrams of the relative size and position of the growing "child" in the uterus, and a description of the birth process that to some extent acknowledges the woman's role as an active one: "With modern anesthetics and skilled medical help the discomforts of childbirth are lightened." Corner discredits the old wives' tale that a woman can transfer a "maternal impression" or physical mark to her unborn baby if she experiences any severe shock or trauma during pregnancy.

Corner advises girls on the differences in sexual attitudes between men and women: "A man's part in sex life and reproduction is only a small part of his activity; the woman's part requires much of her life." Women want love and devotion, but with men and mature boys sex thoughts are "more frank and outspoken." Their urges are "more physical, less vague, and more easily aroused than a girl's." In a passage that foreshadows the sexism that was to be a prominent part of sex education in the fifties Corner counsels girls on choosing a husband: "In the case of a woman who marries, the general rule that a woman's work is done through other people is intensified. In selecting a mate she is choosing the workshop in which she is to do her life's work, selecting the instruments with which to make her mark in the world."

Under "Sex Problems" for girls Corner lists the anxiety of achieving personal attractiveness, self-excitement (masturbation), and crushes. The latter, consisting of passionate attachments between girls "verging on the sexual," "may cause difficulty in making proper adjustments to the other sex." But he does not class crushes with homosexuality, which "may be an inborn trait, a deformity of the instincts; in other cases it is believed to be set up as a result of unfortunate circumstances in youth." Homosexuals can be cured, he maintains. "Many homosexual women, are, moreover, able to control this tendency and turn their energies into useful service." Such tendencies "may be acquired by association," so a girl should take care to avoid a woman who makes physical advances. Other sexual annoyances for young girls are exhibitionists and men who touch or fondle girls in crowds. Neither are dangerous, only pitiful and unpleasant for the girl.

One of many pamphlets by the YMCA was *The Other Sex* (1939), by Dora Hudson Klemer, a "physician, social worker and mother." Imparting the conventional advice about sexual physiology and hygiene, Klemer follows Corner's lead in including a glossary and a diagram of both male and female external genitalia. The pamphlet is characteristic of the time in its emphasis on the need for maintaining chastity, a condition that Klemer defines as "a clean slate, with nothing to unlearn." She enumerates drawbacks to unchastity in two lists, one for each sex. For girls there is the fear of pregnancy (because no birth control used outside marriage and without the clinical advice of a doctor is safe); the dangers of abortion; guilt, which spoils the thrill of marriage; and the fact that boys don't marry unchaste girls. The list for boys points out that sex is not necessary for health; prostitutes have venereal disease; and there is risk of pregnancy for the girl. Above all, promiscuous young men have unhappy marriages and never experience the supreme expression of love or learn the discipline of self-control, which is necessary in all areas of life.

Several relics of the past were issued in new editions at the end of the decade. In 1936 the Self and Sex series was reprinted (for the last time) almost unchanged from its revision ten years earlier. Irving Steinhardt's *Ten Sex Talks to Girls and Ten Sex Talks to Boys*, first printed in 1914, were reissued as *Sex Talks to Girls and Sex Talks to Boys* in 1938 and 1940, respectively. The advice to young men is little updated—boys are still warned of the dangers of the public toilet and assured that "venereal diseases are well-nigh incurable" and that masturbation produces insanity. They are urged to dissuade girls from immodest dress and paint and to check their sisters' wardrobes frequently to make sure that they are not being given extravagant gifts by ill-intentioned men.

As Steinhardt explains in the preface, *Sex Talks to Girls* also has few changes from the first edition "because decency and right living and the ways of avoiding diseases of the sexual tract do not change." His book, he brags, "has outlived the lurid, exciting, arousing and vicious books on this subject because it was clean but instructive." In a gesture toward modernity he does include a diagram of the female external genitalia in which the clitoris appears but is not labeled. However, he still maintains that the hymen is rarely destroyed in any other way but by an attempt to introduce something into the vagina and advises girls that a signed statement should be secured from a doctor if it is necessary to interfere with the hymen. The ghastly photo of a syphilitic baby remains, as does his plea to girls to "endeavor to bring back to the 'straight and happy path' of virtue those girls who have strayed from it."

Steinhardt continues to attack the corset as a "fashionable" contraption (in 1939) and further scolds young girls for sporting immodest modern dress: "If a man came up to you in the street and, without speaking to you, merely reached down and raised your skirts in order to see your lower limbs, you would think him insane, or grossly insulting. Yet that is what your present mode of dressing would suggest that you wanted, except that you freely expose yourself to view without giving any man the trouble of having to lift your clothing." Other targets of his wrath are "paint," "dances whose poses or steps are suggestive," drinking, flirting ("You cannot act like a 'fallen' woman and not expect to be treated as such"), accepting rides from strangers, meeting men on street corners, and "pick-ups."

Institutional Books of the Forties

As World War II approached, sex education became a minor issue indeed. Young men in their late teens, sent off to war and the possibility of an early death, abandoned traditional sexual codes as meaningless. These lapses society found excusable, if not totally acceptable, but the seeds of change had been sown.

For these reasons, and because shortages of paper curtailed civilian printing, there were very few sex education books printed during the war years. Those that did appear were sponsored by schools or churches and were meant to be used in those institutions. The one exception is *Love at the Threshold* (1942), by Frances Strain (author of *Being Born*), a book that was addressed to college-age young people and emphasized conventional morality in a setting of romantic love and early marriage—but without mentioning the war in any way. There was a large gap between the advice of Strain and other older sex educators and the advice handed out by the U.S. Army with free condoms—"If you can't be good, be careful!"

A Boy Grows Up (1940), by Harry C. McKown, is an example of the institutional "teen life" book of the forties. The author, editor of *School Activities*, writes in a pompous and didactic style but adopts a phony veneer of teen slang. The book is typical of those designed for supplementary reading in social-hygiene courses called "Senior Problems" or "Life Adjustment." There are many chapters on problems of gaining social maturity—managing finances, education, recreation, etiquette, friendships, nutrition, health, alcohol, and tobacco—and one chapter on sex, which is largely devoted to discouraging masturbation. "Even though, if practiced moderately, masturbation does not cause insanity or disease, it is hardly advisable" because it is "done secretly and is, therefore, generally accompanied by a feeling of wrong-doing." In the time-honored manner McKown gives a list of twelve ways to avoid not only masturbation but even erections: keep the bowels clear, have a hobby, exercise self-control, change position frequently when seated, and so on.

The controversy among librarians as to their responsibilities in sex education had become heated by 1941. In that year Frances Strain was invited to be the featured speaker at the Illinois Library Association's annual conference. She told the assembled librarians that the circulation of sex education books should not be restricted except in the case of definitely technical works. She also urged the profession to develop a better understanding of sex education and to have in mind some reliable suggestions to offer parents and teachers—presumably including *Being Born* and *Love at the Threshold*.

An example of the pamphlet meant to be used by biology teachers in a unit on reproduction is *Life Goes On* (1942), by Jessie Williams Clemensen and others. (A trio of educators collaborated in producing the pamphlet's thirty-five pages—Clemenson and Freda Buckingham Daniels, both high-school teachers, and William Ralph La Porte, professor of physical education and chairman of the division of health and physical education at the University of Southern California.) The authors proposed to counsel the young facing the puzzling question "How can I maintain a wholesome relationship with the opposite sex?" The answer, couched in dry and stuffy prose, has much to say about mitosis and Mendel's law but very little about making love. (A chart of the male sex organs, with Victorian reticence, ignores the penis.) Inspirational quotes head each chapter ("'Sex is never low and unworthy unless it is made so by a low and unworthy person'—Dr. Florence Meredith"). A section on venereal disease states that syphilis is now curable if treated early and that gonorrhea is spread mostly by intercourse and almost never by door knobs, food, towels, or toilet seats. However, the authors remind boys that 90 percent of prostitutes have gonorrhea.

A discussion of the stages of personality growth leads to the subject of petting (under "Special Problems"). This practice the authors describe as "a selfish experiment in sexual sensation by two people who have little true interest in the future welfare of each other." There are serious dangers in petting: (1) The possibility of contracting syphilis or other diseases spread by kissing, (2) overstimulation of the ductless glands, (3) acquisition of a reputation as a "petter" or "necker," and (4) loss of control. The intimate sex relations that may follow loss of control "nearly always" have tragic results, including one or more of the following: serious psychological conditions caused by fear, distrust, jealousy, shame, remorse, or loss of self-respect; blocked emotional maturity; infection with venereal disease; forced marriage; illegitimate children; illegal abortions, which often cause death or invalidism; decreased chances for marriage; and decreased chances for happiness in marriage. How, then, to control the sex instinct? The authors suggest yet another list: (1) stay in groups, (2) avoid suggestive books, magazines, and movies, (3) avoid vulgar conversation, (4) keep the mind occupied with wholesome things like school, church, home duties, and hobbies, (5) exercise, (6) avoid alcohol, and (7) follow one's best impulses.

Around this time a few churches also began to prepare sex education pamphlets for use in Christian education classes. A fairly conservative example is Alice M. Hustad's *Strictly Confidential for Young Girls*, published in 1944 in Minnesota by the Board of Parish Education. Speaking from a "background of Christian philosophy," Hustad takes on such topics of interest to teenage girls as personality, grooming, and mental health through Christianity. She wastes no time equivocating on questions like how to prevent venereal disease—just don't have sex before marriage: "God promised punishment to those who abuse the sex life by sinful, impure desires of lust" so those who contact venereal disease get what they deserve. Questions and answers on dating focus on the hazards of blind dates, going steady, dutch treats, drinking, and smoking.

Hustad disapproves of the ballroom: "Since dancing removes many barriers to intimacy, a girl may be easily led to permit intimacies which she will later regret." Girls are forearmed to resist these intimacies if they are aware of the arguments a boy may use "to convince a girl to gratify his sex 'desires.'" He might call her old-fashioned, break down her resistance with petting and alcohol, tell her nobody will know, assure her of his love, ask her to prove their compatibility, and accuse her of frigidity. Nor is there safety in contraceptives—they "fail repeatedly." Girls should also beware of "homo-sexualists": "If any girl wants you to be her friend alone, and if she insists upon 'cuddling' or other physical contacts, avoid her entirely." Madame Chiang Kai-shek is held up as a shining example of womanhood. Wise girls will emulate her and use the teen years to prepare for marriage responsibilities. The ideal girl will "study the art of pleasing a husband and learn to taste of the sweetness of humility and submission"—a theme that was soon to become the basis for the next phase of repressive sex education literature in the fifties.

■ BIBLIOGRAPHY

Banning, Margaret Culkin. "The Case for Chastity." *Reader's Digest*, August 1937. Reprinted July 1962.

Cady, Bertha Louise (Chapman). *The Way Life Begins: An Introduction to Sex Education*. New York: American Social Hygiene Association, 1917; rev. ed., 1939.

Clemensen, Jessie Williams, et al. *Life Goes On*. New York: Harcourt, 1942.

Corner, George Washington. *Attaining Manhood: A Doctor Talks to Boys About Sex*. New York: Harper, 1938.

———. *Attaining Womanhood: A Doctor Talks to Girls About Sex*. New York: Harper, 1939.

De Schweinitz, Karl. *Growing Up: The Story of How We Become Alive, Are Born and Grow Up*. New York: Macmillan, 1928; rev. ed., 1945.

Dickerson, Roy Ernest. *Growing into Manhood*. New York: Association Press, 1933.

———. *So Youth May Know: New Viewpoints on Sex and Love*. New York: Association Press, 1930; rev. ed., 1948.

Drake, Emma Frances. *What a Woman of Forty-five Ought to Know*. Self and Sex Series. Philadelphia: Vir, 1928.

———. *What a Young Wife Ought to Know*. Self and Sex Series. Philadelphia: Vir, 1928; rev. ed., 1936.

Hustad, Alice M. *Strictly Confidential for Young Girls*. Minneapolis: Board of Parish Education, 1944.

Klemer, Dora Hudson. *The Other Sex: A Frank Statement, Addressed to Both Boys and Girls, of the Essential Facts that Young People Want and Need to Know About Sex*. New York: Association Press, 1939.

Lamson, Armenouhie Tashjian. *How I Came to Be (My Birth)*, 2nd ed., rev. and enl. New York: Macmillan, 1926.

Lindsey, Benjamin Barr. *Companionate Marriage*. Garden City, N.Y.: Garden City Publishing, 1929.

———, and Wainwright Evans. *The Revolt of Modern Youth*. New York: Boni and Liveright, 1925.

McKown, Harry C. *A Boy Grows Up*. New York: McGraw-Hill, 1940; 2nd ed., 1949.

Moore, Harry Hascall. *Keeping in Condition: A Handbook on Training for Older Boys*, rev. ed. New York: Macmillan, 1924.

Rice, Thurman Brooks. *How Life Goes On and On: A Story for Girls of High School Age*. Chicago: American Medical Association, 1933.

———. *In Training: For Boys of High School Age*. Chicago: American Medical Association, 1933.

Sanger, Margaret. *What Every Boy and Girl Should Know*. New York: Brentano's, 1927.

Spaller, Louise Frances. *Personal Help for Boys*. Marietta, Ohio: Mullikin, 1921.

———. *Personal Help for Girls*. Marietta, Ohio: Mullikin, 1918.

Stall, Sylvanus. *What a Man of Forty-five Ought to Know*. Self and Sex Series. Philadelphia: Vir, 1928.

———. *What a Young Boy Ought to Know*. Self and Sex Series. Philadelphia: Vir, 1926; rev. eds., 1928, 1936.

———. *What a Young Husband Ought to Know*. Self and Sex Series. Philadelphia: Vir, 1928; rev. ed., 1936.

———. *What a Young Man Ought to Know*. Self and Sex Series. Philadelphia: Vir, 1928; rev. ed., 1936.

Steinhardt, Irving David. *Sex Talks to Boys*, rev. ed. Philadelphia: Lippincott, 1940.

———. *Sex Talk to Girls (Twelve Years and Older)*. rev. ed. Philadelphia: Lippincott, 1938.

Stopes, Marie Carmichael. *Sex and the Young*. New York: Putnam, 1926.

Strain, Frances Bruce. *Being Born*. New York: Appleton-Century, 1936; rev. and enl. 1954; 3rd ed. Hawthorn, 1970.

———. *Love at the Threshold*. New York: Appleton-Century-Crofts, 1942.

Swabacker, Leslie J. *Letters to My Daughter*. Chicago: Atwood and Knight, 1926.

"What to Do with the Youngster Who Asks for a Book of Sex-Information?" *Wilson Library Bulletin*, 8 (January 1934): 276–286.

Wood-Allen, Mary. *What a Young Girl Ought to Know*. Self and Sex Series. Philadelphia: Vir, 1928.

———. *What a Young Woman Ought to Know*. Self and Sex Series. Philadelphia: Vir, 1928; rev. ed., 1936.

Chapter 6

The Dating Manuals

After the agonies and uncertainties of World War II America turned with relief to the stability of home and marriage and social conformity. In the literature of the period male and female role behavior and relationships between the sexes became rigidly defined and were subject to prescribed expectations. During the war many women had taken on such jobs as welding and truck driving and had learned to make decisions for themselves. Now that the men were back home, it was necessary to return all the players to their accustomed places on the board so that the game of life could proceed as before.

Teenagers, with their natural desire for conformity, were especially vulnerable to these pressures. Boy-girl interaction was codified into the intricate ritual known as dating, and every adolescent was expected to participate. The rules were complex and exact and covered every possible variation. In 1950 Evelyn Duvall, the leading authority on dating, laid out the basic pattern in *Facts of Life and Love for Teenagers:*

> John calls for Mary at her home at the appointed time. Mary is ready for John and answers the door herself when he rings (he has come to see her, not some other member of her family). She greets him pleasantly and leads him into the living room where her parents are waiting to meet him.
>
> Mary introduces John to her parents by saying something like this: "Mother, this is John. Dad, you remember John plays center on the team." This little lead as a part of the introduction gives Dad and John something to talk about at once. Dad may ask a simple question on how the team is going this season. John is put at

his ease and answers, while Mother and Dad relax and enjoy getting acquainted with him.

In a few moments Mary picks up her coat and, smiling at John, indicates that they had probably better be on their way. If John holds the coat for Mary, she accepts his assistance graciously; if he does not, she slips into her coat without comment and prepares for departure.

As the couple is about to leave, Mary turns to her parents and says, "We are going to the Bijou for the double feature (or whatever), you know. We should be home before midnight (or whatever hour seems reasonable)." This declaration of plans and specifying of time for homecoming has a double purpose. It lets her folks know that she is taking responsibility for getting in before it is too late, and prevents them from putting down the parental foot too hard. Further, such initiative on Mary's part lets John know what is expected of him in getting Mary home. If Mary has already talked over their plans with her parents before John has arrived, her last-minute announcement is simply a confirmation for all four of them.

The couple leave, with John opening the door for Mary, while she accepts the courtesy with a smile. When they reach the box office, Mary steps back and looks at the display cards while John buys the tickets. Inside, if there is an usher, Mary follows him while John follows her down the aisle. If there is no usher on duty, John goes ahead and finds seats while Mary follows. Once seated, John helps Mary slip out of her coat and get settled. They enjoy the show without annoying their neighbors with talking, giggling, or other disturbing behavior.

Out of the theater, John may suggest something to eat or he may conduct Mary to the place of his choice. When he asks her what she would like to have, she thoughtfully hesitates until she sees what price range he has in mind. She says something like this: "What is good here, John?" or "What do you suggest?" If John recommends the steak sandwich with French fries, or the double-gooey sundae with nuts, this gives Mary the general idea of what he is prepared to spend. If she is friendly and shrewd she may note that John, in his desire to do the right thing, is suggesting something extravagant. If so, she will ask for something that she knows costs a little less. But if John says, "Which do you like better, coke or root beer?" Mary graciously keeps within these bounds. Over their food, John and Mary talk about the movie they have just seen or friends they have in common or anything that is of mutual interest. As they leave the restaurant, John pays the

> check and Mary thanks him by saying simply, "That was good; thank you, John."
>
> Once back at Mary's house, Mary gets out her key, unlocks the door, and then turns to John with a smile. She says, "It's been a lovely evening. Thank you, John," or something similar that lets John know she has enjoyed the date. John replies, "I have enjoyed it, too. I'll be seeing you." Then she opens the door and goes in without further hesitation. Since this is the first date, neither John nor Mary expect a goodnight kiss. So Mary is careful not to linger at the door, which might make John wonder what she expects him to do.

Two purposes lie behind these elaborate social instructions. One is to limit the possibility of any expression of physical sexuality in a situation that is inherently sexual. The other is to train the girl to defer to and bolster the male ego at every turn. Thus society began to remind girls of their traditional feminine roles and to encourage them to put aside the new freedoms and responsibilities they had assumed while the men were away at war. That the pattern of early dating led to early marriage and the conventional integration of young men and women into society was the expected and desired end. To ensure this outcome, however, it was necessary to prevent the couple from finding satisfaction within the dating pattern, so that their sexual tensions moved them inexorably toward a wedding.

Evelyn Duvall was the leading exponent of this intricately plotted dating ritual. Her *Facts of Life and Love for Teenagers* (1950, 1956, 1963) dominated the fifties in teen sex education and in its latest edition continues to appear on conservative reading lists. It is the book that many women now in their forties—the age group that has provided most of the leadership of the women's movement—read and revered in their teens. Duvall was an eminently respectable doctor of sociology (although she was usually referred to as *Mrs.* Duvall). Early in her career she began to specialize in marriage and the family—her doctoral thesis was entitled "Conceptions of Parenthood"—and was executive director of the Association for Family Living and subsequently executive secretary of the National Council on Family Relations. She lectured and taught widely, and for many years her voice was ubiquitous not only in the professional journals but also in popular magazines like *Coronet*, *Reader's Digest*, and *Parents' Maga-*

zine. Her picture in the 1947 *Current Biography* annual shows a slim, pleasant-faced woman, impeccably groomed and coiffed and wearing a ladylike string of pearls at the neck of her tailored suit.

Duvall was a prolific writer. In addition to the three editions of *Facts of Life and Love for Teenagers* she addressed young people's sexual problems in *When You Marry* (1945), *The Art of Dating* (1958, 1967), *Why Wait Till Marriage?* (1965), and numerous pamphlets and articles. For children she wrote *About Sex and Growing Up* (1968), and for parents, *Today's Teen-agers* (1966). With her husband, a college professor (the *Dr.* Duvall) whom she had married immediately upon graduating from Syracuse University, she coauthored two books: *Sense and Nonsense About Sex* (1962) and *Sex Ways—In Fact and Faith* (1961). Sylvanus Duvall alone wrote *101 Questions to Ask Yourself Before You Marry* (1950), which was changed to *Before You Marry* in the 1959 edition. But it was *Facts of Life and Love* that remained the classic for teenagers in the fifties. Because it was the model for middle-class teen behavior for an entire generation and because the other sex education books of that period echo its dictates point for point, it is worth looking at in some detail.

▪ Duvall and the Dating Ritual

Not since *What a Young Boy Ought to Know* had there been a teen sex education book that so exactly caught the mood of its times. Duvall's advanced degrees won her the trust of the fifties establishment, just as Stall's clerical background had done in his time. Both authors agreed on the essential message: sex is extremely dangerous unless rigorously controlled. Duvall compares it to electricity, which, when harnessed, can light homes, cook meals, and warm feet, but when left to run wild as lightning, can "hurt and destroy and leave forever scarred all that you hold dear."

Duvall's writing is thoughtful and moderate, sprightly but not cute. "Lively" is the word that was most often applied by her contemporaries. Her work shows serious research (although her bias sometimes keeps her from completely assimilating new facts), but the tone is always human and warm. Perhaps Duvall's most serious limitation, other than the rigid concept of correct male/female behavior imposed by her times, is a certain naive lack of humor. However, her dignity and good sense save her from attempts at teen slang—a mistake that made some other books quickly out-of-date and ridiculous.

The first two chapters of *Facts of Life and Love*, one for boys and one for girls, go over the physical facts of puberty and internal reproductive anatomy. Girls are advised on menstruation, bras and girdles, and skin problems, and boys are told that although "our grandfathers feared that the loss of semen somehow meant the loss of manhood," wet dreams are no cause for alarm, nor is it necessary to have intercourse to develop normally. A new interest in "grown-up matters" for girls is equated with "relationships with boys, hairdos, fashions, and love stories." This implied narrowness of female interests is emphasized in a paragraph on "Learning to be a woman." According to Duvall, femininity means learning to love and be loved, to enjoy boys and men as persons, and to enjoy the fine arts of being a real woman. Masculinity, by contrast, involves learning to establish oneself with other boys and men as an accepted member of the male community, learning to love girls, attaining secure economic and social status as an adult male, and searching for the meaning of life and the answer to the question "Who am I?"

In the next chapter Duvall takes up the more easily answered question "Where do babies come from?" This information, she feels, was formerly hard to find: "Books may be written on the subject, but often the library does not have them, or they are kept out of sight in conformity with the taboo that still exists in some places against reading or discussing such things." Duvall remedies the apparent lack with a brief description of pregnancy, birth, and heredity. The illustrations in this section are photographs of an exhibit on human reproduction from the Museum of Science and Industry in Chicago. Although earnest in attempting to depict these processes accurately, they are not entirely successful; they lack contrast and the print is too small for easy reading. The photographs seem especially cumbersome in comparison to the bouncy little sketches from teen life that illustrate the rest of the book. Drawn by Ruth Belew, these cartoons make up for Duvall's lack of humor; they were widely imitated and probably had a great deal to do with the book's success.

Duvall turns next to the problems that can come from the

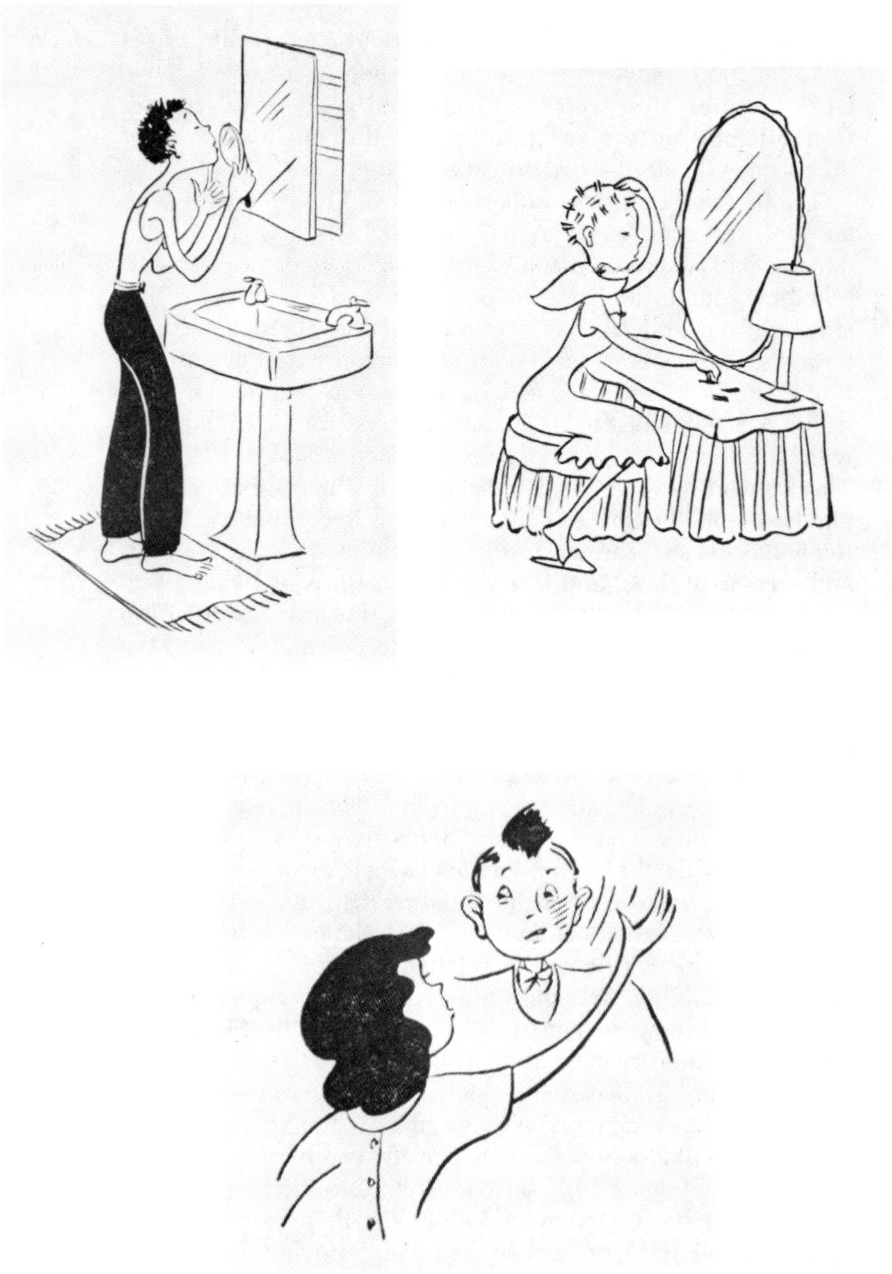

Figs. 8-10. Scenes from teen life drawn by Ruth Belew. From *Facts of Life and Love for Teenagers*, by Evelyn Duvall.

misuse of sexuality. The first of "Sex troubles and worries" ("Sex problems and promises" in the 1956 edition) is "getting into trouble," that is, illicit pregnancy. In the 1956 edition she quotes a study by Leontyne Young that showed that many girls deliberately allow themselves to get pregnant in order to get back at parents, or in imitation of a promiscuous mother or sister, or because they are starved for affection. Other girls, says Duvall, may be the victims of older men, or have sex on impulse, or lack knowledge of the workings of their bodies. Once a girl has conceived, she will have to go through with the pregnancy because abortion is illegal and dangerous and is considered immoral by many religious groups. However, her parents and social-welfare agencies can help her. Regarding contraception, Duvall admits that "several methods work satisfactorily when prescribed by a competent physician," but she doesn't recommend or describe any of them and notes that preventing conception is not only a personal issue but a social question—the Catholic Church, for instance, considers it a mortal sin.

Other "Sex troubles and worries" are prostitution, venereal disease, homosexuality, and masturbation. The first she condemns for social rather than moral reasons: "Not only is it bad in itself, in that it capitalizes on the exploitative impulses of man and enslaves woman, but it also is a basic factor in civic corruption and a common breeding place for venereal disease." The symptoms of syphilis and gonorrhea are briefly described; both can be cured by early diagnosis and care, she admits, but the "only sure protection is in restricting sexual intercourse to marriage."

Alfred Kinsey's *Sexual Behavior in the Human Male* had appeared in 1948, two years before the first edition of *Facts of Life and Love for Teenagers*. Duvall was too good a social scientist to pretend she was not aware of Kinsey's finding that at least one-third of American men had had a homosexual experience at some time in their lives, but in her writing for teenagers she displayed a cautionary ambivalence about this topic. Kinsey's influence is evident in Duvall's admission in *Facts of Life and Love* that "most people at some time in their lives have experienced some kind of homosexual tie" and in her explanation of sexual behavior as a continuum, or scale, from homosexuality to heterosexuality: "At the homosexual end of the scale are persons whose sexual interests involve members of the same sex exclusively; at the other end of the scale are men and women who are interested in members of the other sex only; in between is the large number of persons of both sexes who at some time in their lives and to some extent find their own sex appealing, but whose capacities for responding to the other sex are also well developed."

Like many teen sex educators who wrote in the years immediately following the release of Kinsey's findings, however, Duvall still saw homosexuality as a disease—"Sometimes our earliest experiences with people give us little faith in them or in ourselves or in love itself, and so we may develop twisted feelings about others and distorted ways of responding to them"—and a menace—"The boy who has been approached by an older man in ways that do not seem quite right to him should avoid further opportunities to be alone with this particular individual. Sound counseling help is also needed by the boy who has been inducted into homosexual activities and has become deeply involved emotionally." Her conclusion is that "we" should get over our anxieties about it, and "understand it as a not unusual part of growing up, although its overt forms are not to be actively sought."

Masturbation can be another anxiety-causing subject. "Not long ago," she reminds boys, people thought masturbation caused insanity, and some persons still think it is a sin. Others believe it can be detected by circles under the eyes, pimples, or a peculiar look in the eye. All nonsense, she maintains stoutly, "Today we know that the tendency to relieve sexual tension by rubbing the genital area to the point of release is a very common practice. Statistical studies and clinical findings indicate that between 80 and 90 percent of teen-age boys report that they masturbate, and that somewhat fewer teen-age girls also report the practice." However, masturbation can exaggerate a tendency to be withdrawn and solitary, and "some authorities report that a history of masturbation on the part of the woman, and in some cases of men too, makes more difficult the adjustments to the marriage partner later. Some girls who have stimulated themselves to the point of release for years before marriage may require exactly the same type of frictional excitation from their husbands after marriage in order to achieve full release from sexual tension." In the final analysis, Duvall decides that "one finds it hard to say that masturbation, therefore, is right or wrong, harmless or harmful; it all depends upon the many interrelated factors in the individual involved."

The main body of *Facts of Life and Love* is devoted to the minutiae of the dating ritual. Duvall has no doubts that every teenager will and should date, and she offers no comfort to those who do not. Indeed, she makes it plain that she considers such failure to participate as willful and demolishes excuses in a paragraph headed "If I only had. . . ." She advises that if things are a bit slow in getting started, girls may (subtly) have to take the initiative at first, because boys mature more slowly. The novice dater can expect to feel awkward, but expertise soon develops—"You learn how to do it by doing it. At first you will feel somewhat uncomfortable in new situations and embarrassed in unexpected predicaments. But with experience you polish off the rough edges and become smooth."

Duvall explores correct dating technique in all its aspects: telephone etiquette, accepting and giving gifts, how to ask a girl out (never say, "What are you doing Friday night?"), last-minute invitations, accepting a date graciously, being stood up, what to do and where to go on a date, conversation on a date, costs, responding to a "line," introductions, being friendly to a date's grandparents, brothers, and sisters, what to wear ("stockings or socks, long dress or short, dress or skirt and sweater . . ."), hogging the bathroom when preparing for a date, borrowing clothes from other members of the family, deciding how late is all right, using the family car, and blind dates and double dates. Most parents "would prefer that their young people date those with the same general background—national, religious, social—as their own," she explains and hints delicately at interracial dating problems: "Issues of tolerance, democracy, brotherhood, and fair play may seem more important to you than conforming to some tradition." Throughout, Duvall upholds the importance of conformity, as in her careful advice on the thin-ice situation of ridding oneself of a bad reputation or dating a serviceman.

Although the problem of "that goodnight kiss" can be a matter of regional custom, according to Duvall the general agreement is that the first date is too soon. But for necking and petting, never is too soon. The former she defines as "any love-making above the neck" and the latter as "the caressing of other more sensitive parts of the body in a crescendo of sexual stimulation." Petting is habit-forming, she warns, because "these forces are often very strong and insistent. Once released, they tend to press for completion." To help daters know exactly when to apply the brakes she provides a list of danger signs: the boy will react first, with flushed face, rapid breathing, pounding heart. "Changes in his sex organs are obvious" and his hands perspire. At this point "some girls experience an all-over relaxation." Duvall explains that stopping is a girl's responsibility because women are less easily excited and more slowly moved to demand sexual contact: "If two lovers are swept off their feet, it is the girl that is blamed. . . . 'She should have known better,'" people will say. However, it is important that a girl know how to make a boy stop without hurting his ego. Several suggestions are incorporated in little anecdotes—for instance, the girl who firmly removes the boy's hand "as she says with mock surprise, 'Why, this isn't Tuesday, is it?'"

How to say no in other difficult situations is the subject of the next chapter—not only how to say no but how to say it with grace and tact so that the smooth surface of social acceptance is not disturbed. Duvall shows how to turn down a drink or a cigarette so that everybody else is still comfortable drinking and smoking, how to refuse to go along with the gang to a questionable night spot without seeming like a prig, how to ask a date to stop drinking so nicely that he will ask for another date, how to handle unwelcome advances or refuse a date without rejecting the person—all useful and appropriate tactics in the context of the times.

"Love under a cloud" explores the pain of loving inappropriately. Crushes on members of one's own sex—which Duvall explains as resulting from delayed emotional development—and on other love objects that parents will not accept (no examples) can be unhappy situations. In a passage remarkable for its rarity in teen sex education Duvall explores the trauma of falling in love with a married man (the picture shows a babysitter with her employers) or woman. Duvall displays an unusual candor in admitting that this kind of love is quite common and discusses its understandable appeal and inherent heartache with calm good sense.

Going steady was an inevitable outcome of dating, and one that Duvall and other sex educators looked at askance. Although she acknowledges the benefits of going steady, including the comfort of social security, she is wary about the possibility of the couple becoming "too involved" or the pain of the inevitable breakup. Practical advice for recovering from a broken heart and getting back in circulation is offered to the ex-steady.

Further chapters on the nature of love, getting engaged, and preparing for marriage complete the book. Not until she can set it properly in the context of marriage does Duvall describe the sex act itself and then only in the most straightforward terms: "Physically it is a relatively simple procedure. After an initial period of sexual excitation, the penis becomes erect and is thrust into the vagina. A series of in and out movements eventuates in the ejaculation of semen from the penis. The woman may or may not have a climax in which her sex tension is released. Following the sexual climax is a period of relaxation and usually sleep."

The first two editions of *Facts of Life and Love* (1950 and 1956) differ in only minor ways. The later edition adds an index, changes the paragraph and chapter headings, and rearranges the material on dating, but the content remains the same. There are a few tiny deletions, such as a reference to "enjoying" a shady reputation and a sentence implying that engagement adjustment predicts marriage adjustment (possibly removed because it might be interpreted as sanctioning sex for engaged couples).

The 1963 edition, however, looks entirely different and has a new title: *Love and the Facts of Life*. The page is larger, and the cartoons by Ruth Belew have been replaced with more subtle and dignified drawings. The book opens with a new chapter on feelings and emotional maturity, in which we are told a sad story about a girl who married the first man who came along and found herself a drudge at eighteen. This change of attitude toward early marriage is expanded in the final chapter, where Duvall explains that early marriage (or sex) is unwise and better deferred for ten or twelve years while a young person gets an education: "Too early involvement in irresponsible sexuality stunts growth as a complete human being." A change of attitude is also apparent in the passage on petting. While Duvall still does not approve, she does qualify her disapproval. In answer to "What's the harm?" she allows that it depends on circumstances, such as whether the two people know and love each other or are strangers; whether they are the same age or he grown and she young; and whether "they have high standards of conduct or see themselves as creatures of impulse."

A few minor changes are the inclusion of a caution against carrying "anti-pregnancy pills" for emergencies and the removal of the equivocal passage about the harm of masturbation. Definitions of lesbian, hermaphrodite, and sex change are provided, as are a number of slang terms for prostitute—"easy make," "call girl," "B-girl." The discussion of dating techniques is preserved intact from ten years earlier.

One interesting new feature of the 1963 edition is a chapter called "What do you want to know?" which gives a statistical analysis of the sources of sex information for teens for the years 1938 and 1960. The analysis showed that in 1938 thirty percent of teenagers got most of their sex information from parents; by 1960 that had risen to forty percent. Sex education in a religious setting accounted for the knowledge of only one percent in 1938 and three percent in 1960. The schools were the source for eight percent in 1938 and (in spite of the furor over sex education classes) exactly the same percentage in 1960. Peers counted for sixty-six percent of boys' knowledge and forty percent of girls' in 1938; while the figure for boys declined to thirty-three percent in 1960, it rose to fifty percent for girls.

The most striking change came in the amount of sex information that was gained from books. In 1938 only four percent of young people learned the facts of life from the printed page. By 1960 thirty-three percent of girls and twenty-five percent of boys claimed books as their major source of information about sex. Duvall credits this to an increase in the quality and availability of the literature: "A generation and more ago, a young person had a hard time digging out of dictionaries and medical books what he wanted to know about himself and the process of growing up. Now there are a number of books that clearly answer young people's questions about these things in good, wholesome ways." Librarians routinely stock such materials, she explains, for the use of responsible students. Duvall's many titles and editions made up a large section of that stock.

Although the 1963 *Love and the Facts of Life* was popular, it never attained the classic status of *Facts of Life and Love for Teenagers*. Librarians in conservative communities are often still faced with requests for that title from teachers who feel that the 1963 changes are just a bit racy for their reading lists.

A Uniform View

What about the other sex education books of the fifties? Had Duvall swept the field? We have seen that repressive times spur an increase in the production of cautionary-advice literature, and this was true of the postwar years. The increased willingness of libraries to purchase sex education books probably also inspired publishers to take advantage of the new market. In any case, there were at least thirty books and countless pamphlets produced between 1948 and 1960.

Although style and format varied, a surprising degree of unanimity prevailed in the content of these works. A brief description of male and female reproductive anatomy was obligatory, as was an explanation of the mechanics of conception, pregnancy, and birth. Most authors expressed at least token approval of natural childbirth. A perfunctory description of sexual intercourse was usual, but only in terms of the male dynamic. Boys were reassured that nocturnal emissions and involuntary erections were normal and that they should not feel guilty about the sexual imagery in wet dreams. Girls were told that menstruation was not normally painful but that they should be careful about getting chilled or exercising violently. Sex educators were quick to deny the old tales about masturbation, but just as quick to warn that there is danger in excessive indulgence and in the resulting guilt and shame. They were still horrified at homosexuality but considered it a sickness curable by psychotherapy. Although there was occasional mention of lesbians, homosexuality was seen as primarily male behavior, and it was usually attributed to fixation at an immature stage of emotional development. Writers continued to warn young boys against the possibility of homosexual seduction and urged them to "report" any older man who approached them.

Dating received warm approval throughout the fifties' literature, which described the ritual in varying degrees of detail. Going steady, however, made the sex educators distinctly uneasy, and they pointed out its perils at length. Kissing and necking received reluctant sanction, but petting did not. Petters were warned of the danger of being swept away and the consequences of losing control: pregnancy, venereal disease, abortion, forced marriage. Contraception was mentioned, but only to stress its riskiness, and not until the end of the decade were specific methods described. Girls were invariably reminded of their responsibility for setting limits, not only because they bear the risk of pregnancy but because they were thought to be less easily aroused. In the main, early engagement and marriage were encouraged, although a reaction against this trend began to set in toward the close of the fifties. At that time, too, a few street words—in quotes—began to creep in. There was, of course, almost no acknowledgment of sexual pleasure, although the possibility of orgasm for women was occasionally suggested. However, sex educators remained opposed to premarital intercourse under any circumstances.

▪ Kinsey's Findings

The overwhelming uniformity of the sex education books of the fifties seems to indicate that they were an accurate reflection of current sexual attitudes. Evidently this was how middle-class American parents expected their children to behave and most likely believed they *did* behave. But what was the reality of teenage sexuality? The publication of Alfred Kinsey's monumental *Sexual Behavior in the Human Male* in 1948 and *Sexual Behavior in the Human Female* in 1953 caused a great furor. The disparity between the assumptions of the sex educators and the reality of teen sex behavior as documented by Kinsey was shocking to America's puritanical sensibilities. While teenagers were being told that premarital sex would inevitably lead to terrible consequences, fifty percent of the married women Kinsey interviewed had not been virgins when they married; the figure for married men varied from sixty to ninety-eight percent, depending on educational level. Kinsey reported that one half to three quarters of premarital coitus occurred in teenagers' own homes. What is more, sixty-nine percent of the nonvirginal brides had no regrets later, and thirteen percent had only minor regrets. Eighty-three percent who became pregnant out of wedlock were not sorry, nor were sixteen percent of those who had contracted venereal disease.

Kinsey also found evidence that a significant increase in female sexual activity had taken place during the 1920s; among women born before 1900 fourteen percent of those unmarried by age twenty-five had had sexual intercourse; among women born in the next decade thirty-six percent of those unmarried by age twenty-five were experienced. Frequency of male intercourse had remained unchanged from Victorian times—the shift took place quite suddenly in women's behavior only. This new trend had not continued to increase but had remained on the same level from 1930 to 1953. Frequency of petting followed a similar pattern, although it was found to be far more common for men among those with higher education. According to Kinsey, masturbation and petting to climax had a clearly beneficial relationship to the degree of satisfaction girls achieved in marital sex: "A major factor in orgasmic marriage for females is premarital orgasmic experience." Among girls who had experienced orgasm before marriage forty-five percent were orgasmic with all marital coitus in the first year of marriage; among the nonexperienced only twenty-five percent. Most shocking of all, Kinsey found that thirty-seven percent of American males and twenty-eight percent of American females had had or would have at least one homosexual experience between the onset of adolescence and old age. "The facts are complex," he explained carefully, "and can only be understood by focusing on *homosexual behavior* rather than on *homosexual people*."

America roared with outrage. Energetic attempts were made to discredit Kinsey's methods and motives, and the House Committee on Un-American Activities accused him of espousing the communist doctrine of free love. Like Evelyn Duvall in *Facts of Life and Love*, the sex educators coped in their own way. Many of them reinterpreted Kinsey's findings to their own satisfaction. Regarding homosexuality, for instance, some of them posited a false distinction between normal homosexuality (the kind most people experience) and abnormal homosexuality (the kind that results in perverts). The evidence linking petting to better-educated people was taken to mean that college men were too intelligent to risk premarital intercourse. What the sex educators could neither accept nor distort was conveniently ignored and forgotten. Some of Kinsey's data—especially those relating to women's sexual pleasure—have not been fully absorbed into teenage sex instruction to this day.

▪ Variations on the Fifties Theme

Despite Kinsey, then, the sex education books of the postwar years continued to project a view of normal and acceptable sex behavior that the researcher's finding had largely invalidated. As we have outlined, these books showed a remarkable uniformity of content. A number of titles, however, reflected marginal differences in style and emphasis that throw further light on the attitudes of the times. Let us look at points where some of these books vary, bearing in mind that the similarities far outweigh the differences.

Teen Days (1946), by Frances Strain, the author of *Being Born* (1936), is remarkable for its sexism, even in a sexist era. Writing two years after World War II, Strain looks askance at the new independence women had gained by working in defense industries: "As for girls in general they do seem to be edging up on the boys what with their slacks, their flat shoes, their war jobs, the handling of machinery, the driving of trucks, street cars, and other he-man occupations. And how they do love their pay envelopes!" Girls seem to have forgotten, she laments, that there are distinct differences between the sexes: "Many women are not ready to admit these differences. In their desire for equality with men they do not want to recognize them. Again and again a girl will say in speaking of grievances between herself and a sweetheart, 'I wouldn't have done that to him!' Of course she wouldn't because she is a woman and he is a man." To clarify current thinking about male and female qualities Strain delineates the "Differences between Boy and Girl Nature":

BOYS	GIRLS
Think less of dress	Spend more time and thought on clothes
Are less emotional	Are more stormy and tearful
Adhere more strictly to principle	"Break over just this once"
Keep a secret better	"Don't tell anyone . . ."
Have broader interests	Neglect newspapers
Are more loyal (even after separation)	Indifferent or resentful after break
Are less talkative	Are chatterboxes
Are more content in solitude	Can't bear to be alone
Have more respect for rights of others	All's fair in love and war
Endure pain less well	Seem to have more endurance for pain

BOYS	GIRLS
Are not inclined to nag	Can't stop talking about it
Are better spenders	Watch their pennies
Are more tolerant	Want to "make over" a person
Are more jealous	Are more possessive
Like conservative dress	Like people to notice dress
Are more conceited	Watch the looking-glass
Are less demonstrative	Are more affectionate
Are more direct in approach	Are more tactful
Are less orderly around the house	Are more orderly
Are more aggressive	Are more yielding
Are more forgiving	Hold a grudge longer
Are physically more modest	Like to display their charms
Love more than one	Love "one and only"
Forget about birthdays and anniversaries	Are more sentimental
Are more businesslike	Allow personal feelings to enter transactions
Stand on their rights	Are more self-sacrificing
Make up their minds	Change their minds

Girls' athletics, Strain feels, should be used to train women in cooperation rather than aggression: "After school, inter-class games take the place of practice for competitive games, the objective being not victory over an adversary but individual development, release from tension, and good-fellowship." Passivity should prevail even in childbirth, the essential female activity: "There are gay little capsules of all colors and kinds which ease the way or put one to sleep. Usually a mother need not concern herself with choices of these medical aids. Her part is to choose a physician whom she can trust . . . and then leave details and methods to him."

Strain is heartily in favor of early dating, feeling that it is good practice for success in marriage. She projects a pyramid of dating progress, "a structure built by American boys and girls themselves in the last few decades," which begins at the base with group dating and proceeds through the stages of double dating, single dating, going steady, courtship, and engagement toward the acme of marriage. Although "there has been too much talk about 'petting' and 'smooching,'" Strain presents a list of "Rules for Conduct" that is more practical than most: do not go drifting off into cozy corners and lover's lanes, avoid blackouts and dimouts, seat the boy in a chair and not on the couch, have interesting things to do, and do not succumb to sighs and tears and ask for comforting.

Dates and Dating (1948), by Esther Emerson Sweeney, copyrighted by the National Board of the Young Women's Christian Association, is typical of the pamphlets of courtship etiquette that were produced by many social agencies during this period. Dating is "a testing ground for marriage" and a way to increase one's understanding of people. "Today's dates are tomorrow's brides," but petting and necking are not for the unmarried: "These are actually preparatory love-making steps leading to the complete physical and emotional union of two persons. They are not complete acts in themselves. They can terminate only in tension and frustration."

The Stork Didn't Bring You! (1948, 1961), by Lois Pemberton, is distinguished by sporadic and awkward attempts at teen slang. Describing the courtship practices of the previous generation, she writes, "Saturday night jam sessions were strictly ham from the family's own vocal cords with pop or mom beating a wheezy accompaniment on the old pianola." Following a glossary of scientific sexual terms, she explains that there are other words "no printer prints" and that are not found in any dictionary, so "be good kids then, and stick to the accepted ones, huh?" Pemberton drops the jazzy syntax, however, when she gets down to serious matters—for instance, in defining orgasm: "The climax or ultimate gratification in sexual intercourse. In men, it is the moment of seminal emission. In women, satisfaction is signified by the expansion and contraction of the vaginal walls."

Pemberton is scornful of anyone who does not conform to the approved stereotypes of male and female teenage behavior, characterizing deviants as the overly sex-conscious, the wolf, the wallflower, the clinging vine, the gushing goon, the tomboy, the sissy, and "other creeps." She sees such nonconformity as the cause of homosexuality: "Sex and self-consciousness is carried to perverted degrees" by those who are "physically unattractive or have grotesque disabilities. . . . Their twisted minds may lead them into all kinds of unnatural sexual relations with those of their own sex." Nonconformists are also the ones who most often succumb to the temptations of petting: "Over-indulgence in kissing can lead only to the dark corners and the progressive gruesome twosome stages. . . . And it's almost always the unpopular ones who are guilty, and they smooch in defiance at being cast aside socially." As a further deterrent to premarital sex Pemberton offers this description of abortion: "The curette operation, illegally performed by unethical doctors and untrained midwives at an exorbitant fee . . . consists of opening the cervix and scraping the embryo from the womb. A fearfully painful performance. It'll be done primitively with half-sterilized instruments, in drab surroundings. No anesthesia or kind word accompany it to ease the fears and pain."

Letters to Jane (1948), by Gladys Shultz, is a series of missives written by a mother to her daughter at college at the point when "sex rears its ugly head." Jane had been necking with her boyfriend one night when "it turned into something else again. All of a sudden I wasn't myself any more." She tells her mother that although she is still a virgin, she is shocked and surprised at "learning I am not the nice girl I always thought I was." Through the letters Jane's mother sends to her daughter Shultz works in most of the expected advice on the physical and emotional aspects of sex. Jane shares these letters with the other girls in the dormitory, including one named Shirley, a thin, dark, intense girl with an unhappy face. Shirley advocates free love and a woman's right to have an illegitimate child. Mother, however, sees through this façade and reveals Shirley's underlying insecurity. One kindly letter explains to Shirley and Jane that when a man really loves a woman he wants her for his wife, not as a "make," and that a man wants to feel that he doesn't have to watch his wife all the time. When Jane gets Shirley a date with a friend of her own boyfriend, Shirley's radical opinions melt away. After several more letters Jane gets engaged, and all ends happily in expectation of a wedding.

Toward Manhood (1951), by Herman Bundesen, was evidently meant to be a male counterpart of *Letters to Jane*. Although the format differs, both books were published by the same publisher and both use the same drawings of the male and female reproductive systems. Bundesen, who was health commissioner of Chicago, had strong opinions about vice. Sex, he felt, "like hunger, is one of the driving forces of life. It will not be denied. . . . There is no primitive impulse that can work more lasting harm on others, if uncontrolled, than the sex urge." Young people can have a hard time squelching this power: "The boy who wants to be as clean in mind as he is in body may sometimes feel that he is obsessed by lewd devils, which he cannot fight off no matter how hard he tries." Seductive girls—"round-heels" or "teasers"—are "definitely dangerous, however sympathetic one may be because of the origin of their warped and twisted attitudes." Homosexuality is also a menace—"a sign of a sick and twisted personality." Furthermore, "women with a concealed homosexual tendency are incapable of warm, motherly feelings. Their love is selfish."

Like Pemberton, Bundesen emphasizes the dangers of abortion, which, of course, was to remain illegal for another twenty years: "To dislodge a strong, healthy embryo or fetus from the mother's womb is a risky business. Death is very much more likely to result from an operation of this kind than from childbirth." A young woman who has had an abortion may "all the rest of her life blame herself for having done a great wrong, refrain from marriage, and forfeit all chances for a happy family life." There may be suicide attempts or a "black market" adoption of the baby by an unsuitable couple. A young man is also in for rough going if he "should betray his ideals and has acquired a venereal disease in consequence."

In a first mention of drugs Bundesen deplores the "unspeakably vicious drug traffic" and the power of those substances to destroy inhibitions. Nor is it much better to frequent "beer joints and bootleg hangouts" (an unlikely event in 1951). Early marriage is a solution to all these problems, even though "in many cases it means that the young wife must drop her college work. The girls don't seem to mind it however. They usually report that they would rather have their baby than a college degree."

A pair of books by Frank Howard Richardson, *For Boys Only* (1952, 1959) and *For Girls Only* (1953, 1960), stand out in their use of particularly affected prose. Each employs the format of a fictionalized set of chats; the "fellows" are treated to talks at a school chapel by a figure called the Doctor ("We always have a big time at these parties"), and the girls are instructed around the bonfire at summer camp by a misty person called Lady. Lady has little to tell the girls other than the facts of menstruation and how to be clean and charming, and her advice about men is restricted to warnings, as exemplified in her story about a "fast" camper who "goes for a ride" with a boy who drives the camp truck. Lady conveys her information about venereal disease in one sentence: "There are certain diseases that are known as the 'social diseases' because they are usually, although not always, the direct result of immoral association between men and women." At the end of the book Lady sits by the dying campfire, well satisfied with her summer's work: "There was a prayer in her heart that each one would grow into womanhood fully equipped to make the world a better place, and to create a home that America could be proud of."

The Doctor, on the other hand, provides much more anatomical detail for the boys, but in an awkward, conversational fashion. In talking about the sperm's role in conception: "Pretty big jump from a speck so small you can't see it without a microscope, to a big lug like one of you, wasn't it? Now what do you suppose the womb does so that it can take care of such an egg, if it gets fertilized?" In this atmosphere of manly camaraderie the boys get up their courage to ask some questions, such as, "I say, doctor, just what is the fun in what the older fellows are always beating their gums about—petting, or necking, or boodling? Is it the same as what the older people used to call spooning?" Another boy asks, "What makes older fellows try to get boys to let them do things to them they know they ought not to do?" to which the Doctor answers that these people are "mentally 'off'" and should be reported to the authorities. "After all, fellows," the doctor confides as he ends his talk, "there's a lot of satisfaction in being decent, and a good sport, and having the feeling toward girls and women we all know the right sort of boys and men have. We know they're not as strong as we are and so are entitled to our protection: and it just isn't cricket to harm them or make trouble for them. . . . There are lots of ways of having good times with girls. Let's not choose the wrong ones."

Your Dating Days (1954), by Paul Landis, is an excerpt from a larger work by the same author entitled *Your Marriage and Family Living*. Landis, who was a professor of sociology at the State College of Washington, is primarily interested in discussing preparation for marriage, and his book includes some startling statistics on teen dating from the Purdue Opinion Poll for Young People. Compiled at a time when sex educators were picturing

American teenagers as almost unanimously involved in dating and were describing nonparticipants as social outcasts, this poll revealed that forty-eight percent of boys and thirty-nine percent of girls rarely or never went out on dates.

Research findings that indicated frequent premarital intercourse among teenagers were also studiously ignored by many writers. Lester Kirkendall, professor of family life at Oregon State University, prominent sex educator, and cofounder of the Sex Information and Education Council of the U.S., researched and wrote a serious adult study on the subject, *Premarital Intercourse and Interpersonal Relationships* (1961). Yet, in his pamphlet for teenagers, *Understanding Sex* (first printed in 1947, revised in 1957, and included in the 1954 and 1966 editions of *How to Be a Successful Teen-ager*, by William C. Menninger), he invoked the dangers of pregnancy, venereal disease, and loss of respect as deterrents, warning young people that "practically all dating relationships in which premarital intercourse occurs fail to continue into engagement and marriage." This warning and advice remained essentially unchanged throughout the successive editions. However, Kirkendall's pamphlet is unique in one way. For the very first time teenagers are told (after the usual warnings) that it might be all right to be friends with a homosexual: "Many people have homosexual desires, yet know how to control their impulses and never seek to bring others into homosexual practices. Such persons may make as good citizens and as good friends as anyone else."

In 1955 Gladys Shultz, author of *Letters to Jane*, wrote another book, *It's Time You Knew*, addressed to Jane's younger sister. The book has a peculiar glossary, not of scientific terms but of words and phrases that Shultz thought might be puzzling to young girls, such as *illicit relations* ("less blunt sounding than fornication"), *mistress* ("As you get older, you will realize how very many complications are possible in the relations between the sexes. In this country such arrangements are not condoned or excused"), *promiscuity* ("more is found the lower one goes in the social scale—it is often associated with ignorance"), and *prostitute* ("just about the worst thing a human being can do"). Although Shultz tells Jane's sister that "it is not usual for a girl in the early or middle teens to have very strong sex feelings," this statement is carefully qualified in another chapter: "If a girl at or after puberty is troubled by strong sex drives—an urge to have more than friendly relations with the boys she knows, or to do a good deal of masturbating—then she, too, should seek help. This is not the usual picture for girls in the early or middle teens, and a sympathetic, up-to-date doctor ought to be consulted. Conceivably, some disturbance of the glands may be responsible, such as overactivity of the pituitary or thyroid."

In 1956 two works that previously had been issued as pamphlets by the American Medical Association and the National Education Association were published in book form—*Learning About Love* and *What's Happening to Me?* by Marion Lerrigo and Helen Southard. Although the stated objective of these works was "to support the teen-ager in his intention and desire to live up to ideals of good sex conduct and to avoid actions that may make him feel guilty and unhappy," the books were entirely conventional in content. No one asked why sex was expected to make a teenager feel guilty and unhappy.

Religious sex education books generally followed the thinking of the secular sex educators. Marginal differences in liberality or conservatism reflected the stance of the sponsoring denomination. And, of course, these writers were able to employ the authority of religious dogma and scriptural interpretation to reinforce the fading threats of pregnancy, venereal disease, and social ostracism. *From Teens to Marriage*, by Reuben Behlmer, was published in 1959 by Concordia (Lutheran) and is fairly typical of midline Protestantism. The first sentence—"You have been wonderfully made by the divine Creator (Psalm 139:14)"—sets the biblical tone. The author extols the virtues of home, family, school, and religion. "The story of life" suffers from a lack of diagrams to clarify the anatomical description (just where *is* the inguinal canal?). After the usual information on birth, menstruation, and masturbation a detailed guide to dating includes this directive: "If you are one who has never dated, the fault might be yours; if so, correct it." Behlmer interprets the admonition from Exodus 20:14 ("Thou shalt not commit adultery") to forbid both extra- and premarital sex relations, but he reminds transgressors that God forgives all sins (John 8:1–11). A discussion of love, engagement, and marriage cautions against the high divorce risk of marriages between people of unlike faiths, and warns in detail against marrying a Catholic—even giving the full text of the agreement required in such cases.

Some other sex education books with a religious orientation

were *Growing Up: A Book for Girls, by a Catholic Woman Doctor*, by Mary Kidd (1946); *Life and Love: A Christian View of Sex*, by Clyde Marramore (1956); and *God, Sex and Youth*, by William Hulme (1959).

▪ TOWARD THE SIXTIES

It was not until 1958 that a sex education book was written that began to reflect the sexual revolution that had begun to overtake American society—*Sex and the Adolescent*, by Maxine Davis. The author, a magazine writer, was not a member of the sexology establishment, and she brought a fresh perspective to the subject. As a journalist Davis did not attempt to ignore the facts, but there is a certain schizophrenic quality to her work; time and again she verges on new insights, which she then qualifies with older attitudes. Davis puts her subject in historical perspective, as in her discussion of the development of attitudes about masturbation, and her style is warm and anecdotal. In spite of this, the book was never very popular, possibly because of its slight unorthodoxy.

Right at the beginning Davis breaks with tradition by explaining that although she "employs the vocabulary the doctor uses" for clarity, there are other perfectly good Anglo-Saxon words. Examples are *pee, screw*, and *come*. "For personal use, any term that expresses clearly what one wants to say is a good word." Her description of intercourse, which she explains is "a mere diagram of action," is followed by a passage that gives the first hint of sex as a highly civilized pleasure that increases with skill and care: "Sexual love is a much longer, more complicated experience than just the above. It is an art which good men learn later on." The usual advice on masturbation is proffered, with two interesting additions. Davis points out approvingly that a young man may learn to delay his orgasm by masturbating with fantasies. She also raises the problem of religious disapproval—the Roman Catholic Church states specifically that masturbation is "intrinsically evil, being contrary to the Divine and Natural Laws." This can be a problem for the individual who "must reconcile his religious convictions, his sex life, and his whole self." Davis reluctantly acknowledges Kinsey's data on homosexuality—"Today we shudder at new sets of statistics showing how many true homosexuals there are in the country and how many other people have had homosexual experience"—but copes by making the distinction (unfounded in Kinsey's work) between "normal" homosexuality and perversion.

Davis is forthright about women's sexual pleasure. She defines the clitoris as "a small organ designed solely for enjoyment of sexual activity," explaining further that the clitoris "has no other purpose. In times past women either did not know (or else pretended not to know) that it existed." Orgasm, while "not absolutely essential to health or happiness," enables a woman "to share her husband's pleasure." She notes (Kinsey's finding) that although girls are only mildly stimulated from erotica and visual stimuli, some kinds of "personal contact will arouse a surge of desire so intense that it requires expression and release." She describes techniques of female masturbation, such as finger and thigh pressure, and warns that girls who masturbate without climax may form the habit of self-suppression and be unable to find satisfaction in married sex. About petting she is generally disapproving but admits that it is something that "everybody does"—"an almost universal practice" that "helps a young person learn about his own desires and those of the opposite sex," adding that this is "especially important for girls."

Unlike earlier sex educators, Davis discusses (albeit negatively) the possibility of petting to orgasm: "Steadies who pet may develop techniques for finding gratification and reaching orgasm without intercourse and thereby establish a sexual pattern that may interfere later with the far deeper satisfaction of complete union in marriage." She owns up to the findings of "responsible studies" that many women have sex before marriage and allows that "girls who do" are no longer outcasts. Because in illicit sex boys are liable to be hasty and inconsiderate, however, "for a girl it is not likely to be genuinely pleasurable."

Although Davis warns that contraceptives give "a sense of security for which there is very little foundation," she does describe the condom, the diaphragm, the rhythm method, and withdrawal in some detail. She credits Kinsey for some statistics indicating that the consequences of abortion "may not be so dire as supposed" and states that although these operations are illegal, some abortionists may be competent and responsible. Still, at this point, she cannot resist including a vivid horror story about a visit to an abortionist. However clearly such passages locate *Sex and the Adolescent* within the literature of its decade, Davis's book unmistakably points toward the relaxation of attitudes that would become increasingly evident in the sex education books of the sixties.

■ BIBLIOGRAPHY

Behlmer, Reuben D. *From Teens to Marriage*. St. Louis, Mo.: Concordia, 1959.

Brecher, Edward M. *The Sex Researchers*. Boston: Little, Brown, 1969.

Bundesen, Herman N. *Toward Manhood*. Philadelphia: Lippincott, 1951.

Davis, Maxine. *Sex and the Adolescent*. New York: Dial, 1958.

Duvall, Evelyn Ruth Millis. *About Sex and Growing Up*. New York: Association Press, 1968.

———. *The Art of Dating*. New York: Association Press, 1958; rev. ed., 1967.

———. *Facts of Life and Love for Teenagers*. New York: Association Press, 1950; rev. ed., 1956.

———. *Love and the Facts of Life*. New York: Association Press, 1963.

———. *Today's Teen-agers*. New York: Association Press, 1966.

———. *Why Wait Till Marriage?* New York: Association Press, 1965.

———, and Sylvanus Milne Duvall. *Sense and Nonsense About Sex*. New York: Association Press, 1962.

———, eds. *Sex Ways—In Fact and Faith*. New York: Association Press, 1961.

Duvall, Evelyn Ruth Millis and Reuben Hill. *When You Marry*. New York: Association Press, 1945; rev. ed., Lexington, Mass.: Heath, 1953; high-school eds., 1962, 1967.

Duvall, Sylvanus Milne. *Before You Marry: 101 Questions to Ask Yourself*. New York: Association Press, 1959.

———. *101 Questions to Ask Yourself Before You Marry*. New York: Association Press, 1950.

Hulme, William Edward. *God, Sex and Youth*. Englewood Cliffs, N.J.: Prentice-Hall, 1959.

Kidd, Mary. *Growing Up: A Book for Girls, by a Catholic Woman Doctor*. New York: Benziger Bros., 1946.

Kinsey, Alfred C., et al. *Sexual Behavior in the Human Female*. Philadelphia: Saunders, 1953.

Kinsey, Alfred C., Wardell B. Pomeroy, and Clyde E. Martin. *Sexual Behavior in the Human Male*. Philadelphia: Saunders, 1948.

Kirkendall, Lester Allen. *Premarital Intercourse and Interpersonal Relationships*. New York: Julian, 1961.

———. *Understanding Sex*. Chicago: Science Research Associates, 1947; rev. ed., 1957.

Landis, Paul H. *Your Dating Days: Looking Forward to Happy Marriage*. New York: McGraw-Hill (Whittlesey House), 1954.

Lerrigo, Marion Olive, and Helen Southard. *Learning About Love: Sound Facts and Healthy Attitudes Toward Sex and Marriage*. New York: Dutton, 1956.

———. *What's Happening to Me?* New York: Dutton, 1956.

Marramore, Clyde M. *Life and Love: A Christian View of Sex*. Grand Rapids, Mich.: Zondervan, 1956.

Menninger, William C., et al. *How to Be a Successful Teen-ager*. New York: Sterling, 1954, 1966.

Pemberton, Lois Loyd. *The Stork Didn't Bring You!* New York: Hermitage, 1948; rev. ed., New York: Nelson, 1961.

Richardson, Frank Howard. *For Boys Only: The Doctor Discusses the Mysteries of Manhood*. Atlanta: Tupper and Love, 1952, 1959.

———. *For Girls Only: The Doctor Discusses the Mysteries of Womanhood*. Atlanta: Tupper and Love, 1953, 1960.

Shultz, Gladys Denny. *It's Time You Knew*. Philadelphia: Lippincott, 1955.

———. *Letters to Jane*. Philadelphia: Lippincott, 1948.

Strain, Frances Bruce. *Teen Days*. New York: Appleton-Century-Crofts, 1946.

Sweeney, Esther Emerson. *Dates and Dating*. Whiteside, N.Y.: Woman's Press, 1948.

Chapter 7

The Sexual Revolution

While the youth of the sixties were exploring the outer limits of reality with LSD, protesting the Vietnam War, marching in civil-rights demonstrations, and making love not war, the sex educators of that decade wrote dozens of books that attempted to keep the lid on a sexual revolution that was already well underway. The one significant difference between the books of the sixties and those of the fifties was a growing but reluctant recognition of women's sexuality, as cautious references to the clitoris as the source of sexual pleasure for women became more frequent. However, there were still a few last gasps from the proponents of the repressive attitudes toward women so characteristic of the postwar years.

One such writer was Dr. Bernhardt Gottlieb. Although his 1960 book for young men, *What a Boy Should Know About Sex*, is unremarkable except for the unconscious echo of Sylvanus Stall in the title, Gottlieb's book for young women, *What a Girl Should Know About Sex* (1961), is exceptional in its emphasis on "a feminine characteristic called passivity." With warm approval Gottlieb describes the deliberate muffling of a young girl's humanity: "The first impulse of the young adolescent girl is opposition to everything and everybody, . . . a display of aggression, a protest against discipline and control. But then something happens. The girl quietly changes and somehow loses her battling attitude. Gradually she becomes sweet, docile, and agreeable. From the active, assertive adolescent she gradually changes into a passive young woman." Furthermore, "her feminine trait of self-effacement is ever present. It gives her satisfaction." This becomes important later in meeting the demands of a husband:

"His mother attended to the household chores and to his personal needs. Now that he has a home of his own, he expects his wife to take on many of the tasks that his mother performed."

In fact, as Gottlieb sees it, women's maternal functions dominate not only their relationships with their husbands but everything they do in life: "Their first interest is to become a mother. Every other interest in life becomes less important. A woman's motherliness is ever present even in her interests of college, job, or professional career. Her place of employment becomes a second home to her. She thinks how nice it would be to have flowers on the desk and appropriate pictures on the walls, so that others who come to her little nook will feel her warmth." On the subject of childbirth he declares, "It is as though woman instead of man was made to suffer in order to obtain certain satisfactions and pleasures." And, in closing, "Maternal love demands nothing, sets no limits, makes no reservations."

In contrast, *What Teenagers Want to Know* (1962), by Florence Levinsohn, is forthright about discussing the confusion women face in making new role choices and meeting society's traditional expectations for them. Like other sex educators of the time, she deplores the new climate of sexual indulgence: "Advertising, television, movies, and novels often lead an adolescent to think that sexual experience must be the key to glamour and romance, the road to a new world of importance and strength." But the rules say wait, she reminds teenagers. Peer-group pressure is a strong influence on sexual attitudes, but parents want their sons and daughters to remain virgins until married. Levinsohn acknowledges the strain created by these conflicting pressures and notes that they may produce extreme attitudes on either end of the scale: "All the circumstances may combine to create strong inhibitions, to prevent [a young man or woman] from any sexual experimentation at all. At the other extreme the circumstances may combine to lead to a great deal of sexual experience, to promiscuity, often in the form of conquests." Both attitudes call for professional help, she says.

▪ Sex Prevention in the Sixties

In 1963, the year that saw the third edition of Evelyn Duvall's *Love and the Facts of Life*, Ann Landers organized her opinions on the subject in a book that was based on her syndicated newspaper column. *Ann Landers Talks to Teen-agers About Sex* is studded with anecdotes, examples, and object lessons from her mailbag. From the statistical sampling that her correspondents provided Landers must have been well aware that many teenagers were no longer automatically following the behavioral codes they had inherited. The introduction addressed to parents speaks of teenagers "pulled and hauled by biological urges on the one hand and fear of the consequences on the other." Yet, in the body of the book, she offers teenagers no help with the conflict. Sex outside of marriage is "unacceptable in our society" and "it isn't worth the risks." Sex on the sly makes a girl feel "cheap, dirty and disgusted with the boy," and teenage boys are "undisciplined and awkward" lovers.

She has sharp words for those who feel that some practical advice might be in order: "Every now and then I get a letter from some knuckle-head who tells me if I really want to befriend teenagers, I should give them some helpful hints on how to avoid pregnancy instead of being so doggone puritanical and unrealistic." There is no foolproof method of birth control anyway, Landers retorts. By way of a "helpful hint" she suggests sublimation—athletics for boys and housework for girls. An abstainer from alcohol herself, Landers emphasizes the evils of drink, but she is humane and wise in discussing kind ways to break up with a steady without causing too much pain. Her advice on venereal disease is also practical and sympathetic for 1963; she advises teenagers to go to a family doctor or city or county health department for treatment and ask them not to contact their parents; they might not, although there is no guarantee, because some states require that parents be notified.

The many desperate letters Landers had received from boys who suspected they were homosexual had made her aware of the emotion surrounding that subject. In her book she explains that nobody understands the cause of homosexuality but details several lurid case histories illustrating popular theories about it. She admits that transvestites and child molesters are not homosexual and adds that "many homosexuals are content as they are and have no wish to change. They are not a problem to society or to themselves." However, Landers concludes that "most homosexuals yearn to be normal" because they are "twisted and sick"; unfortunately, only about four out of one hundred can be made heterosexual. "God meant sex to be pleasurable, beautiful, filled with wonder and rich in reward," she rhapsodizes, "but—only if it is used properly." To the girl who wrote that her amorous boyfriend was "fed up with the broken record" of her resistance Landers replies, "That broken record produces darned fine music. Just keep telling him to behave himself . . . behave himself . . . behave himself. . . ."

Two books that were also far behind the times were *Moving into Manhood* (1963) and *The Way to Womanhood* (1965), by William Bauer, who was then the director of health education for the American Medical Association. Bauer begins his advice to young men by expounding the Victorian doctrine of seminal conservation: "Your sex is what makes you a man. Its influence upon you is not only physical, but spiritual and emotional. Physically, your sex makes you strong and ambitious. Your sex also makes you a leader because it gives you the impulses and the qualities which make for leadership." Masturbation, he states, is "almost always accompanied by an instinctive sense of guilt or at least of shame." Regarding drugs Bauer warns: "The smoking of so-called 'reefers' is practiced in certain areas by some young people and is admittedly a serious evil. Marijuana users become irresponsible and get themselves into trouble by doing things which they would never have dreamed of doing in their right senses. This includes sexual misconduct. Often the body's demand for drugs leads to robbery, blackmail, or even murder."

In *The Way to Womanhood* Bauer is joined by his wife, Florence, as coauthor ("Just call us Polly and Bill"). They agree that "marriage and motherhood is woman's most important role in life. A career should be secondary." To that end the way to attract boys is to be nonchalant and save physical expression of affection for special moments, as "when he really does delight you." At these times a girl should show her feelings "in unexpected ways, such as grabbing both his hands and whirling around with him, or giving him a quick hug and dancing away." This exercise of restraint should not be too hard because "sexual desire in a girl may not come until after her marriage. In some women it never comes. Such a lack is rarely known to a boy or man."

According to the Bauers, painful menstruation may be caused by "a girl's unconscious rebellion against being a girl." They are stern about abortion—it is "cold, calculated murder of the child and often endangers or takes the life of the mother"—and they take a firm stand against premarital sex and other violation of traditional sexual mores: "The real reason that any irregular sexual life should be avoided is that it is wrong. It is wrong morally, religiously, socially, medically, and biologically; in every one of these fields it violates the fundamental experience of the race through many centuries."

Similarly, Bertrand Glassberg writes in *Barron's Teen-age Sex Counselor* (1965) that "even the Godless Communists are becoming doubtful of the wisdom of permitting free sexual relationships." In answer to the question "Is the hymen ever broken without intercourse having taken place?" Glassberg is not reassuring ("very rarely" he says), and when asked "Why can't teenagers use contraceptives?" he declares that "contraceptives are intended for the use of husbands and wives." Other books of the same year and type were *Youth Considers Sex*, by William Edward Hulme; *Love, Sex, and the Teenager*, by Rhoda Lorand; *Not While You're a Freshman*, by Helen Walker Puner; *Adolescent Freedom and Responsibility*, by Gerald J. Taylor; and the third edition of *The Stork Didn't Bring You!*, by Lois Pemberton. In addition, two religious sex education books were published in 1965—*Learning to Love*, by Marc Oraison, and the revised edition of *Sex and the Whole Person*, by Frank Wier.

Another sex education book published in 1965 was a different matter. This was *Love and Sex in Plain Language*, by Eric W. Johnson. With its spare and simple style and emphasis on human communication it can be seen as the first of the modern sex education books. Frequent later editions (1967, 1973, 1977, 1985) kept abreast of rapid changes in attitudes and scientific knowledge, and the last edition (to be examined in detail in Chapter 9) is still in use. In 1965 Johnson was headmaster of the Friends' Central School in Philadelphia. Although *Love and Sex in Plain Language* is not radically different in content from most books that preceded it, Johnson's clear writing, his empathy for teenagers' feelings, and his sense of organization make it outstanding.

The book is addressed to junior-high teenagers, but, as Johnson points out, it could be used by bright ten-year-olds as well as college-age youth. The chapters proceed logically from "The man's part in love and sex" and "The woman's part in love and sex" to "Sexual intercourse," The baby from fertilization to birth," "How a baby is born and what a newborn is like," through chapters on the differences between human sex and animal sex, birth control, and love. In sixty-eight pages Johnson conveys more information than other books three times its size. The sepia ink drawings by Edward C. Smith are informative and often beautiful: one illustration depicting three nude boys of vastly different stages of sexual development demonstrates "normal teen-age boys of the same age"; another pair of drawings shows the moment of fertilization and the path of the egg to the uterus.

Like his contemporaries, Johnson calls homosexuality a sickness (although he does not associate it with child molesting) and is sure that the frequent masturbator will be prey to guilt, shame, and social isolation. Although he does dwell on the unfortunate circumstances of illegitimate pregnancy and venereal disease, his primary reason for urging teenagers not to undertake sexual intercourse too lightly is a respect for people, who, he emphasizes," are not made to be used." Sex without deep caring can also cause guilt and shame, which may spoil later experiences.

Johnson lays out rigid role expectations for the sexes: "A typical boy is vigorous and aggressive; a typical girl is sweeter and gentler than he and has a greater desire to please others. A father is expected to earn a living for his family and to provide manly companionship for his wife and children. On the other hand, a mother, even if she helps to earn a living for the family, provides loving care for her children, manages the household and is a source of tenderness and womanly love."

The greatest fault of *Love and Sex in Plain Language*, but one that was remedied in later editions, is the inadequate description of female sexuality. There is no drawing of female external genitalia and no explanation of the function of the clitoris. Although Johnson does say that intercourse is "one of the greatest pleasures mankind enjoys," he offers a description that, while admirable in other ways, is entirely from the male point of view:

> Some couples may have sexual intercourse several times a week, others perhaps only once or twice a month. Intercourse may take anywhere from a few minutes to half an hour or more. The couple come together and usually kiss, embrace and caress each other. Often they tell their love for each other. After a time, the woman's mind and body become prepared for the act of coitus; her vagina becomes moist and soft. Meanwhile, and much more quickly, the man's penis has become erect so that it enters the vagina easily. After a time of moving back and forth, the husband and wife reach the climax of sexual pleasure, called an *orgasm*. For the hus-

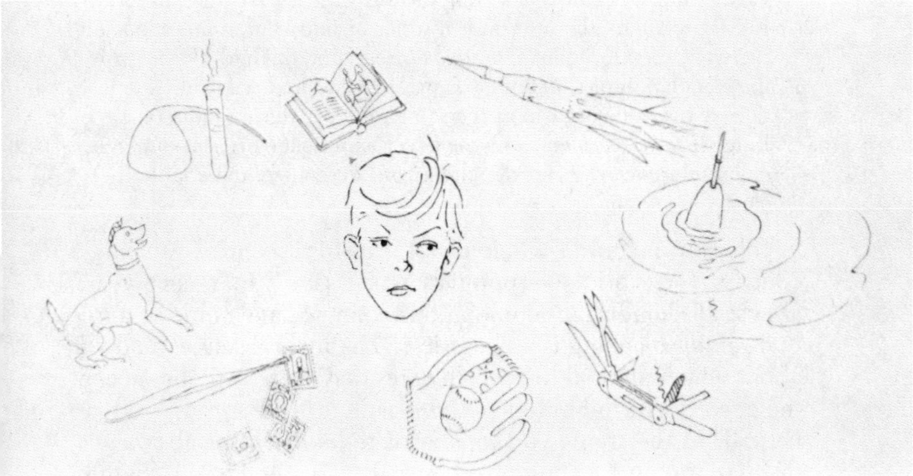

'ig. 11. A boy's world. Drawing by Edward C. Smith. From *Love and Sex in Plain* *.anguage*, by Eric W. Johnson (1967 edition).

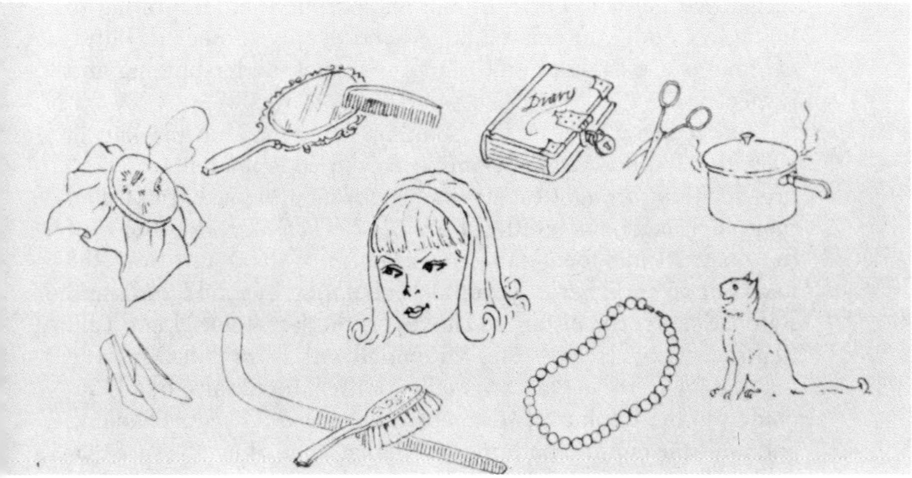

'ig. 12. A girl's world. Drawing by Edward C. Smith. From *Love and Sex in Plain* *.anguage*, by Eric W. Johnson (1967 edition).

> band, this is the moment when the semen is ejaculated inside the vagina in a series of quick spurts toward the neck of the uterus. For the woman, the orgasm is a series of muscular contractions of the walls of the vagina. There is no secretion of fluid like that of the ejaculation of semen in a man. Husband and wife rather seldom experience orgasm at the same moment during intercourse. Indeed, some women rarely or never experience orgasm but still enjoy intercourse. After the climax of intercourse, the couple feel close, loving and relaxed.

Johnson devotes a whole chapter to birth control. Voicing a concern for world overpopulation, he says, "In recent years, almost all thoughtful people in this country have come to agree that family planning is a necessity." The main discussion now is about which method to use. He notes that even Catholics accept the need for birth limitation and permit it if the means used are natural. In the framework of marriage he discusses abstinence, the diaphragm, the condom, chemicals, the pill, the coil, rhythm, and sterilization and notes that it is important to follow a doctor's advice to ensure the effectiveness of most birth-control methods. In a final chapter on love Johnson reiterates his theme: "Never forget that human beings are not made to be used, but rather to be understood, appreciated, loved and deeply respected. Physical love is a part—but only a part—of such understanding and respect."

Taking advantage of the booming sex education market, in 1966 the Public Affairs Committee, an independent research organization, brought together seven of its previously published pamphlets in a book entitled *Teen Love, Teen Marriage*. Some of the material included dated back as far as 1950 and bore the marks of an earlier era—pamphlets on dating by Paul Landis and Ralph Eckert, for instance. However, the last item, "Let's Talk Sense about Sex!," by Lester Kirkendall with Elizabeth Ogg, is an unusual piece that was originally written for adults but is included in the book as if for teens. The authors discuss changing and multiple cultural patterns that make "none of us . . . sure that our traditional sex code is 'right.'" The central moral issue, they tell grownups, is the quality of the relationship, not the degree of genital activity.

Also in 1966 a book appeared that challenged many long-held beliefs and assumptions about human sexuality. *Human Sexual Response*, by William Masters and Virginia Johnson, was a monumental collection of observed data on the sex act. Among other things Masters and Johnson's research indicated that women's capacity for sexual enjoyment was much greater than earlier studies had found; the book fundamentally changed the way women regarded their bodies and their sex lives. The following year, when researchers at the Kinsey Institute at Indiana University were employed by the Chicago-based National Opinion Research Center to survey the sexual behavior patterns of a random sample of college students, they found that the patterns of the forties and fifties had remained almost unchanged, with one significant difference: in the sixties a much larger proportion of girls were *enjoying* their first experience with coitus.

Nevertheless, warners and doomsayers continued to be heard. A rambling and uninformed book by Wade V. Lewis, *Sex: In Defense of Teen-agers* (1967), blames the drug scene for the breakdown of moral standards: "*U.S. News and World Report* describes a recent drug craze and its dangers. It is not confined to 'beatniks' but is permeating the colleges, even the high schools." Lewis implies that even a girl who drinks soda is not safe—her date may sneak knockout drops into her drink for nefarious sexual reasons.

Even more peculiar is *Young People and Sex* (1967), by Arthur H. Cain. The book was one of a series of titles by Cain covering "young people and . . ."—just about every topic, from smoking to jobs. In *Young People and Sex* Cain offers his eccentric opinions on some of the most complicated and controversial aspects of sexuality. Sexual customs and attitudes have been changing at an unprecedented speed, he states. The resulting confusion has been "expressed in a tendency to close the gap between the sexes." It is becoming hard to tell the boys from the girls—especially since the latter are turning into "intellectual eunuchs." Petting, he claims, can cause infection in the girl and strain the sexual organs of the boy. Postponement of sex is "infinitely preferable."

A chapter on "Sexual customs and attitudes in other countries" soon deteriorates into a superficial look at the status of prostitution in the world's major cities. Cain declares that the most moral states are those where prostitution is legal; in areas where women have been instrumental in getting the practice outlawed sexual chaos reigns. He holds up Switzerland as an example of a country where there is good sexual order, because the women are beautiful and don't vote. He defines normal sexual behavior as mutual orgasm in the act of intercourse and then launches into an unconsciously lascivious examination of "abnormal" behaviors and conditions: vaginismus (painful contractions of the vagina), impotency, oral-genital sex, sodomy, coprolalia (involuntary use of obscene language for sexual gratification), and group sex. His fiercest scorn is reserved for homosexuals. "No homosexual behavior can under any circumstances or from any point of view be regarded as normal," and he dismisses the "alleged sex education" that condones homosexuality. Cain describes the "sissified 'pansy' or 'swish'" and points out indignantly, "To most normal men the objectionable thing about these unfortunate people is that they almost always insist perversely on flagrantly intruding their incongruous behavior into societies that regard it as fundamentally insulting." For the problems of pornography he offers a novel solution—high-school seniors should take a course in the subject so that they become thoroughly weary of it and it ceases to be forbidden fruit.

More traditional in its approach to sex prevention was *Sex Before Twenty: New Answers for Youth* (1967, 1971), by Helen Elizabeth Southard. The author had written a number of sex education pamphlets for the American Medical Association with coauthor Marion Lerrigo and was a psychologist and family-life specialist for the Young Women's Christian Association. Southard admits that "a woman can have a climax also, although she does not always experience it because her sexual responses are different from those of men." She finds masturbation infantile, and homosexuality a normal developmental stage that confirmed homosexuals "might grow out of if they didn't feel that they were born that way." But Southard gives her greatest attention to the perils of premarital sex, which she relates to almost every subject she takes up.

Published in 1967, the misnamed *Every Girl's Book of Sex*, by Arlette Fribourg, was actually a stilted gynecology primer for women of all ages. Its vocabulary ("brassière," "toilette," "swim in the sea") suggested that the author may have been European. Just as odd, but in a refreshing way, was *Dear Doctor Hip Pocrates: Advice Your Family Doctor Never Gave You* (1968). The author, Eugene Schoenfeld, had written a column of medical advice for the underground newspaper the *Berkeley Barb* during the height of the sexual and political turmoil in that college community. The book is a collection of letters to that column, many of them poignant, funny, startling, or simply weird. Mixed in with queries about the hallucinogenic properties of various substances, descriptions of bizarre sexual problems, and treatments of mace poisoning is some sound sexual advice. Whether discussing the legal status of abortion, the effectiveness of various contraceptive methods, the long-term results of going braless, or the use of masturbation as a remedy for menstrual cramps, Dr. Hip provides bits of information unavailable in other sex education books for teenagers. In an uncharacteristically serious moment he sums up the sexual situation of the late sixties: "Two views prevail today. One is to concentrate on loving the person. The other holds that the act itself should be paramount. The most fulfilling and difficult way is to do both."

As the decade drew to a close, most sex educators held to their established themes or opinions or changed them only slightly. The jazzy pink cover of *A Girl's Guide to Dating and Going Steady*, by Tom McGinnis (1968), belied the book's contents—a diatribe against sexual expression outside marriage, with no physiology at all and very little other information that did not focus on the moral. The author of *The Stork is Dead* (1968), Charlie Shedd, was an elderly minister of a large church in Texas, who for several years had written a column on sex and love for *Teen* magazine. In his book he stresses the differences between the ever-ready male and the emotionally needy female and gives examples of "lines guys use to get a young thing to go further." Shedd lists reasons (none he considers justifiable) why girls give in and draws a sorry picture of what it is like to be married at seventeen. In a chapter on "Strange things that might happen" he talks of petting to orgasm as "almost too weird to describe" and warns that participants might get "fixated" and never be able to enjoy intercourse. Oral sex is all right in marriage but "does more harm than good in pre-marital relationships," and anal sex is neurotic. As for homosexuals, "turn them over to God" and walk away. Masturbation can be very bad when it is compulsive, but "teenage masturbation is preferable to teenage intercourse," and seen in that light it can be regarded as a gift of God. If you must have sex, he says—bowing to the inevitable—use birth control. He recommends foam and a condom. But if a relationship has reached that point, it would be far better for the couple to stop seeing each other entirely.

Helen Jean Burn, head writer for the Maryland Educational Cultural Broadcasting Commission, revived the question-and-answer format in her 1969 *Better than the Birds, Smarter than the Bees: No-nonsense Answers to Honest Questions About Sex and Growing Up*. Some of Burn's supposedly no-nonsense answers would not have been out of place in the books from the turn of the century. When asked the best method of birth control, she replies, "Don't have sexual intercourse." Girls are told that an "illegal abortionist may use a rusty coat hanger or a knitting needle or anything else he has handy." Regarding the temptation to masturbate Burns advises teenagers to use that "push" to excel in other things; spending time alone in one's room is a waste, anyway—better to have a hobby.

An unusual but chilling and Machiavellian book was Ellen Peck's *How to Get a Teen-age Boy and What to Do with Him When You Get Him* (1969). This had little to say about physical sex but a great deal to say about the relations between the sexes. Peck provides girls with a detailed guide to the techniques of manipulating conversation and using psychology in order to "get" boys. Girls are taught to lie, dissemble, double deal, and betray their friends in order to get next to an interesting male. Peck's position on petting is thoroughly expedient—go slow on "making out," she advises, because that will keep a boy interested longer.

Religious Texts

Throughout the decade, as secular authorities became more accepting of masturbation and birth control, Catholic educators reacted by issuing a number of books that stressed the sinfulness of these activities. *The Catholic Youth's Guide to Life and Love* (1960), by the Very Reverend Monsignor George Kelly, is fairly typical. The book carries the nihil obstat and the imprimatur of the church, certifying it "free of doctrinal or moral error." "By following the teachings of the Church, you can always know that you're on the right path," says Monsignor Kelly. A chapter on physical sex by James T. Geddis, M.D., explains, "It's a fact that acts of self-love cause great spiritual and emotional harm in addition to being sins against the Sixth Commandment." Remedy for this temptation can be sought by "receiving the sacraments daily and saying your daily prayers." A description of the transmission of venereal disease blames not only intercourse but towels and glasses or cups in a public place (although the shared communion vessel is not mentioned).

Kelly stresses the importance of chastity to the family and home. He discourages early dating and especially kissing, because there is "a real danger that the friendship you feel will burst out and overwhelm you, leaving your defenses open to sin." Other chapters examine "Why artificial birth control is wrong" (he quotes Pope Pius XI, who called it "shameful and intrinsically vicious"), "Do you have a religious vocation?" "The spiritual and emotional dangers of marrying a non-Catholic," "Marriage for life," and "The single vocation."

A second book by George Kelly, *Dating for Young Catholics* (1963), was extracted from a series of articles written in 1961 for *Hi-Time*, a religious magazine. Here he exhorts young people to date only Catholics and to struggle with the temptation to commit sins of impurity. He considers the use of birth control to be selfishly motivated, although he allows that the rhythm method is acceptable for very pressing reasons, such as health. Other Catholic sex education books included a translation of Marc Oraison's *Learning to Love* (1965), which contained a thoughtful attempt to put the dogma on birth control into perspective, and *A Boy's Sex Life: A Handbook of Basic Information and Moral Guidance* (1969), by William J. Bausch.

Protestant groups were also producing their own sex education texts during the sixties. The Methodist point of view, for instance, was presented in *Sex and the Whole Person: A Christian View* (1962, 1965), by Frank E. Wier, and *Love, Sex, and Life* (1964, 1966), by Marjory Bracher, discussed the Lutheran position. The Concordia Sex Education series, also Lutheran, included *Take the High Road*, by A. J. Bueltmann (1967), and *Life Can Be Sexual*, by Elmer N. Witt (1967). Richard Hettlinger spoke from the liberal Episcopal perspective in *Living with Sex: The Student's Dilemma* (1966), a book for older teenagers and college students, and the Unitarian Church was represented in *Commonsense Sex: A Basis for Discussion and Reappraisal*, by Ronald Mazur (1968).

▪ A New Approach: Positive, Nonjudgmental

The more modern and less didactic sex education books of the seventies were anticipated in 1969 by Paul Bohannan's *Love, Sex, and Being Human.* An anthropologist, Bohannan made an attempt to show teenagers how to "devise their own moralities." "I am not advocating any specific moral behavior," he says, but "I have some values of my own that sometimes show." Using examples from other societies and frequent quotes from Masters and Johnson, he explains that the association between sex and love is not natural and "normal" but a learned cultural value. Furthermore, he points out that "masturbation is a source of consolation, pleasure, and relief of tension before it is possible to link one's sexuality with love and with a loved person." He has an unusual theory about the origin of homosexual patterns: "Confirmed, constant, and habitual homosexuality . . . always arises from some difficulty in the formation of the learned capacity to love, or from inability to esteem one's self highly enough to think one is lovable." The book never gained wide readership, perhaps because of Bohannan's formidable style.

A truly radical work from the same year, and the first book that really approached sex for teenagers in a positive way, was Dr. Eleanor Hamilton's *Sex Before Marriage: Guidance for Young Adults, Ages 16–20.* In spite of its ground-breaking nature, the book failed to create a furor because teachers and librarians chose to dismiss it as being meant for the college student, ignoring the clear indication in the title that it was also addressed to younger people.

Hamilton's perspective in *Sex Before Marriage* is to consider sex as an integral part of the whole spectrum of bodily pleasures. Masturbation, she writes, has an important function in the ongoing process of developing sexual awareness and responses while growing up. It is "nature's way of preparing you for the later enjoyment of sexuality with a partner" and is a useful release from tension. Furthermore, it is not really possible to masturbate "too much," because the body sets its own limits: "A person who has learned how to come to orgasm through masturbation is much more likely to be a good sex partner in marriage than one who has not." Her objection to petting is not that it is done but that it is not done well: "If two teenagers do decide to pet, they would be wise to see to it that each comes to orgasm." A pattern of arousal without satisfaction can set bad precedents; girls, for example, can be adversely affected by always having to switch on the red light. However, many women, she reveals, find manual orgasms more satisfying than intercourse, and there is nothing wrong with this: "The word clitoris comes from the Greek word for key, and the clitoris is, indeed, like a magic key to sexual satisfaction for the female."

Hamilton is forthright in explaining that adults have deliberately instilled a fear of sex in young people: "It helps in dissipating guilt if you realize that many of the religious precepts denying sex pleasure to the unmarried are based on conditions which existed at a time long in the past. Their continuance into the present is superstition and reflects not only ignorance of scientific technology but faulty knowledge of the social psychology of today." She tells teenagers quite bluntly that "virginity is about as useful in a prospective wife as an appendix" and adds that "ninety-five percent of the dangers of premarital sex could be eliminated if parents would make their homes and their own knowledge available to their children as they would in all other areas of life."

In addition to giving the facts about birth-control methods, Hamilton explores what was then known about the complex psychological factors involved in its use. She is adamant about the need to change abortion laws and feels that it is preferable to spend money on a trip to Japan or England for a legal operation rather than chance an encounter with an illegal abortionist in the United States. She provides a sympathetic chapter of helpful advice for the unmarried girl who decides to go through with her pregnancy. In a discussion of drugs (an inexplicably rare topic in most other sex education books in that decade of chemical experimentation) she frowns on LSD for good reason but, in referring to the most common drug, says, "If marijuana is legitimized (as many people believe it will be), it may be added to the list of mild pleasures enjoyed by man—sensual, though not necessarily sexual." She minimizes the risk of venereal disease—there is very little chance of contracting it, she says, if partners are selective—but is more concerned about the common and seldom discussed female genital infections of monilia and trichomoniasis. Hamilton's comforting words were spread further when *Sex Before Marriage* appeared in paperback in 1973, followed by another book for younger teenagers, *Sex, with Love* (which is described in Chapter 9).

A third landmark book after Stall's *What a Young Boy Ought to Know* (1897) and Duvall's *Facts of Life and Love for Teenagers* (1950) was *Boys and Sex* (1968), written by Wardell Pomeroy with collaborator John Tebbel. Pomeroy was uniquely qualified to speak to teenagers about sex. As Alfred Kinsey's associate, and later as director of the Institute for Sex Research, he had conducted thousands of interviews on the subject with young people. His research had made him aware of the hiatus between accepted sexual attitudes and actual sexual behavior in our society. Consequently his approach in *Boys and Sex*, and its companion volume *Girls and Sex* (1969), was to talk to teenagers in a helpful way about the behavior he knew perfectly well was going on but to remind them that while they were entitled to their own choices and their own privacy, they would have to deal with the disapproval of adults unless they were discreet.

In the introduction to *Boys and Sex*, intended to reassure parents, Pomeroy states his purpose. Other books for teenagers on sex, he explains, have been "too moralistic, too judgmental, or lacking in forthrightness." Proposing to remedy that lack, he says soothingly, "I am not suggesting in these pages that your sons engage in sexual behavior of any kind. The reality, of course, is that the vast majority of them have already engaged in sex behavior of one kind or another. Once this reality is acknowledged and faced, the next question is, What's going to be done about it!" He encourages parents to talk to their children about sex casually and often and lists the range of possible attitudes toward sexuality. Fitting himself into that scale, he lays out his own credo: "Sex is pleasurable, and . . . it cannot be denied until we are in our twenties or later. One must show a concern for the other person who may be involved in an act and, moreover, one must learn to live in our society, which is basically antisexual.'" He declares his own belief in marriage and his advocacy of sexual attitudes and behavior that "help us to make the best possible sexual adjustment in marriage." Helping teenagers to develop healthy attitudes, he feels, is more important than providing them with detailed biological information, and this is what he plans to concentrate on in *Boys and Sex*.

Not claiming to be an authority, Pomeroy gives the young readers permission to think for themselves in the very first pages. People disagree about sex, he says, and that's all right. It's even all right to disagree with him—this is not a book of advice. The most important thing to get clear right at the start is "a fundamental fact which often seems to be overlooked by those who talk about sex—that sex is one of the most pleasurable activities available to human beings." In the obligatory chapter on anatomy and physiology that follows he is "deliberately sketchy" (he uses scientific terms here but defines the street words in a later section). Pomeroy is more interested in behavior and soon gets down to discussing the kinds of sexual activity with which most boys are already familiar from experience. People are born sexual beings, he explains, and even babies have sexual feelings. Almost everybody has been involved in episodes of sex play before adolescence (he gives statistics), and it is nothing to be ashamed of, even though parents usually disapprove strongly.

Pomeroy attempts an objective approach to masturbation, giving a list of pros and cons, but it is immediately apparent where his sympathies lie, and he soon gives up the pose and admits that it is "not only harmless, but is positively good and healthy, and should be encouraged because it helps young people to grow up sexually in a natural way." He explains the variations in technique, for both boys and girls, and praises it as a way for a boy to learn to delay his orgasm—a skill that is useful later in intercourse.

Homosexuality also is given thoughtful and informed consideration. He traces the historical origins of Judeo-Christian attitudes toward it and points out that it is prohibited by law everywhere in the United States. However, the practice is biologically normal, because all mammals show some signs of homosexual behavior. Pomeroy disagrees with the still widely accepted Freudian theory that homosexuality is the result of fixation at a normal developmental stage, preferring to see it in terms of Alfred Kinsey's view of human sexuality as a range or scale, with those who are only heterosexual at one end and those who are only homosexual at the other and most people somewhere in between. He explains that most Americans tend to perceive the situation in opposites and extremes. "We are only beginning to understand this extremely complex problem," says Pomeroy, "and anyone who says he has 'the' answer must be taken with a grain of salt." In the meantime he urges tolerance for those who are different.

In discussing dating, Pomeroy spends a great deal of time on every adolescent's fear of rejection and analyzes the differences in the expectations and sexual patterns brought to the experience by the two sexes. Girls think of dating as primarily a social good time, while boys probably think of it as a means of having some sort of physical contact with a girl. Petting is something almost everybody does before marriage. It is pleasurable, a learning experience, a form of communication. To relieve frustration he recommends masturbation afterward or petting to orgasm if both parties want it. The real morality of petting is that it should be mutual—a boy should never force a girl to go further than she desires. The same is true of the decision to have intercourse or not. Again he gives a detailed list of pros and cons; in the last analysis a person who feels comfortable about a decision to have sex should be able to be discreet or to face society's disapproval. *Boys and Sex* remains one of the most sensible and careful sex education books yet written, and in its 1981 revised edition it is useful today.

Girls and Sex, on the other hand, is invalidated by sexism in Pomeroy's acceptance of the roles society imposes on women. Published in 1969, it is completely different from *Boys and Sex*. Unlike most other authors of companion volumes, who simply lifted whole chapters from the first work and made only minor adjustments to adapt it to the other sex, Pomeroy carefully rewrote nearly every word. In an introduction for parents he addresses the special anxiety fathers and mothers feel over their daughters' sexuality.

> Parents tell me they are teaching their daughters to be "ladylike." That means the social amenities—to be feminine, demure, nonaggressive, to keep their dresses down and their legs crossed, and not to chase the boys. In the society we live in these are generally considered desirable attributes, but they are not attributes which lead toward a good sexual adjustment in marriage unless they are accompanied by teaching her to be a warm, open, responsive, sexually unafraid person. A young woman must unlearn her ladylike conduct in the bedroom and there revert to her more unrestrained nature in order to become a sexually responsive wife.

His message for the girls themselves is similar. In the first chapter he again presents his own credo, which he has clarified since writing *Boys and Sex* the year before. Whether to engage in sexual activity must be an individual's own decision and should be based on as much information as possible, he begins. The purpose of *Girls and Sex* is to provide that information:

> My feeling is that sexual behavior for both girls and boys is something both pleasurable and desirable as long as certain rules are fol-

> lowed. The rules are simple: 1. Nothing is done to hurt someone else or to go against their wishes and desires—in brief, responsibility for the other person. 2. Whatever is done is not done so openly that it will get a girl or a boy into trouble with society. On the other side of the coin, I would respect those who choose *not* to engage in any sexual experiences. That is their right.

Pomeroy examines in some detail the common differences in attitude between the sexes. Boys, with their earlier experiences with orgasm, tend to be genital-oriented, while girls react to the romantic ambience of sex. A girl needs to understand these differences, because

> a girl will come to understand she must be something of an actress in life. It will be clear that she has been given three roles to play. One is her role in society, first as a young girl growing up, then as a wife and mother, or as a career girl, or both, whatever the case may be. The second role is her relationship with boys, in which, as I have said, she must learn to be both ladylike and, eventually, unladylike when that kind of behavior is required. The third role is perhaps the most difficult—the role she must play as herself, an individual responsible to herself.

The chapter on physiology deals with girls' worry about the size of their breasts and has more extensive information on menstruation than that provided for boys. The section on childhood sex play is also adapted for girls' information needs. In addition to the reassurance about the normality of such play, Pomeroy deals with the troublesome but seldom-mentioned topic of sexual advances from older men—often uncles or fathers of friends, as well as strangers.

Dating can be less of a problem for girls if they keep in mind those important differences between the sexes. It is unfortunate that society makes it necessary for a girl to be constantly concerned with her reputation: "As long as it is necessary to play the ridiculous game of 'good girl,' 'bad girl' and 'prude,' I suppose the best thing a girl can do is confront squarely the kind of face she wants to present to the world and develop her dating behavior accordingly." With this caution in mind petting receives qualified approval as a preparation for intercourse at a later stage. Girls may not enjoy it particularly when they first begin but will soon find out what stimulates them best. Here Pomeroy offers a more sensible reason for a girl to slow the boy down—not because petting is bad in any way but because she needs time to catch up to his level of arousal. Pomeroy again stresses mutuality as the measure of petting morality.

Perhaps the most important precedent set by *Girls and Sex* is a factual and informed chapter on "The female orgasm." Tackling a subject that had been nearly unmentionable in teen sex literature, Pomeroy carefully undoes the myth of the vaginal orgasm and explains the physiology of stimulation and response of the clitoris. He refers often to the findings of Masters and Johnson and to statistics from his own research—telling girls, for instance, that although parents may not like to hear it, "it is demonstrably true that girls who have orgasm when they are young—that is, up to fifteen—are those who have the least difficulty having one in marriage later on." He describes what was then known about multiple orgasms and defines a nymphomaniac as "a woman who has a higher rate of sexual outlet than the person who calls her that name." Orgasm is a learned response, and girls should not be disappointed if they do not have one the first time they try. "Orgasm should not be viewed as a tyrant"; the important thing is the feeling of closeness and the shared pleasure of intercourse. The rest of the book presents information on masturbation, homosexuality, birth control, and the decision of whether or not to have intercourse with the same objectivity that was given to boys.

The sexist tendencies of *Girls and Sex* are inevitable for a book written in 1969—Pomeroy was far more sympathetic and fair-minded toward girls than most of his fellow sex educators at the time. Twelve years later he showed his ability to grow with the times by correcting these faults in the revised editions of 1981, thus making these landmark books helpful to yet another decade of teenagers.

▪ BIBLIOGRAPHY

Bauer, William W. *Moving into Manhood*. Garden City, N.Y.: Doubleday, 1963.

———, and Florence M. Bauer. *The Way to Womanhood*. Garden City, N.Y.: Doubleday, 1965.

Bausch, William J. *A Boy's Sex Life: A Handbook of Basic Information and Moral Guidance*. Notre Dame, Ind.: Fides, 1969.

Bohannan, Paul. *Love, Sex, and Being Human: A Book About the Human Condition for Young People*. Garden City, N.Y.: Doubleday, 1969.
Bracher, Marjory Louise. *Love, Sex, and Life*. Philadelphia: Fortress, 1964; rev. ed., 1966.
Bueltmann, A. J. *Take the High Road*. St. Louis, Mo.: Concordia, 1967.
Burn, Helen Jean. *Better than the Birds, Smarter than the Bees: No-nonsense Answers to Honest Questions About Sex and Growing Up*. Nashville, Tenn.: Abingdon, 1969.
Cain, Arthur H. *Young People and Sex*. New York: Day, 1967.
Duvall, Evelyn Ruth Millis. *Love and the Facts of Life*. New York: Association Press, 1963.
Fribourg, Arlette. *Every Girl's Book of Sex*. New York: Arc, 1967.
Glassberg, Bertrand Younker. *Barron's Teen-age Sex Counselor*. Woodbury, N.Y.: Barron's Educational Series, 1965.
Gottlieb, Bernhardt S. *What a Boy Should Know About Sex*. Indianapolis: Bobbs-Merrill, 1960.
———. *What a Girl Should Know About Sex*. Indianapolis: Bobbs-Merrill, 1961.
Hamilton, Eleanor. *Sex Before Marriage: Guidance for Young Adults, Ages 16–20*. New York: Meredith, 1969; New York: Bantam, 1973.
Hettlinger, Richard Frederick. *Living with Sex: The Student's Dilemma*. New York: Seabury, 1966.
Hulme, William Edward. *Youth Considers Sex*. New York: Nelson, 1965.
Johnson, Eric W. *Love and Sex in Plain Language*. Philadelphia: Lippincott, 1965; rev. eds., 1967, 1973, 1977, 1985.
Kelly, George. *The Catholic Youth's Guide to Life and Love*. New York: Random House, 1960.
———. *Dating for Young Catholics*. Garden City, N.Y.: Doubleday, 1963.
Landers, Ann (pseud. of Esther P. Lederer). *Ann Landers Talks to Teen-agers About Sex*. Englewood Cliffs, N.J.: Prentice-Hall, 1963.
Levinsohn, Florence. *What Teenagers Want to Know*. Chicago: Budlong, 1962.
Lewis, Wade V. *Sex: In Defense of Teen-agers*. Boston: Christopher, 1967.
Lorand, Rhoda L. *Love, Sex, and the Teenager*. New York: Macmillan, 1965.

Masters, William H., and Virginia E. Johnson. *Human Sexual Response*. Boston: Little, Brown, 1966.

Mazur, Ronald Michael. *Commonsense Sex: A Basis for Discussion and Reappraisal*. Boston: Beacon, 1968.

McGinnis, Tom. *A Girl's Guide to Dating and Going Steady*. Garden City, N.Y.: Doubleday, 1968.

Oraison, Marc. *Learning to Love: Frank Advice for Young Catholics*. Trans. by Andre Humbert. New York: Hawthorne, 1965.

Peck, Ellen. *How to Get a Teen-age Boy and What to Do with Him When You Get Him*. New York: Geis, 1969; New York: Avon, 1974.

Pemberton, Lois Loyd. *The Stork Didn't Bring You!* 3rd ed. New York: Nelson, 1965.

Pomeroy, Wardell Baxter, with John Tebbel. *Boys and Sex*. New York: Delacorte, 1968: New York: Dell, 1971.

———. *Girls and Sex*. New York: Delacorte, 1969; New York: Dell, 1973.

Public Affairs Committee. *Teen Love, Teen Marriage*. New York: Grosset and Dunlap, 1966.

Puner, Helen Walker. *Not While You're a Freshman*. New York: Coward-McCann, 1965.

Schoenfeld, Eugene. *Dear Doctor Hip Pocrates: Advice Your Family Doctor Never Gave You*. New York: Grove, 1968.

Shedd, Charlie W. *The Stork is Dead*. Waco, Tex.: Word, 1968.

Southard, Helen E. *Sex Before Twenty: New Answers for Youth*. New York: Dutton, 1967; rev. ed., 1971.

Taylor, Gerald J. *Adolescent Freedom and Responsibility: A Guide to Sexual Maturity*. New York: Exposition, 1965.

Wier, Frank E. *Sex and the Whole Person: A Christian View*. New York: Abingdon, 1962; rev. ed., 1965.

Witt, Elmer N. *Life Can Be Sexual*. St. Louis, Mo.: Concordia, 1967.

Chapter 8

Instant Obsolescence in the Seventies

As the gigantic love-in of the sixties romped on and wound down into the seventies, sex educators tried desperately to make sense of it all even before the smoke had cleared. The social and political upheavals and the advances in scientific sexual knowledge of the previous decade were bewildering in their far-reaching impact. For the first time, thanks to the pioneering work of Masters and Johnson, a body of observed empirical data existed on the physiology of the sex act itself. The Pill had made it possible to separate coitus from the procreative function, and women were now able to have sexual adventures as casually as men if they wished. Experiments in communal living and group marriage had suggested that the nuclear family might not be the only valid way to set up long-term sexual unions. A new concern for the equality of women had opened up exploration of what it really means to be female—and male. Homosexuality, formerly considered an illness, was being redefined as acceptable sexual behavior. The right to legal abortion was gaining acceptance. Newly interpreted freedoms of speech made it possible for sex education books to use words never before seen in their pages, to illustrate birth-control methods with drawings and photographs, and to show realistic nudes.

Writers of teen sex manuals adopted three different stances toward the sexual turmoil of the decade. The first response was to dig in, look backward, and pretend nothing had happened. At the beginning of the seventies many sex educators continued to reflect the residue of old taboos and fears. Venereal disease and unwanted pregnancy, both now avoidable, were still often presented as punishments and deterrents to any sexual activity at all rather than as mishaps of a badly managed sex life. Instead of providing more detailed and realistic advice on the cure and prevention of disease and methods of contraception, writers emphasized the worst effects of both conditions. In the face of a mass of statistics showing a high incidence of premarital intercourse, some writers continued to insist that the only socially acceptable sex took place within marriage. Others modified the limitation; they approved sex in relationships characterized by "deep caring" but maintained that casual sex was manipulative and psychologically harmful—at least to girls. Despite the growing acceptance and visibility of the gay lifestyle, they continued to cling to the idea of homosexuality as a perversion and a sickness, albeit a curable one.

The second attitude toward the new ideas and behaviors was enthusiastic and uncritical acceptance. Some writers leaped feet first into the raging sea of pop sexuality, only to find their books swept away in a year or two by the changing tides of fashion. Authors who cheerfully urged hip and carefree sex found themselves embarrassed and out of print very soon. Some of these ultraliberal manuals explored the boundaries of the genre, not only in content but also in form and style.

A third contingent was made up of respected sex education professionals who tried their best to write thoughtful guidebooks to the new sensibilities but found themselves needing to update their books continually to stay ahead of major changes in social attitudes. Legislation and official opinion toward homosexuality, abortion, and the status of women were in particularly rapid metamorphosis during the decade, and knowledgeable writers found that they repeatedly had to eat their words and rewrite their chapters on these sensitive topics.

In spite of this confusion, or perhaps because of it, the seventies were a prolific time for sex education manuals. But very few of the many titles examined in this chapter survived the decade. Most died immediately or in a couple of years, and those that outlasted the commotion did so in the shape of revised, second, third, or even fourth editions. We shall examine an example of that adjustment process in detail later in this chapter.

■ Looking Backward

Among the sex education books published in 1970 three were markedly old-fashioned in style, if not unforgivably so in content: *Understanding Sex*, by Alan F. Guttmacher; *The Facts of Sex: A Revolutionary Approach to Sex Instruction for Teenagers*, by John James (a pseudonym); and *A Teenager's Guide to Life and Love*, by Dr. Benjamin Spock. *Understanding Sex* has opening passages that come perilously close to the antiquated "birds and bees" approach. Guttmacher, a retired obstetrician and president of the Planned Parenthood Federation, was seventy-two at the time of its writing, and while his attitudes are remarkably liberal for a man of his generation, his style is best described as kindly but garrulous. The book tells far more than any teenager wants to know about obstetrical procedures, for instance, or the details of reproductive anatomy. Guttmacher is opposed to anything more than kissing between casual friends: "To make serious petting justifiable behavior there must be the element of feeling, of emotional involvement, of commitment to each other. In essence, in our culture mature and healthy people care deeply before becoming involved in sex whether heavy petting or sexual intercourse." Guttmacher sees sexuality as part of a behavior continuum, with heterosexuality spanning the greatest part of that range; he estimates that only 4 percent of men and 1 or 2 percent of women are homosexuals, with bisexuals making up "a relatively small group." He freely admits that there is "no clear-cut cause" for homosexuality but offers "disturbed parent-child relationships" ("the combination of an overattached, seductive mother and an absent, weak, or rejecting father") as a possible explanation. He sees lesbianism as a "safety valve" for girls who are afraid of heterosexual contacts. Such a life is "certainly not to be encouraged" because it carries "dreadful penalties." Guttmacher, as might be expected from the head of Planned Parenthood, is informative about birth-control methods (although here, as in the rest of the book, there are no diagrams or photographs). He emphasizes that the use of contraceptives should be a moral obligation for couples who have no desire to produce a child.

The books by James and Spock were not really addressed to young people, in spite of their titles. Nor did James's *The Facts of Sex* represent a "revolutionary approach" to sex education as the title claimed, being little more than a superficial essay on various aspects of sexuality. Although in *A Teenager's Guide to Life and Love* Spock does make occasional attempts to speak to young readers, for the most part he merely offers advice and comfort to parents. In a section on the rivalry between the sexes Spock's Freudian bias and his theories on the proper care of small children lead him into some resounding sexism. He implies that women compete with men because of penis envy and suggests that contemporary women are overeducated: "Quitc a few women nowadays, especially some of those who have gone to college, find the life of taking care of their babies and children all day boring and frustrating. I think that the main reason so many mothers are bored is that their upbringing and their education have made them somehow expect to get their satisfaction and their pride as adults from the same occupations outside the home as men." Dr. Spock was soon to rue these and similar words, when such remarks were vehemently attacked by leaders of the women's movement.

Several authors of older books issued new versions in 1971. Helen Southard, whose *Sex Before Twenty* had been conservative in 1967, produced an equally conservative update. Gladys Shultz, who had proffered advice to a college daughter via the U.S. mail in *Letters to Jane* (1948), now corresponded with a college granddaughter in *Letters to a New Generation*, to the effect that most recent changes in social thinking and behavior, from the use of drugs to the emphasis on clitoral orgasm, were deplorable.

A pair of new books with a conservative stance that quickly dated them were *Sex and Sensibility: A New Look at Being a Woman* (1974), by Elizabeth M. Whelan, and *Making Sense Out of Sex: A New Look at Being a Man* (1975), also by Elizabeth M. Whelan in collaboration with her father-in-law, Stephen T. Whelan. Both Whelans have M.P.H. degrees from the Yale School of Medicine. In these books they stressed their opposition to any sex whatsoever for teenagers. Homosexuality was described as "definitely not normal" and in the volume for boys was linked with molestation. In the volume for girls the word "homosexual" appeared only in the glossary, and "lesbian" not at all. Birth control was discussed only in the context of marriage, and venereal disease was seen as a punishment for illicit sexual activity. Loss of virginity was equated with promiscuity. Although girls were told they might choose a job or career, marriage was presented as a woman's most important objective. Both books reinforced the traditional masculine and feminine role stereotypes.

Psyching Out Sex (1975), by Ingrid Rimland, a book about the psychological and emotional aspects of sexuality, was marred by a dreary format and a wordy style. The author, a high-school counselor and educational psychologist, wrote thoughtful chapters on the new demands of the women's movement and the homophile movement and exposed the negative effects that traditional role expectations can have on the personality. Unfortunately, few teenagers had the patience to pursue Rimland's argument through her pedantic vocabulary and convoluted syntax.

Straight Talk About Love and Sex for Teenagers, by Jane Burgess-Kohn (1979), which employed the familiar question-and-answer format, was an oddly inconsistent book. The author's attitudes seemed to have changed during its writing. The first chapters read like a dating ritual from the fifties, but the next few chapters examined the morality of "premarital sex" for couples who are engaged or at least in love. Burgess-Kohn's underlying assumption was that boys are predators and girls are preyed upon: a girl who "allows" sexual liberties and then discovers that the boy doesn't love her is disgraced. Yet further on, the author debunked virginity as a desirable condition for brides and discussed cohabitation with only mild disapproval. There was a detailed description of fellatio and a relatively informative chapter on homosexuality. The author deplored the idea that the vagina, rather than the clitoris, is the source of female sexual pleasure, yet she described intercourse as if an internal climax were the expected conclusion for women. The focus was on "thoughts, feelings, and questions that many of you have about love and sex," and very little information was provided about basic physiology. Overall, the mixture of old-fashioned and contemporary attitudes in this book was disturbing and confusing.

▪ Liberal Guides

Youth and Sex: Pleasure and Responsibility, by Gordon Jensen (1973), was an extremely liberal book with a strangely contrasting chapter on homosexuality that perpetuated old myths and stereotypes. The rest of the book was informed, aware, sympathetic, and even somewhat erotic. Jensen began with a list of sexual words followed by "other words that mean the same thing" and their definitions. For "intercourse" he gave thirty-one equivalent terms, most of them vulgar, and then said drily, "Notice that there are a lot of words for this act of sexual behavior. They all mean that the penis is put into the vagina." The illustrations were also extraordinarily frank—photographs of a nude young couple holding hands, closeup photos of the vulva, both closed and spread open to show the internal structure, and a picture of the same young couple examining an unrolled condom. Jensen discussed the benefits of masturbation and provided a detailed and realistic description of intercourse. He approved of petting if both parties were willing, although he advised that a girl should not become more involved sexually than is comfortable for her.

Jensen endorsed the condom as the cheapest, most efficient, and most easily available contraceptive and tried to overcome some of the common resistance to it, even recommending that girls carry one or two of them for emergencies. He did not attempt to discourage premarital intercourse, saying, "Several strong arguments can be made against virginity"—it handicaps initial sexual adjustment in marriage, for one. In general, "Each person has to come to terms with his own moral convictions and conflicts in the matter of premarital intercourse." A chapter on legal abortion discussed methods and costs, the position of the Catholic Church, and possible psychological reactions. In view of Jensen's fundamentally permissive stance in *Youth and Sex* it was surprising to find him insisting that "homosexuals often are quite maladjusted mentally and socially. Almost all of them have short-range goals, and much of their behavior is self-defeating. The life of a homosexual is dismal compared with the life of a normal heterosexual person."

An even more liberal book, perhaps the most liberal teen sex education book yet published, was *The Sex Handbook: Information and Help for Minors* (1974), by Heidi Handman and Peter Brennan. Addressing their book to teenagers under eighteen, the authors provided "practical information that's hard to get—information about your body, about having sex, about getting birth control . . . ," but they said nothing about love because "you already know your own feelings better than anybody else." The style was direct and colloquial, and the stress was on enjoyment and avoiding interference from authority figures: "Parents, schools, churches, and even the government try to make it as difficult as possible to enjoy your own body." There were separate chapters on losing your virginity ("How to have intercourse for the first time—how to make it easier and more enjoyable"), female orgasm, and advanced techniques like oral and anal sex. The chapters on birth control, abortion, and venereal disease discussed not only methods but how teenagers could get advice and care on their own: "The care and feeding of sex organs" explained what to expect of a gynecological examination and the symptoms and treatment of common infections, while a chapter on sex and the law explained such matters as the rights of emancipated minors and the meaning of statutory rape. The book ended with a useful but quickly outdated "directory of services in every state where people under eighteen can get birth control, pregnancy tests, VD tests, general medical care, abortions, abortion referrals, legal help, and counseling with sexual problems." This hedonistic approach severely limited the book's acceptability to most parents and librarians, however, and it was denounced by several reviewers for dealing with sex "only from the neck down."

In 1977 Dr. Peter Mayle, author of two controversial sex education books for children—*Where Did I Come From?* and *What's Happening to Me?* (both 1975)—wrote a teen sex education book called *Will I Like It?* The publisher kept the large-type picture-book format of the juvenile titles and replaced the cartoons that had made them so refreshing with some semipornographic photographs. As the subtitle indicated (*Your First Sexual Experience: What to Expect, What to Avoid, and How Both of You Can Get the Most Out of It*), the book was a how-to guide for teenagers who had decided to have sex and had already picked out a partner. The tone was friendly and not condescending, and some of the advice was highly practical, but the whole was marred by a certain lack of attention to factual detail, especially in the superficial and flip coverage of birth control and VD. The book jacket—a large, voluptuous nude whose likeness extended from the front to the back cover—combined with the big flat picture-book format made an impossibly intimidating package for self-conscious teens.

Three adult books typical of the spirit of the times appeared often in library collections for young people, although the intended audience was older. *Our Sexual Evolution* (1971), by Helen Colton, was a relatively sober and approving once-over-lightly of the new attitudes. *The Young Person's Guide to Love* (1975), by Morton M. Hunt, was one of a series of titles by this author exploiting the media fascination with the sudden availability of a widened range of sexual choices. In this book he explored the variety of human emotions as related to sexual experience. All kinds of love—gay and straight, sadism and masochism, May-December romances—were included, and the author urged readers to be tolerant of other people's relationships, no matter how strange they might seem. *The Sex Book: A Modern Pictorial Encyclopedia* (1971), by Martin Goldstein, was the most sensational of the three. Although the intentions of its original German publisher were probably more scholarly than prurient, in America critics found it hard to be objective about its surfeit of photographs of human genitals and copulating couples in an astonishing variety of activities and positions.

▪ Advice from Grandmother and Sisters

A warm and sensible book that proved useful on into the early eighties was *Ask Beth: You Can't Ask Your Mother* (1972), by Elizabeth C. Winship. This was a collection of answers to letters from teenagers by the author of the newspaper column "Ask Beth." The tone was grandmotherly but aware. Winship came down slightly on the conservative side of such issues as homosexuality and premarital sex, but with humor and compassion. The book outlasted more liberal guides because of the general nature of its advice—the abortion information predated the 1973 Supreme Court decision that made it legal, for instance, but this was only slightly troublesome in context. In addition to the usual sex-related topics, Winship also covered a broad range of other adolescent worries.

Sex guides from the feminist point of view were surprisingly scarce. An outstanding title of this type was Andrea Boroff Eagan's *Why Am I So Miserable if These Are the Best Years of My Life? A Survival Guide for the Young Woman.* First published in 1976, in its 1979 edition this book is still valid and will be discussed in the next section. A small but excellent manual for liberated young women was *Sex and the Teenage Girl*, by *Playgirl* magazine editor Carol Botwin. Inexplicably, it vanished from print very shortly after its release in 1972.

The blockbuster in feminist sex and health books was the monumental *Our Bodies, Ourselves* (1973), by the Boston Women's Health Collective. Originally produced by a feminist group with the help of medical advisers, it was an assemblage of dependable, detailed information and firsthand testimonials about the workings of the female body. For the first time it gave many women a new sense of understanding and control over their physical and sexual selves, and as such it was welcomed joyfully or viewed with dire alarm. The book remains an important work and continues to be a storm center of controversy. Although it was not really addressed to teenagers, the issue of its use with adolescents soon became politicized. Conservatives felt that its explicit photographs and detailed first-person descriptions of intercourse, masturbation, and the lesbian lifestyle were more than any teenager needed to know, while feminists passionately defended the excellence of its information and the warm and comforting humanity of its text. The contents undoubtedly *were* useful in part for young women, but the fight to include it in young adult library collections became less urgent with the 1980 publication of *Changing Bodies, Changing Lives*, a similar and equally excellent book for teenagers by some of the same editors.

▪ Comic Books and Other Adventures

Perhaps the wildest experiment in sex-guide format was *Facts o' Life Funnies* (1972), edited by Lora Fountain and distributed by the Multi Media Resource Center of San Francisco. This was a comic book that presented some cautionary tales about sex with cheerful obscenity. The first story, for instance, was "Fat Freddy Gets the Clap," drawn by Gilbert Shelton, dean of underground comic artists. Our hapless hero, one of the Furry Freak Brothers, discovers some painful symptoms after a weeklong bed-in with his happily round-heeled girlfriend. Yelping in agony, he takes his massively bandaged penis off to the free clinic, where a hefty doctor gives him a shot and then whacks him jovially on the back. "You gotta be careful where you stick that thing, kid!" she advises cheerfully. Although the book was highly effective at communicating basic sexual hygiene to teenagers, spoilsport parents and librarians found it coarse and objectionable.

The use of the comic book as sex education was legitimized by Sol Gordon in 1975 with the publication of a book with the breathless title *You! The Psychology of Surviving and Enhancing Your Social Life, Love Life, Sex Life, School Life, Home Life, Work Life, Emotional Life, Creative Life, Spiritual Life, Style of Life, Life.* The book was built around a collection of previously published comics (including *Ten Heavy Facts About Sex, Protect Yourself from Becoming an Unwanted Parent, V. D. Claptrap, Gut News for Modern Eaters, Juice Use,* and *Drug Doubt*), which Gordon had first distributed independently. Roger Conant had provided the crude but effective drawings and some horrendous puns, and Gordon contributed the serious data. The combination was eye-catching and irresistible to teenagers, and although not as deliberately obscene as *Facts o' Life Funnies*, the comics were raunchy enough to alarm conservative authorities. In 1971, when representatives from Gordon's Institute for Family Research and Education of Syracuse University distributed free copies of one of the earlier titles to teenagers at the New York State Fair, they were soon stopped by the management, and not until Gordon had seen the matter through the courts were they allowed to return to the fair in 1974.

The controversy over these little comic books was all the more surprising considering the impressive academic and professional credentials of their author. Sol Gordon is a clinical psychologist and professor of child and family studies and director of the Institute for Family Research and Education, a program of Syracuse University's College for Human Development. By the early seventies he was already a well-known writer and speaker on adolescent sexual development, and with the publication of *You!* he became the voice of the seventies as Duvall and Stall had been the definitive spokespeople for their times.

You!, with its joyous, nonlinear, free-form style exactly caught the exuberant, let-it-all-hang-out spirit of the psychedelic sixties and seventies. Relating loosely to the theme of being a (sexual) human being, it was a rambling collection of poems, lists, cartoons, engravings, drawings, photographs, observations, personal credos, anecdotes, jokes, aphorisms, and blank pages to write on, plus those outrageous comic books. Teenagers adored

Fig. 13. Cartoon by Roger Conant. From *Ten Heavy Facts About Sex*, by Sol Gordon and Roger Conant.

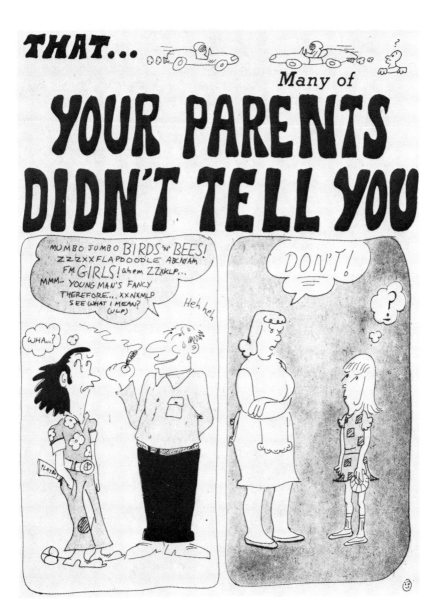

it. Much sound information and advice was painlessly communicated in its flamboyant pages, and the book's overwhelming popularity silenced even the stuffiest objectors.

Sol Gordon quickly became the darling of liberal librarians and teachers. But even he couldn't carry off an ill-conceived little volume called *You Would if You Loved Me* (1978). This purported to be a collection of "lines" that boys use to seduce girls, with the rationale that forearmed is forewarned. Thesc one-liners were oldies but not goodies. They ranged from the oily ("I just want to hold you all night") to the crude ("I would like to get into your pants"). In some cases Gordon supplied peculiarly flat and witless "snappy comebacks" for girls ("He: I've been admiring your rear end for weeks. She: Admiring will get you nowhere!"). Although the basic idea was probably a good one, the project failed in execution. Teenagers objected to the premise that males are always unscrupulous aggressors, and adults found the lines perhaps too close to reality not to be revolting.

▪ Survival by Edition

You! was too faithful to the zeitgeist of the seventies to last much beyond the end of the decade. Gordon's more enduring contribution to the literature of sex education is a small volume that ever since its first printing has been the most useful simple book in the field. *Facts About Sex* lasted through the drastic social changes of the era because Gordon continually rewrote it in a meticulous reflection of shifting current knowledge and attitudes. A detailed examination of these adjustments makes an interesting demonstration of this process, the common survival technique used, as we have seen, by youth-sex writers since Sylvanus Stall.

Facts About Sex was originally published in 1969 as *Facts About Sex for Exceptional Youth*. In this first version it was designed to be used with retarded or learning-impaired teenagers. Quickly realizing from the response that there was a need for such a simple book among normal teenagers who were unskilled or unwilling readers, Gordon adapted the book for more general distribution the next year. In an "Introduction for parents and youth" he explained that "knowing too much" does not lead to sexual misbehavior. Quite the reverse is true: "Most books about sex are written to please parents who have Victorian views." In this book he promised to be brief and limit himself to the physical facts of sex and also to include the "so-called dirty words" where they were relevant. And brief it was—twenty-two pages of text in all, with most chapters only one or two pages of large type.

Facts About Sex was saved from condescension by Gordon's straightforward style and by the exquisite nudes and anatomical charts drawn by Vivien Cohen. The first page got down to basics immediately with a definition of sexual intercourse ("This is when the man inserts his penis into the woman's vagina") and a list of slang synonyms for that function. He outlined conception and birth (with drawings that illustrate the birth process), male and female sexual anatomy, menstruation, wet dreams, and masturbation ("compulsive" masturbation is a sign of tension). He touched on venereal disease and illegitimate pregnancy, explaining in a footnote that abortion, now legal in some states, is a better choice than bearing an unwanted child. Gordon was not permissive about casual sex for the young and emphasized the link between love and sex: "Without love, 'making out' or intense physical contact short of sexual intercourse is often not a pleasant experience. It could lead to an increase of tension rather than provide an outlet for sexual urges. It is better to wait until you are an independent adult and in love before having sexual relations."

Under "Sex problems" he mentioned child molesters, rape, prostitution, impotence, frigidity, and homosexuality, which he pointed out was illegal. He listed some slang terms for homosexual: "faggot," "queer," and "gay." For prevention of pregnancy he suggested the Pill ("not suitable for everyone"), the diaphragm, or the condom but cautioned that contraceptives are not 100-percent effective. The last chapter consisted of the ten most common questions Gordon had been asked by teenagers. In answer to "Do you think it's right to have sexual intercourse at our ages?" he invoked the "risk of unhappy or tragic consequences" but conceded that "older working or college youth who love each other and can easily arrange for contraceptives and privacy may want to make their own decisions about premarital sex." Other questions concerned venereal disease, oral sex, the meaning of "cherry," and the origins of homosexuality and the possibility of cure. It is not caused by any one thing, he answers, and is not uncommon, but a few experiences do not make one a homosexual.

Published in 1973, the third edition, entitled *Facts About Sex for Today's Youth*, shows a considerable number of changes. It was in that year that a U.S. Supreme Court decision legalized abortion in America. Ruling on the cases *Roe v. Wade* and *Doe v. Bolton*, the court declared that all state laws that prohibit or restrict a woman's right to obtain an abortion in the first three months of pregnancy were unconstitutional. Also in that year the American Psychiatric Association changed its official definition of homosexuality from "mental disorder" to "sexual orientation disturbance," a term that was applied only to "those who wish to change their sexual orientation." In a press release on December 15 the association declared that "homosexuality in and of itself implies no impairment in judgment, stability, reliability, or vocational capabilities."

Both events were reflected in Gordon's revision. A reference to the illegality of abortion was removed, and the section on homosexuality (formerly headed "Sex problems," now headed "Sex problems and differences") was expanded. Gordon explained that psychologists no longer "see 'voluntary' homosexuality as a problem or disorder" and added the clarification that "most boys and girls have homosexual thoughts occasionally." The words "lesbian," "dyke," and "butch" were added to the slang vocabulary list, and Gordon explained that religious and professional groups were opposed to laws that interfere with private sexual behavior.

Perhaps the most noticeable change in the 1973 edition of *Facts About Sex* was in the illustrations—black and oriental teenagers were now included in a genre that had previously ignored these audiences. In the "Author's introduction" the "Victorian" parents became "uptight" parents. New research, said Gordon, showed that "many (if not most) teenagers will have sex before marriage without parental knowledge or consent." While he acknowledged this behavior, he assured parents that he did not advocate it. In the first chapter a drawing of the female external genitalia was added, thus introducing the clitoris, and the description of masturbation added the sentence "The clitoris is a source of sexual pleasure for the woman both in masturbation and during intercourse." The age for female puberty was lowered (incorrectly) from twelve to ten or eleven. "Some young people" who have sex before marriage was adjusted to "many young people."

Whereas the first edition had described premarital sex as "something that is not right," Gordon now referred to "enjoying" sex thoughts and shared the new finding that women may have gonorrhea without obvious symptoms. To the list of birth-control methods he added foam and intrauterine devices and some clear pictures of various contraceptive techniques and apparatus. In the question section the query about the meaning of the word "cherry" was removed and in its place was an inquiry about the boundaries of normal and abnormal sex. To the information about venereal disease he added that almost all states now permit treatment of minors without parental consent.

Five years later the changes in the 1978 edition of *Facts About Sex for Today's Youth* were fewer but similarly significant. The book was adorned with completely new drawings by Vivien Cohen that retained the multiracial theme. The words on homosexuality, now appearing under the heading "Sex differences," stressed that such behavior is no longer considered a disease or a disorder. Gordon continued to give the slang terms for homosexuals but distinguished between those words that are "popular" and those that are "negative." Bisexuality and lifelong celibacy as valid sex choices were also mentioned in this section. Other minor changes emphasized that abortion is preferable to teenage pregnancy and that sexual intercourse is not the most important expression of love. Herpes was discussed in the section on venereal disease, and Gordon added the odd observation that immature love affairs are tiring but the real thing is energizing. The bibliography emphasized books, tapes, and filmstrips produced by Gordon himself. In this edition the book is currently useful and will be discussed in a present-day context in the next section.

Another book that went through a series of editions to stay afloat was Eric Johnson's excellent *Love and Sex in Plain Language*. First published in 1965 and first revised in 1967 (see Chapter 7), it underwent another metamorphosis in 1973. This edition was slightly expanded, and the new illustrations by Russ Hoover were not quite as effective as the sepia drawings of the earlier editions. A few other changes in this edition were slight but significant. The chapter on female anatomy now came before that for the male; the function of the clitoris was added to the description of intercourse; orgasm was described as "a glorious spasm"; the chapter called "Husband and wife unite in sexual intercourse" was now titled "Man and woman unite in sexual intercourse"; information on legal abortion was added; and the discussion of fertilization explained principles of heredity and the function of chromosomes.

More important was the inclusion of a new chapter on the differences—and similarities—between male and female sexuality that discussed sex-role expectations: "People have come more and more to want to be free, free to be themselves, whichever sex they may belong to. They are less willing to play unthinkingly the role of man or woman that our society encourages. In other words, we are coming to see that in each of us there is some of what we think of as the masculine and some of what we think of as the feminine." The greatest change was Johnson's complete revision of the chapter on homosexuality. Now entitled "Homosexuality—being 'gay'" rather than "Some special problems of sex," the chapter was a model of compassionate thinking on the subject. Johnson defined a new term here—homophobia: "the strong, unreasoning fear of homosexuality, not unlike racial or religious prejudice." He explained that heterosexuals are called "straight" as distinguished from "gay," that female homosexuals are often called "lesbians," and that there are many people who are bisexual. He spoke approvingly of the gay-liberation movement and said, "Many homosexual men and women are happy and satisfied and are managing to make successes of their lives." A further revision of *Love and Sex in Plain Language* in 1977 made only one change: a rewording of the paragraph on rape made it more sympathetic to the victim. The current usefulness of the book, now in a fourth edition (1985), is discussed in the next section.

An adaptation of *Love and Sex in Plain Language* for preadolescents was published in 1970 under the title *Love and Sex and Growing Up*. A third excellent book by Eric Johnson was *Sex: Telling It Straight*, which first appeared in the same year. Johnson addressed it to "boys and girls who are growing up in places where hardship is one of the facts of life." The book spoke simply to young teenagers growing up in urban ghettos or in isolated rural areas about the basics of sex and love and dealt with many problems then ordinarily considered to be outside the experience of middle-class people (incest, for instance: "If a member of your family tries to have sexual intercourse with you, you should tell someone who can try to get help at once"). Although Johnson stressed the stereotyped male and female role expectations, he was innovative in including a two-way glossary that provided the slang equivalents for standard sex terms, and vice versa. Such a list was an obvious need in sex education, but in 1970 many public librarians were still too shy of four-letter words to add this book to their collections. A 1979 edition soft-pedaled this feature.

A few other books printed in the early and middle seventies managed to remain popular into the eighties by virtue of new editions. *Our Bodies, Ourselves* and *Why Am I So Miserable if These Are the Best Years of My Life?* have already been mentioned. *Sex and Birth Control: A Guide for the Young*, by E. James Lieberman and Ellen Peck, was a long and thorough discussion of modern methods of pregnancy prevention and venereal-disease control that had to go back to the drawing board when the Dalkon Shield IUD was found highly unsafe. Even a conservative sexual-conduct guide, Richard Hettlinger's *Growing Up with Sex*, needed to adjust its 1971 words about homosexuals to fit into the new enlightened conservatism of the early eighties.

After 1977 things began to settle down, and several sound sex guides written in the last years of the decade escaped the instant obsolescence that had previously undone so many who had tried to interpret these tumultuous years. In the following pages these and later books will be discussed in contemporary context as we turn from the historical perspective to a hard look at the urgent sex education needs of the present.

■ BIBLIOGRAPHY

Boston Women's Health Collective. *Our Bodies, Ourselves*. New York: Simon and Schuster, 1973; rev. ed., 1976.

Botwin, Carol. *Sex and the Teenage Girl*. New York: Lancer, 1972.

Burgess-Kohn, Jane. *Straight Talk About Love and Sex for Teenagers*. Boston: Beacon, 1979.

Colton, Helen. *Our Sexual Evolution*. New York: Watts, 1971.

Eagan, Andrea Boroff. *Why Am I So Miserable if These Are the Best Years of My Life? A Survival Guide for the Young Woman.* Philadelphia: Lippincott, 1976; rev. ed., New York: Avon, 1979.

Fountain, Lora. *Facts o' Life Funnies.* San Francisco: Multi Media Resource Center, 1972.

Goldstein, Martin. *The Sex Book: A Modern Pictorial Encyclopedia.* New York: Herder and Herder, 1971.

Gordon, Sol. *Facts About Sex: A Basic Guide.* New York: Day, 1970.

———. *Facts About Sex for Exceptional Youth.* Plainview, N.Y.: Charles Brown, 1969.

———. *Facts About Sex for Today's Youth.* New York: Day, 1973; rev. ed., Fayetteville, N.Y.: Ed-U, 1978.

———. *Ten Heavy Facts About Sex.* Syracuse, N.Y.: Ed-U, 1971.

———. *You Would if You Loved Me.* New York: Bantam, 1978.

———, with Roger Conant. *You! The Psychology of Surviving and Enhancing Your Social Life, Love Life, Sex Life, School Life, Home Life, Work Life, Emotional Life, Creative Life, Spiritual Life, Style of Life, Life.* New York: Quadrangle, 1975.

Guttmacher, Alan Frank. *Understanding Sex: A Young Person's Guide.* New York: Harper and Row, 1970; New York: New American Library, 1970.

Handman, Heidi, and Peter Brennan. *The Sex Handbook: Information and Help for Minors.* New York: Putnam, 1974.

Hettlinger, Richard F. *Growing Up with Sex.* New York: Seabury, 1971; new rev. ed., New York: Continuum, 1980.

Hunt, Morton M. *The Young Person's Guide to Love.* New York: Farrar, 1975; New York: Dell, 1977.

James, John (pseud.). *The Facts of Sex: A Revolutionary Approach to Sex Instruction for Teenagers.* Princeton, N.J.: Vertex, 1970.

Jensen, Gordon D. *Youth and Sex: Pleasure and Responsibility.* Chicago: Nelson-Hall, 1973.

Johnson, Eric W. *Love and Sex in Plain Language.* Philadelphia: Lippincott, 1965; rev. eds., 1967, 1973, 1977; New York: Bantam, 1974; rev. ed., New York: Harper and Row, 1985.

———. *Sex: Telling It Straight.* Philadelphia: Lippincott, 1970; rev. ed., 1979.

———, and Corinne B. Johnson. *Love and Sex and Growing Up.* Philadelphia: Lippincott, 1970; New York: Bantam, 1974.

Lieberman, E. James, and Ellen Peck. *Sex and Birth Control: A Guide for the Young.* New York: Crowell, 1973; New York: Schocken, 1975; rev. ed., New York: Harper and Row, 1981.

Mayle, Peter. *Will I Like It? Your First Sexual Experience: What to Expect, What to Avoid, and How Both of You Can Get the Most Out of It.* Los Angeles: Corwin, 1977.

Rimland, Ingrid. *Psyching Out Sex.* Philadelphia: Westminster, 1975.

Shultz, Gladys Denny. *Letters to a New Generation: For Today's Inquiring Teenage Girl.* Philadelphia: Lippincott, 1971.

Southard, Helen E. *Sex Before Twenty: New Answers for Young People.* Rev. ed., New York: Dutton, 1971.

Spock, Benjamin. *A Teenager's Guide to Life and Love.* New York: Simon and Schuster, 1970.

Whelan, Elizabeth M. *Sex and Sensibility: A New Look at Being a Woman.* New York: McGraw-Hill, 1974.

Whelan, Stephen T., and Elizabeth M. Whelan. *Making Sense Out of Sex: A New Look at Being a Man.* New York: McGraw-Hill, 1975.

Winship, Elizabeth C. *Ask Beth: You Can't Ask Your Mother.* Boston: Houghton Mifflin, 1972, 1976.

—And Now

Introduction

How easy it is to smile knowingly at the quaint assumptions and amusing errors of sex education past. How wrong they were, and how obviously harmful their advice! But now we've got it right at last. *They* were judgmental, controlling, ineffective. Not us. The things *we* tell young people are the right things. The way we try to get them to behave is the right way to act, the way that is—obviously—good for them. Exactly so, Sylvanus Stall would have said in 1892.

The most useful lesson to be learned from the history of sex education is humility. We will never get it right once and for all. Sexual styles and attitudes and behaviors and problems will continue to change, so that what seems to us today to be the ultimate word will appear out of date in ten years and ridiculous in twenty. Advice will continue to lag behind reality, because the people who write it form their sexual opinions twenty years earlier than the people who need it. Nearly a century of adolescent sex manuals show this mechanism at work clearly and inexorably, and there is no reason to think that anything has changed. It is only harder—or impossible—to see it in our own day.

The first step in overcoming the mistakes of the past, then, is to recognize them. The second step is to understand our own times. We live today in an era of oppressive sexual ambiguity. Although there seems to be a great deal of freedom, it is undercut by a hidden residue of guilt from the past. Images and messages of sexual permission are everywhere: in novels, plays, movies, television, advertising, popular music. But in real life the official position is still covert disapproval. The media say go, authority and conscience say stop—especially to teenagers.

Three major social trends have contributed to this ambivalence in sexual attitudes. On a background of permissiveness left over from the sixties and seventies has been superimposed the new conservatism, as the nation has turned massively to the political and religious right. Rampant herpes and AIDS brought about a sudden revival of respect for the value of monogamous relationships. And soaring rates of teenage unwed pregnancy made even liberals rethink the wisdom of approving early sexual activity.

Teenagers *are* sexually active in ever-increasing numbers and at earlier and earlier ages. Many studies have shown this beyond any doubt. The falling age of menarche may be at least partially responsible for these statistics: the average age of onset of menstruation has dropped from 14.5 in the late nineteenth century[1] to 12.9 years at the present time,[2] due to better nutrition and health. But the rate of increase in early sexual initiation is too large to be solely explained by this factor. In 1981 the Alan Guttmacher Institute reported that among unmarried sixteen-year-olds forty-five percent of the males and thirty-two percent of the females were sexually active, and among eighteen-year-olds the rate rose to seventy percent for males and fifty-two percent for females.[3] A 1979 survey of urban teenagers found that by the age of nineteen sixty-five percent of the white women and ninety percent of the black women had had intercourse at least once. This was significantly higher than the findings of a similar survey in 1971, when forty-one percent of the white adolescents and seventy-eight percent of the black were experienced.[4] This earlier study showed that seventeen percent of the sixteen-year-old women were nonvirgins, but that number had increased to thirty-five percent by 1979. Furthermore, there is some evidence that the traditional higher rate of sexual activity for males is disappearing. A Colorado study indicated that the rates for sexually experienced males in tenth, eleventh, and twelfth grades were twenty-one percent, twenty-eight percent, and thirty-three percent, while those for girls were twenty-six percent, forty percent, and fifty-five percent.[5] Peter Scales, former director of education for the Planned Parenthood Federation, summed all these numbers up rather conservatively in an interview for the *Los Angeles Times*: one in five teens has had sex by the age of fifteen, he claimed, and half of the teens in the United States will be sexually active by the time they finish high school.[6] Yet in 1982 thirty-eight percent of American adults still felt emphatically that it was "always" or "almost always" wrong for a man and woman to have sex before marriage.[7]

It is important when analyzing patterns of adolescent sexual activity to point out that while young people may be more experienced, they are not promiscuous. The majority have had only one sexual partner,[8] and most surveys indicate that half have intercourse less than once a month.[9]

But selectivity does not mean responsibility. A 1980 study found that over half of teenage couples failed to use birth control at first intercourse, and one third of them never used contraception at all.[10] The result is ninety-six births annually per one thousand girls aged fifteen to nineteen, the highest rate in the western world.[11] A 1978 study translated the statistics even more strikingly: four out of ten fourteen-year-old girls will become pregnant at least once by age nineteen if current trends continue.[12] Early unwed pregnancy contributes to a multitude of other social problems and has been recognized since 1978 as a target area of concern by the U.S. Public Health Service—and all other thinking American adults.

Venereal disease (now more correctly called "sexually transmitted disease," or STD) is also epidemic among teens. The 1980 rate of gonorrhea was triple that of 1960. Of the one million new cases of STD annually, two thirds are contracted by people aged fifteen to twenty-four.[13] STD is increasing most rapidly among the youngest teens, eleven- to fourteen-year-olds.[14] And the specter of AIDS, the new Black Death, hangs over us all.

Large segments of American society react to these dreary statistics with attempts to impose a return to older values. Evangelical Christian publishing houses produce a flood of "dating" guides that demand complete chastity until marriage, to the tune of sales figures that astonish mainstream publishers. A new caution about explicit sexuality has begun to take hold in young adult fiction, and "squeaky clean" formula romances hark back to the innocent days of the fifties. For the first time organized attempts at suppression are being directed against certain sex education manuals deemed too liberal by the far right. (As we have seen, the genre has to this point been nearly inviolate, protected by its aura of scientific authority and objectivity.) Foes of abortion campaign aggressively for a reversal of *Roe vs. Wade*. The Reagan administration has pushed for a "squeal rule" that would require physicians in government-funded clinics to notify parents if their children request prescription birth control. After the defeat of the Equal Rights Amendment feminists saw the ground they had gained during the women's movement begin to erode.

Throughout all this the mass media continue to present a behavioral norm of casual sexual acting-out. This conflict of cultural ideals, this oppressive ambivalence about sexuality, is experienced most intensely by adolescents. Pressured by their peers into too-early sexual experience, they are apt to feel that "everybody's doing it" except them. And yet, once the troublesome virginity is lost, they are often unable to accept their own sexual activity enough to be able to plan for contraception. Finding themselves pregnant, as many inevitably do, their typical wail is "Now everybody will know what I've been doing!" (This, of course, is only one possible explanation for the complex problem of adolescent pregnancy—but it illustrates the point.) The dilemma is neatly summed up in the film *The Breakfast Club*. Taunted to reveal whether she is a virgin, a young girl says—with more poignance than originality—"That question's sort of a two-edged sword, isn't it? If you say yes, you're a prude. And if you say no, you're a—well, a slut."

To cut through this tangle of sexual cross-purposes, anachronisms, and unfinished business that our mismanaged past has handed them young people desperately need help. But not the kind of "help" they have formerly been offered in so many of the sex manuals. A new approach is needed, one that will first of all regard the sexuality of young adults not as an act-centered problem but as an integral process of their total humanity. Dr. Michael A. Carrera has spoken to his fellow sex educators about the need for the holistic view of adolescent sexuality: "The issues regarding body image, gender and social roles, affection, love, and intimacy must be fully explored at least as much as those issues regarding the understanding of the female and male sexual systems and birth control methods. . . . We must be able to link them to the full and diverse dimensions of a young person's development."[15]

We now know that "the adolescent's interest and preoccupation with sexuality is not something that just happens overnight."[16] Sexuality begins before birth, not at puberty. The Victorian model of a one-shot teaching session, in which the young pubescent person is handed a package of secret revelations, is no longer applicable, but its ghost clings persistently in the shape of the timing of sex ed classes and manuals. Sexuality education should be an ongoing component of all education, and at the very least, as Alex Comfort has said, it should be "pre-need." Can it be that the adolescent sex education book as a genre has outlived its purpose?

However that may be, until our society is comfortable enough with sexuality so that the subject is no longer isolated from other learning, the sex education manual in some form or other will remain one of the most important vehicles for communicating information and attitudes to the young. To increase their effectiveness we need to make sure, first, that they are relevant and solidly grounded in what is actually going on in young adults' lives. When teens are asked what they most want to know from these books, the answers center on the act of intercourse—how to do it, what it feels like, what happens before and after.[17] This has been the very subject that writers have most often treated with a gingerly reluctance to provide detail. But adolescents also need to have the act of intercourse set in a broader context of mutual human respect and caring. Lester Kirkendall has said, "High-quality interpersonal relationships create a moral climate."[18] Sexual skills are not limited to the bedroom. Peter Scales puts it this way: "We're talking about being able to solve problems and make decisions, to identify alternatives."[19]

The manuals also must try to clear away harmful debris from the past, to heal guilt and secretiveness, to debunk popular myths, to expose destructive gender roles. Writers need to make a special effort to address young men. Deryck Calderwood urges: "Their traditional role expects them to be all-knowledgeable about sexual matters and to be the initiators of sexual behavior. Yet at every age for which we have standardized knowledge tests . . . males measure lower than females in the amount of information they possess."[20] And perhaps most important, the guides need to help young people learn to communicate accurately and honestly about sex—with a partner, parents, friends, and themselves—so that they can articulate and solve problems and clarify their own values.

These are the long-range objectives, and with movement toward their accomplishment the urgent short-term goals—to persuade teens to delay sexual activity, to practice birth control, to avoid sexually transmitted disease—may also begin to be achieved. To determine how well the present-day versions of the sex education book measure up to these objectives this second section of *Sex Guides* will examine the form in all its manifestations since 1977. The aim is to help librarians, teachers, youth workers, parents, and young adults themselves choose the best and most appropriate books and films about sexuality.

■ NOTES

[1]Vern L. Bullough. "Age at Menarche: A Misunderstanding." *Science*, July 17, 1981, p. 365.

[2]Joan Lipsitz. "Sexual Development of Young Adolescents." Speech given before the American Association of Sex Educators, Counselors, and Therapists, March 1980.

[3]Alan Guttmacher Institute. *Teenage Pregnancy: The Problem That Hasn't Gone Away*, 1981.

[4]M. Zelnik and J. F. Kantner. "Sexual Activity, Contraceptive Use, and Pregnancy Among Metropolitan-Area Teenagers: 1971–1979." *Family Planning Perspectives*, Sept./Oct. 1980, p. 230.

[5]S. L. Jessor and R. Jessor. "Transition from Virginity to Nonvirginity Among Youth: A Social Psychological Study over Time." *Developmental Psychology*, July 1975, p. 473.

[6]Elizabeth Mehren. "Realistic Approach to Teen Sex Educates Adults on Facts of Life." *Los Angeles Times*, June 28, 1983, Section 5, p. 1.

[7]Arland Thornton and Deborah Freedman. *The Changing American Family*. Population Bulletin. Population Reference Bureau, Inc., October 1983.

[8]M. J. Rogel, M. E. Zuehlke, A. C. Petersen, M. Tobin-Richards, and M. Shelton. "Contraceptive Behavior in Adolescence: A Decision-making Perspective." *Journal of Youth and Adolescence*, Dec. 1980, p. 491.

[9]L. S. Zabin and S. D. Clark. "Institutional Factors Affecting Teenagers' Choice and Reasons for Delay in Attending a Family Planning Clinic." *Family Planning Perspectives*, Jan./Feb. 1983, p. 25.

[10]Zelnik and Kantner, *ibid.*

[11]Alan Guttmacher Institute. "Teenage Pregnancy in Developed Countries: Determinants and Policy Implications." *Family Planning Perspectives*, March/April 1985, p. 53.

[12]C. Tietze. "Teenage Pregnancies: Looking Ahead to 1984." *Family Planning Perspectives*, July/August 1978, p. 205.

[13]Mehren, *ibid.*

[14]Peter Scales. "How We Guarantee the Ineffectiveness of Sex Education." *SIECUS Report*, March 1978, p. 1.

[15]Michael A. Carrera. "Some Reflections on Adolescent Sexuality." *SIECUS Report*, March 1983, p. 1.

[16]Judy A. Shea. "Adolescent Sexuality." In Richard M. Lerner and Nancy L. Galambos, eds. *Experiencing Adolescents: A Sourcebook for Parents, Teachers, and Teens*. New York: Garland, 1984, pp. 51–85.

[17]Judith S. Rubenstein et al. "An Analysis of Sex Education Books for Adolescents by Means of Adolescents' Sexual Interests." *Adolescence*, February 1977, p. 293.

[18]Lester Kirkendall. *Emphasis*, Summer 1982, p. 17.

[19]Mehren, *ibid.*

[20]Deryck Calderwood. "Male Sexual Health." *SIECUS Report*, November 1984, p. 1.

Chapter 9

Modern Manuals on the Old Model

The sex education book as a literary convention is still very much alive. Although the content has grown more sophisticated and the attitudes and information have been adjusted to contemporary thought, sex manuals today remain recognizably connected to the tradition. There is the discussion of sexual anatomy with labeled diagrams, the chapter on the changes of puberty, the chapter on pregnancy and birth, the list of contraceptive devices, the list of venereal diseases, the section of questions and answers, the quotations and anecdotes from teens. The tone remains more cautionary than celebratory, even in these times. (For a sex manual to be erotic or titillating is taboo.) Scientific terminology is used both for exactness and for distance, and the common words for sexual functions are given only once, in quotation marks. Fear of the wicked peer nowadays takes the shape of warnings about sexual learning from popular culture: television, films, pornographic magazines, rock-music lyrics. Even the birds and the bees sometimes still show up as otherwise irrelevant passages describing animal mating. Some contemporary sex educators work closely within the established form; others acknowledge the conventions more freely. But always, however remotely, the pattern from the past can be discerned.

This is not necessarily bad; in fact the solidity of a traditional structure saves explanations between writer and reader and leaves energy for originality of content and style. The astonishing range of the present-day adolescent sex manual can be seen by comparing, say, the amusing little picture book called *Am I Normal?* with the encyclopedic sweep of *Changing Bodies,*

Changing Lives. Modern manuals are written for a variety of readers, rather than the monolithic middle-class sixteen-year-old who was the target in former years. Today a book might be aimed at preteens, young teens, or older teens, or it might be written for reluctant readers or skilled readers, or for a specialized audience, such as gay or handicapped young people. Editorial position can be conservative or liberal or somewhere in between. People who work with young adults, then, should be familiar in some detail with the whole spectrum of sex education manuals, not just one or two titles, so that they can recommend not only a *good* book, but the *right* book for a particular young person or parent.

▪ First Books for Preteens and New Teens

Beginning with the books written for young adolescents or even preteens, a title-by-title examination shows several excellent manuals that follow the traditional model rather closely. *Boys and Sex* and *Girls and Sex* are the old warhorses. These are the books that librarians are most likely to recommend and that bookstore clerks automatically hand to an inquiring parent. They exude respectability, partly because of the distinguished reputation of their author, Wardell Pomeroy, and partly because they have been around so long. When they were first published, in 1968 and 1969, they were considered extremely liberal for their bold recognition of early sexual activity and for their enthusiastic and graphic recommendation of masturbation for both boys and girls. Now the times have caught up, and *Boys and Sex* and *Girls and Sex* in their 1981 editions are serviceable middle-of-the-road classics.

The earlier versions are discussed in some detail in Chapter 7. The heavy emphasis on traditional gender roles is a major flaw that makes these older works no longer usable. In the 1981 editions Pomeroy (and his collaborator, John Tebbel) corrected this to some degree, although traces of the earlier attitudes remain. In *Girls and Sex* young women are now encouraged to develop independence and self-respect (although they are still told that being asked on a date will give them "a sense of status").

In both books the chapters on homosexuality have been extensively rewritten to include a positive description of the gay-rights movement and to remove the implication that lesbians are motivated by a need to reject males. The implied expectation of marriage has been broadened to include "other circumstances of regular intimacy." The phrase "premarital sex" has been replaced in most cases by "early sex." Legal abortion is acknowledged and herpes and NGU have been added to the section on venereal disease. And boys are told a great deal more about love and relationships than was deemed appropriate in 1968.

Although sex educators generally agree on the excellence of *Boys and Sex* and *Girls and Sex*, there are aspects of the chapter on homosexuality that many find troubling. In the earlier editions Pomeroy had based this section on his own experience in taking thousands of sexual case histories and also on Kinsey's finding that homosexuality and heterosexuality are the end points of a behavior continuum in which most people fall somewhere in the middle. In the newer edition Pomeroy continues to regard homosexuality as a voluntary and correctable state, rather than—as most experts now agree—an inborn condition. Deryck Calderwood, in a review in the September 1982 *SIECUS Report*, said:

> Pomeroy presents homosexuality as a matter of choice, and, for boys who feel they are homosexually inclined, he advises beginning active relationships with girls. Parents are also advised to encourage heterosexual social contacts for their sons (yet curiously, in the following chapter they are advised not to prod a boy into dating if he is not interested in girls!). . . . He urges tolerance for homosexual individuals but offers little support for that percentage of his readership that may, in fact, be gay or bisexual.

This failure to clarify the distinction between sexual orientation and behavior was also true of the "Lesbianism" chapter in *Girls and Sex*.

Calderwood also felt that Pomeroy had not gone far enough in reflecting the social changes spearheaded by the women's movement.

> The double standard is still evident here and there. Girls are encouraged to help "train" boys in the social amenities of dating. They are told that boys "ought to know how to stimulate a girl properly" and that "girls should know what it is to be stimulated" and that once they have intercourse they "will never again be a virgin."

In addition, Calderwood regretted that Pomeroy continued to rely on Kinsey's statistics on female sexual behavior rather than update them, "since what change there has been in the sexual behavior of Americans has been largely among females."

Given the general accuracy and reliability of most of the information in this pair of books, an odd and inexplicable shortcoming is the general incorrectness of the descriptions of sexual positions. The female superior position, for example, according to Pomeroy is one in which the woman "lies on top of the male, with her legs together between his"—an arrangement that is anatomically extremely awkward both for insertion and for thrusting. Or his versions of "dog fashion": "the girl lies on her stomach with the male over her, or on her side with him behind her, or on her back with the male beneath her." The popularly accepted meaning of that term is none of the above.

Another puzzling question is why John Tebbel, whom Pomeroy credits in his preface with having "done the actual writing," does not appear on either title page. Too, there are those who feel that the aggressive purple and orange colors and the blatant titles are intimidating to self-conscious young readers.

However, these are minor criticisms in light of the books' virtues. Pomeroy's warmth, lack of condescension, and honesty are unequaled in the literature of sex education. Even more heartening is his vision of human sexuality as a great and positive good. "Maybe we could begin," he says in the first chapter of *Boys and Sex*, "with a fundamental fact with which everyone should be able to agree, which is that sex is one of the most pleasurable activities available to human beings. It ought to be one of the happiest parts of our lives, from our earliest days until we're old." It is Pomeroy's steady grasp of the importance of that vision and his clear understanding of the difficulties of its achievement in a pluralistic, generally sex-negative society that make *Girls and Sex* and *Boys and Sex* worthy of their status as classics.

Another book that deserves the designation of "classic" is *Love and Sex in Plain Language*, by Eric Johnson. First published in 1965, it has come a long way for a book whose first edition deplored frequent masturbation and called homosexuality a sickness. This original version is discussed in Chapter 7 and subsequent revisions in Chapter 8. The 1985 edition, its fourth revision, is impeccably contemporary and reflects the author's impressive growth over the years in social and historical awareness, scientific knowledge, and literary skill. An occasional lapse into preachiness is the book's only fault, and that can be forgiven because it is in the good cause of love, respect for persons, and the intelligent and thoughtful self-determination of sexual values.

Love and Sex in Plain Language has always been outstanding in the sheer quantity of information it contained, and the 1985 edition is rich in interesting facts, often the result of recent findings or research, that seldom appear in sex education books for this age level. The text has been carefully rewritten throughout, even down to the smallest details, to bring it into line with current understanding and social attitudes. For instance, where in 1977 Johnson had said that homosexuality comes from "how we are treated by our parents," in 1985 he has grown to understand that "certainly it is not a simple matter. There is fairly general agreement, however, that a homosexual or heterosexual orientation is a way of being that is established very early in life, possibly before we are born."

Johnson has markedly changed his attitude toward early sex. Formerly permissive, he now comes down heavily on the side of abstinence and postponement, even removing a reference to mutual petting to orgasm. A sensible section on "saying no to sexual intercourse" gives practical help in refusing gracefully—for both sexes. For those young people who are wondering how they will know when the time is right for them to become sexually involved, Johnson quotes a thoughtful and helpful self-quiz from Elizabeth Winship's *Reaching Your Teenager* that lists "the important questions to which you ought to be able to answer yes before you have intercourse."

He offers equally practical and nonjudgmental help to those who choose to be sexually active (although he begins by saying "abstinence can be considered the best method of birth control for teenagers") in a much-expanded section on contraception. This passage includes, in addition to the usual information on devices and methods, a detailed and interesting description of some recent developments in techniques of natural family planning (NFP).

Johnson has greatly expanded his treatment of a number of other subjects. The chapter on STD, for example, includes new paragraphs on nongonococcal urethritis (NGU), or chlamydia, pelvic inflammatory disease, herpes, AIDS, and trichomoniasis—although the author has removed the traditional reassurance about toilet seats. The section on rape has been completely rewritten to reflect current thinking. A passage on teenage pregnancy reveals Johnson's concern, and the pages on abortion have been redone to respect the controversy. The appendix includes a thorough glossary of formal and scientific terms (no street words), a "Mastery Quiz" of sexual knowledge, and an acknowledgment list of "people who read all or parts of the manuscript" that reads like a Who's Who of adolescent sex education.

Eric Johnson's strength lies in his careful discussion of sexual values and ethics. Scrupulously fair to all points of view, he shows young people how to measure the morality of their sexual actions by the yardstick of their effect on others and on themselves and how to relate their decisions to the absolute of the personal worth of each human being or a religious absolute, if one wishes:

> The major religions in the United States teach that it is morally wrong to have sexual intercourse outside of marriage. Fortunately, many churches today provide sex and family-life education programs to help young people deal responsibly with their sexuality. When people's religions do teach that premarital intercourse is wrong and people disregard the teaching, they may very well feel guilty, and this feeling may isolate them from a source of strength, comfort, and confidence that would help them. . . . The decisions that people make about sexuality will differ with different individuals. The decisions will depend upon the beliefs and teaching each person has been exposed to and how each has reacted to them, as well as the social situations they are in and the values and convictions they develop.

To acknowledge the plurality of sexual values in our society and to remain warm and involved but still objective—this is a masterful feat, and Johnson carries it off superbly.

A comparison with *Boys and Sex* and *Girls and Sex* inevitably arises. Is *Love and Sex in Plain Language* a better book for younger teens? In the 1985 edition the answer is probably yes, at the moment. In spite of the reputation of the Pomeroy books for respectability, the Johnson guide may be more acceptable, on close reading, to conservative parents because of its recognition of their values (and others) and its strong support for abstinence or at least postponed sexual initiation. Pomeroy's tone is a trifle more comfortable for teens, but Johnson includes more information and is more up-to-date. Although a parent buying only one book may want to give a bit more preference to Johnson, both authors should certainly appear side by side in school and public libraries.

A newcomer to the business of classic sex education manuals is Lynda Madaras. She has written a pair of outstanding books for young adolescents—*What's Happening to My Body? A Growing Up Guide for Mothers and Daughters* and *The What's Happening to My Body? Book for Boys: A Growing Up Guide for Parents and Sons*. Both are meant to be read together by parents and their nine- to thirteen-year-old sons or daughters. Because these books are intended for such young adolescents, they have only the briefest and most general information about birth control, venereal disease, homosexuality, rape, and making decisions about sexual intercourse. Madaras refers her readers to other books for these subjects and concentrates on explaining the changes of puberty.

Her style is informed but wonderfully easy and conversational. Madaras has written several books on women's health care, but it is her experience in teaching sex education classes for teens and preteens that she draws on here to make her books so comfortable. Early in these classroom sessions she discovered to her discomfort that a roomful of giggly preadolescents and a lecture about penises and vaginas and sex added up to total chaos. So, she says, "I decided that if we were going to get all silly and giggly in class when we talked about these things, we might as well get *really* silly and giggly." She startled the first class of the year by giving everyone photocopies of drawings of the male and female sex organs and letting them color each part as she talked about it—blue polka dots for the scrotum, red and blue stripes for the shaft of the penis, and so on—while they called out all the slang names for those parts that they could think of. By the time they'd finished coloring both the pictures, everyone had giggled off most of the embarrassment and was ready to listen to what she had to say. Her first chapter tells this story and encourages readers to color in the pictures themselves—unless, of course, what they have in hand is a library book.

The technique is typical of Madaras's style. Rather than write from the traditional distance, she puts herself and her young readers in the picture. She often illustrates a point with stories from her own body's functioning—even embarrassing ones like the day in high school when she walked around all day not knowing there was a big spot of menstrual blood on the back of her skirt. The text is liberally sprinkled with observations, worries, and questions from her students. To make sure she is really in touch with the adolescent viewpoint she enlisted the help of teenage coauthors: her own daughter Area for the girls' volume and Dane Saavedra, the fifteen-year-old son of a friend, for the boys' volume.

A valuable feature of *What's Happening to My Body?* is Madaras's orientation toward active rather than passive sexual health care. She encourages girls to make friends with their own bodies not only by looking at their external genitalia in a mirror but also by exploring their internal organs with a finger. She teaches the breast self-examination technique and suggests that girls and their mothers might do it at the same time. Boys are taught testicular self-examination, an important hygiene measure that seldom appears in other books. She gives a chart, for both sexes, for keeping track of puberty changes so that young people can feel on top of the process. But the pelvic exam is never mentioned, perhaps because Madaras feels that such young girls have no need yet to be prepared for this procedure.

The "Introduction for parents," a different one for each book, is funny and wise and real and reassuring to parents who may feel uncomfortable about talking to their own offspring about sex. In the book for mothers and daughters the author begins by telling of her own search for a book to tell Area about menstruation. Going to the library, she found that "there were one or two books for young girls that briefly mentioned the topic, but they were hopelessly out of date, and the tone was all wrong"—a complaint that has appeared in the introductions of sex guides since 1900. So, like many before her, she wrote her own book. The introduction for parents of boys starts out with a hilarious account of an assignment Madaras gives her classes, in which each student is given a raw egg to "parent" for a week as if it were a live baby. She then goes on to make a poignant case for the often ignored needs of young boys for help in understanding the disturbing changes that are happening to their bodies.

Although Madaras is often amusing, she is never flip, and the quality of her information is first-rate. Her books make excellent introductions for just-pubescent youngsters who may be embarrassed to read more advanced guides. However, it is important that their exposure to information not stop with these books but be supplemented with more sophisticated information in a year or two when they are ready for it.

Another pair of books for early adolescents (ten to twelve) are *Am I Normal?* and *Dear Diary*, both by Jeanne Betancourt. Based on films by Debra Franco and David Shepard (films that Madaras mentions using in her classes), these are amusing but slight. Both deal with the embarrassments of puberty—the girl's problems center on her first bra and first menstruation, and the boy's dilemma is a lack of information about wet dreams and penis size. The young actors in the many stills from the films that illustrate the storyline are appealing and the situations are recognizable. Although a modicum of information is worked into the plot, this serves primarily as a discussion opener.

A combination of humor and sex information can be tricky, expecially in books for young teens, and although Madaras and Betancourt carry it off nicely, others have fallen flat in the attempt. *Growing Up Feeling Good* (1983), by Ellen Rosenberg, is a good try that doesn't quite make it. The author has conducted sex education programs in public schools for the last eight years, and the book contains her responses to the thousands of questions asked by her audiences. In the process she seems to have picked up the ten-year-old's funnybone. For instance:

> Wet dreams don't mean you're sickly,
> Just cause they're a little sticky.
> So be cool if you wake up one morning to see
> A "funny" spot that you know is not pee.

Although at first glance the book would seem to be appropriate for junior-high level, the juvenile humor, plus Rosenberg's frequent references to "children" and anecdotes about eleven-year-olds, the apparent age of the people in the illustrations, and, most important, the focus of the text (menstruation, for example is discussed in terms of getting ready for a first period), make it clear that this is a book for fifth and sixth graders, not teens.

Two more books for early adolescents that can be given only lukewarm recommendation are *Threshold*, by Thomas and Lorelie Mintz, and the 1979 edition of *Sex: Telling It Straight*, by Eric Johnson. There is nothing actually wrong with the Johnson book except that the discussion of VD is limited to syphilis and gonorrhea and there is no warning of possible bad effects from an IUD. But it covers the same ground and presents the same attitudes as the author's *Love and Sex in Plain Language* (1985) and does so in a much more terse and less contemporary way.

Threshold: Straightforward Answers to Teenagers' Questions About Sex is a fairly conservative and basic guide for junior-high teenagers, written by a psychiatrist at the University of California Medical School. Each topic is given a brief introduction, which is then followed by twenty or thirty questions and answers, presumably extracted from Mintz's experiences in teaching a sex education class for adolescents. An inordinate number of the questions are fearful: "What if I'm afraid to masturbate?" "Does it hurt to menstruate?" "How old will I be when I start to ejaculate?" and "What do you do if you grow up and discover you just don't like having sex?" There are only a few questions on homosexuality, and the answers imply that some homosexuals can get cured through psychoanalysis. Although the publisher advertised the 1984 printing as "an updated edition," actually it is identical to the 1978 version except for a slight change in the subtitle and the addition of Lorelie Miller Mintz as coauthor.

Don't Worry, You're Normal: A Teenager's Guide to Self-Health, by medical writer Nissa Simon, is like a visit to an informal but not very personable doctor. In a flat but fact-crammed style Simon covers the essentials about health-related topics like nutrition, skin, hair, teeth, posture, sleep, drugs, infectious diseases, emotional concerns, and also basic sexual anatomy and STD. A section on "Sexual questions" touches on birth control. A final chapter describes what a teenager has a right to expect from a complete physical, including, for girls, a brief but not very comforting description of the pelvic examination.

▪ More Sophisticated Books for Early Adolescents

Facts About Sex for Today's Youth, by Sol Gordon, was discussed at some length in its various editions in Chapter 8. In its 1978 and 1985 versions it remains the best guide for unwilling or unskilled readers, both in early adolescence and on up into the late teens. A short and deceptively simple book, its concise text presents all of the essential information in an attractive and dignified format without stuffiness. The handsome illustrations

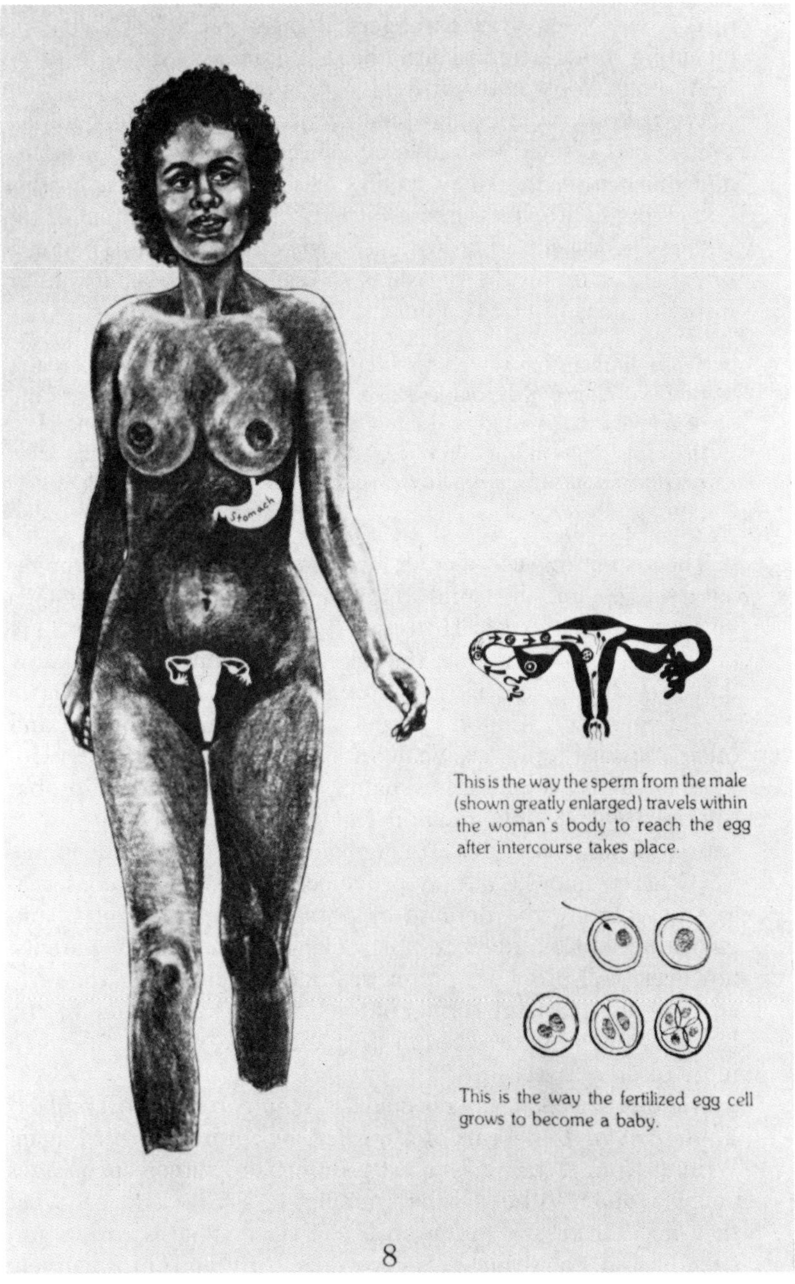

Stomach
This is the way the sperm from the male (shown greatly enlarged) travels within the woman's body to reach the egg after intercourse takes place.
This is the way the fertilized egg cell grows to become a baby.
8

Fig. 14. Young woman. From *Facts About Sex for Today's Youth*, by Sol Gordon (1985 edition).

by Vivien Cohen show teenagers of many racial backgrounds, including some extraordinarily beautiful nudes.

Another book noteworthy for wonderful drawings is *The Facts of Love*, by Alex and Jane Comfort. The simple, compassionate text is filled with lovely pictures by Howard Pemberton and Bill Prosser that show young people caring for each other and enjoying life, but without the explicitly erotic content of the authors' hedonistic adult work, *The Joy of Sex*. Rather *The Facts of Love* celebrates the pleasures of responsible sexuality. In an inspired piece of clarification the Comforts explain:

> Sex in humans has three uses—reproduction, relation, and recreation (in other words, babies, love, and fun). And this is the origin of a lot of the crossed wires and worry which have made one of the best things in life into one of the most anxious for humans. *You need to know which of these three you are after, and which your partner is after.*

The responsible use of contraception is a major theme throughout the book, and the Comforts are adamant in condemning teen love-making without it. However, when proper precautions are taken, sex for play is fine, they maintain, if both people know they are playing and if each is concerned that the other has a good experience. Anatomy, venereal disease, masturbation, and other standard topics are dealt with adequately but briefly. Homosexuality is presented as a matter of preference, since "probably the ability to love anybody, of either sex, physically . . . is natural to humans anyway, though our society doesn't encourage it." Other opinions that may prove controversial with conservative parents are the defense of pornography as harmless and enjoyable and an advocacy of social nudism. Liberal parents, however, will probably prefer this book to any other for early adolescents. The large format of the hardcover is a bit inhibiting, but this fault was corrected in the paperback, which comes in a more discreet size.

Another excellent liberal guide is *Why Am I so Miserable If These Are the Best Years of My Life?*, by Andrea Boroff Eagan. Writing from a strong feminist position, the author encourages young women to be self-determining, to ask for and get what they need from sex and from life. Eagan's tone is strong and friendly but not strident. She writes clearly and informatively about sexual physiology, menstruation, birth control, and STD but also provides sensible guidance on relationships with both boys and girls and on getting along with parents. The chapter on legal rights gives vital facts on rape, juvenile law, the emancipated minor status, and legal rights at school and at home. The 1976 edition has aged surprisingly little and contains nothing that would make it invalid. In the paperback edition of 1979 a few bits of new medical information and an updated bibliography on feminist sexuality were added. A Spanish-language version is available also: *Por Que Me Siento Tan Mal Si Estos Son los Mejores Años de Mi Vida?*

A teen sex manual from television's wise and adorable Dr. Ruth Westheimer should be full of the sparkle that has made her cable TV program, *Good Sex!* and her radio show, *Sexually Speaking*, so popular. Unfortunately, *First Love* (written with educator Dr. Nathan Kravetz) is as flat and dull as yesterday's champagne. Sloppy organization and a tendency to repetitiveness give an impression of hasty composition to take advantage of television's fleeting fame, and Kravetz's attempt to echo the motherly enthusiasm of Dr. Ruth's conversational style succeeds only in being graceless.

More surprising, the advice to young people from the woman who has taught exuberant bedroom athletics to all America is cautious and conservative. Certain passages read as if someone had leaned over her shoulder with a blue pencil, carping, "You can't say *that*! You'll offend the parents!" The effect is schizophrenic. On the one hand Dr. Ruth describes sexual positions and compares the technique of fellatio to licking an ice cream cone, and on the other she repeatedly urges young people to stay at least "technical virgins." She heartily endorses the right to sexual privacy in masturbation for both boys and girls but tells them that if they catch a venereal disease they *must* tell their parents before they get medical help. She also fails to tell young people that they have the right to privacy in seeking birth-control information from a clinic. The chapter on homosexuality is so ambiguously worded that those who disapprove can read their own reactions into it.

On her programs Dr. Ruth often reminds her viewers that she is not a medical doctor; so it is not too surprising to find that although she warns teens about VD, she does not list the diseases or describe the symptoms except in the most general way. But surely it is excessive pussyfooting for a book written in 1985 to avoid even naming chlamydia or AIDS.

Libraries get faint praise in *First Love*: "Often, librarians do not have enough money to buy the books on sexual matters that ought to be in their collections. Therefore, you should also get to a good bookstore and see what books they have on this subject. Libraries may get out-of-date. Bookstores have the long-term good books, and they are also very up-to-date."

However, much of Dr. Ruth's good sense comes through in other places, especially in the discussions of healthy relationships and good communication with parents. And it is certainly appropriate in these times to encourage adolescents to postpone full sexual intercourse. The book will probably be more widely read than other, better sex guides without the magic of a media tie-in. It could have been worse, but with the power of Dr. Ruth's name it's too bad it isn't better.

A catastrophic typographical error sneaked into the first printing of *First Love*. On page 195, in a discussion of the rhythm method of birth control, Westheimer and Kravetz wrote: "The safe times are the week before and the week of ovulation." These days are, of course, exactly the period during which a woman is most likely to conceive, and the passage should have read: "The *unsafe* times are . . ." The error was finally caught by a librarian in New Jersey, having escaped the attention of a number of reviewers (including the author of this book). In a panic, the publisher recalled all copies and ran an urgent advertisement in *Publisher's Weekly* to round up the strays. The second, corrected printing bears a new ISBN number (0-446-34294-7) and a red cover rather than the original white. Librarians and teachers should make sure that this is the version in their collections.

Another sex guide that had its origins in the popular media is *The Teenage Body Book*. As an editor of *Teen* magazine author Kathy McCoy was exposed to the urgency of young readers' questions about sexuality and other problems of coping with adolescence. Drawing on her files of those questions, she has written four books in letter-to-the-editor format that give thoughtful and well-researched answers to these often-desperate queries. *The Teenage Body Book*, written with adolescent-medicine specialist Charles Wibbelsman, uses this Dear Abby style to put sexuality in a perspective of total mind and body health. Beginning with "Dear Doctor: Am I Normal?" the topics range through woman's body, man's body, the changing feelings of adolescence, weight control, exercise, sports injuries, plastic surgery, health habits, psychosomatic illness, and special medical needs of teenagers, such as advice on anorexia nervosa, scoliosis, and Osgood-Schlater disease, as well as the more usual subjects of birth control, STD, abortion, and pregnancy. A broad spectrum of research and attitudes on homosexuality is presented, with quotes from the findings of prominent sex researchers and a testimony from a young lesbian. (In the final analysis "the real question is not whether you're gay or straight, but how you manage your relationships.") In the discussion on intercourse the authors reassure nonparticipators, "As a free—and certainly acceptable—choice virginity is definitely OK," even if "there are times when you begin to feel like the last virgin on earth over the age of 14." Perhaps the most valuable feature of the book is the extensive list of resources: Planned Parenthood clinics, departments of adolescent medicine, gay services, and help centers for special problems, such as alcoholism, asthma, epilepsy, drug abuse, and rape.

A companion volume, *The Teenage Survival Guide*, covers social and emotional problems in more depth than the health orientation of the first book allows. The subjects range from etiquette to pop psychology to career guidance. Only a few pages can be called sex education (in the narrow sense, anyway), but worth mentioning is the thoughtful list of "Honest questions to ask yourself" for the young person who is wondering if he or she is ready for sexual involvement. Unfortunately, the lack of an index hampers the usefulness of both this and the *Body Book*.

Two more books by this author (and probably more to come) replow this fertile field, in some cases repeating older material or—as is more often the case—updating and rewriting it for more effectiveness. In *The Teenage Body Book Guide to Dating* and *The Teenage Body Book Guide to Sexuality* McCoy, while keeping the lively question-and-answer format, extracts, expands, and improves. Many of the changes are stylistic. Given the opportunity to rethink and rewrite, she has tightened and honed her prose without actually changing the content, and second thoughts have led to subtler ideas and insights. Other significant changes are the addition of new medical and statistical data. The section on STD is one of the best in the literature for teens, describing symptoms, treatments, and dangers of ten diseases in some depth and adding "a special note about hepatitis" and "a special warning to gays." All four of these books show responsible research, are highly readable and appealing to teens, and deserve a prominent place in library collections.

McCoy's *Teenage Survival Guide* should not be confused with Sol Gordon's *Teenage Survival Book*. This was a misguided attempt in 1981 to revive *You*, the self-consciously super-hang-loose sex and life manual that had been so popular in the seventies. Little was changed, although at first glance it seemed that the inside of the book was as new as the title because the author had scrambled the contents around. Gordon also dropped much of the most valuable part of the original: four of those six notorious and raunchy comics. The leftover space was filled in with a lot of Gordon's own poetry, a long piece on Margaret Sanger by Toby Clinch, an inappropriate article entitled "Toward a successful marriage," and some updated book lists. What had seemed like so much fun in 1975 now looked merely sloppy and random.

Boys have special sex education needs that are complicated by social pressures to pretend that they already know everything. As Deryck Calderwood has written (*SIECUS Report*, November 1984): "Boys' development of sexuality is presocial, while girls learn to be sexual within the context of social relationships. The experience of masturbation for boys contributes to this more genitally oriented view of sexuality." In other words, girls worry about whether they're doing the right thing and boys worry about whether they're doing the thing right. Or if they're ever going to get to do the thing at all.

One of the few books that has made a realistic attempt to address these dilemmas is *A Young Man's Guide to Sex*, by Jay Gale. His style conveys real understanding of what it is like to be an adolescent male today. His writing is warm and often humorous. The first chapter, for instance, is woven around a Bill Cosby monologue about a terrified kid who tries to find out from his bluffing friends how to do it "The Regular Way." As Gale tells young men, "*As long as you compare your actual sexual performance against that of your fantasies, or against what you believe to be the sexual experiences of other boys, you will feel sexually inadequate.*" It is refreshing to see topics like contraception and abortion treated from the viewpoint of male responsibility. Gale's information on these and other topics is complete and dependable without being clinical.

Unfortunately, the book is seriously flawed by the author's orientation as a sex therapist toward what can go wrong—which is almost everything, according to his anecdotal evidence. Malfunctions and mistakes are anticipated at every turn, and a heavy pall of negativity lies over all. The description of sexual intercourse is followed by two pages of questions all beginning, "I'm afraid. . . ." Although his factual treatment of homosexuality is impeccable, a worrisome story about a boy whose life was nearly ruined by an early same-sex encounter appears twice in other places in the text. And worse, there are ludicrous instructions for little step-by-step exercises in sexual communication, sensate focusing, and masturbation that read like homework assignments from a sex therapist. In final analysis Gale seems to create as much anxiety as he alleviates.

Another book that is seriously flawed is *Loving Sex for Both Sexes*, by Dale Carlson. The author, a young adult and children's novelist, has no qualifications for the subject other than enthusiasm, and her lack of expertise leads her into some peculiar errors and assertions (sexuality, she claims, "is programmed by the unconscious child voice of the parent of the opposite sex"). A general air of uncertainty pervades her discussions of anatomy and sexual functioning. Although Carlson is on firmer ground with feelings and emotions, she has a tendency toward alarming neo-Freudian arabesques, such as her definition of love as a result of interlocking neurotic behavior patterns between two needy personalities.

▪ Guides for Literate Middle Teens

A liberal book for thoughtful young adults who will not be put off by an old-fashioned style is *Sex, with Love*, by Eleanor Hamilton. The first two chapters read as if they had been written by Great-Aunt Sarah ("Make no mistake about it, you are in for *fun* as you move forward into the wonderful topsy-turvy time of puberty"), but later the book settles down into a pleasantly sex-positive tone.

The emphasis is on understanding sex as an activity between two people who want to give each other pleasure. Repeating the then-radical philosophy first expressed in her 1969 book *Sex Before Marriage*, Hamilton approves of masturbation as a way to learn the body's responses, and she suggests petting to orgasm as the preferred method of lovemaking for young people up to the age of about seventeen, both because it trains the mind and body for leisurely sex and because it avoids the difficulties of birth control. Hamilton describes intercourse in terms of both male and female patterns, with emphasis on the more complex female response.

The chapter on same-sex relationships starts with the assumption that everybody is capable of loving both sexes; the way that people choose to express that love is a result of society's pressures and their own life experiences. "Deviant" sex is divided into those behaviors that exploit other people—rape, exhibitionism, voyeurism, child molesting—and those that Hamilton suggests are nobody's business but the participants—transsexuality, transvestism, fetishes, and brother-sister incest.

Recognizing that sexuality encompasses not just genital contact but a person's whole joy in life, Hamilton urges young people to touch each other with affection and to learn the giving art of massage. In a throwback to the birds and the bees, but with a modern twist, there is an intriguing chapter on bizarre animal mating behaviors. Although the section on VD is limited to syphilis and gonorrhea and there are no photographs or diagrams in the book, essential factual data are otherwise adequate. But Hamilton's primary interest is communicating sexual values, and this she does with warmth and intelligence and a degree of sophistication that contrasts oddly with her rather elderly style. A sensible suggestion, but one that might prove controversial with conservative parents, is her idea that young people should initiate a frank talk at home (she gives exact directions) in which they ask for the right to have comfortable and safe sex with their partners in their own rooms behind locked doors. "Here they have to 'put their money where their mouth is,'" Hamilton crows, "or else acknowledge to themselves and to their children that sex is *not* good after all (which they know to be a patent lie)."

For older young adults who read well and who are ready to consider mature concepts of love and relationship Gary F. Kelly's *Learning About Sex: The Contemporary Guide for Young Adults* remains an excellent guide in spite of its 1977 publication date. Kelly, a sex counselor, clearly and objectively explains many of the complex psychosocial aspects of sexual behavior. Without offering advice, he presents the moral issues within the perspective of our pluralistic society and provides self-quizzes and discussion questions to help young people think through their own positions. The author explores newly evolved concepts of masculinity and femininity; his information on the clitoral function is helpful and accurate; and he discredits the theory that girls are slower to become aroused and therefore should be responsible for limiting the couple's sexual activity. A thorough and sympathetic discussion of homosexuality appears in the chapter "Different strokes for different folks." Kelly examines changing attitudes toward marriage and describes alternative ways of structuring a committed relationship, paying attention to their potential benefits and pitfalls. He gives well-selected lists of further reading at the end of each chapter and a glossary of "four-letter and other words." Although the emphasis is on the interpersonal aspects of sex, biology is not neglected.

As might be expected from its age, the book reflects the seventies consciousness rather more than the new conservatism, but not in a trendy or dated way. The discussion of VD, as might also be expected, omits herpes, AIDS, and NGU. But this is relatively untroublesome because the main thrust of the book is toward establishing loving relationships of all kinds in a broad context of social responsibility.

In *Learning About Sex* Kelly avoids the fault, so common to other sex counselors, of unduly stressing malfunction; he lumps all of this material in a chapter on "Sex problems" and allows the rest of the book to concentrate on healthy patterns. Medical sexual therapists who write are often not so capable of rising above the immersion in pathology of their daily practice. We have seen this in Jay Gale's *A Young Man's Guide to Sex*. Another example of this morbid orientation is *Making Sense of Sex: The New Facts About Sex and Love for Young People*, by Helen Singer Kaplan. The author is a highly respected sex therapist and head of the Human Sexuality Program of the Payne Whitney

Clinic at New York Hospital/Cornell Medical Center. As might be expected, she provides a thorough discussion of sexual problems—dysfunctions, variations, and gender disturbances—but also gives scrupulously detailed and accurate material on the internal and external physiology of sex and the biology of reproduction, including much that has been only recently discovered. Her style is cool and meticulous, if somewhat distant, except for the surprisingly erotic description of coitus that opens the first chapter. She makes no moral judgments on behavior other than to affirm that "sex is a natural human function which we have a right to enjoy."

A review of *Making Sense of Sex* in the March 1980 *SIECUS Report*, written by fellow sex educator Gary Kelly, found that "some of Kaplan's fundamental approaches do not represent sound sex education." Although he admitted that from a factual standpoint the book had much of value and "a very positive outlook on many aspects of human sexuality," he criticized her use of technical jargon and the discussion of "subtle relational concepts, much of which is simply too high powered for the average adolescent." More seriously, he claimed that the book "reflects some specific value stances, ranging from the psychoanalytic orientation in discussing the life cycle (Oedipal period, latency period) to the psychiatric judgment that exclusive or intense variant sexual behavior grows out of psychological conflict." In other words, he was wary of Kaplan's statement that "most authorities believe that homosexuality usually results from a disturbed emotional relationship between child and parents." All of these objections are serious enough to limit severely the book's usefulness, even with older teens.

Another nonrecommended title is *Like, Love, Lust: A View of Sex and Sexuality*, by John Langone. This book was completed when its author was a Fellow at the Center for Advanced Study in the Behavioral Sciences at Stanford, California. As such it is typical of the worst aspects of academic pseudo-scholarship. The heart of the book is made up of three essays on pornography, prostitution, and homosexuality that are a pastiche of undigested quotes from a mishmash of sources, without relevance or unifying point of view. The chapter on homosexuality is obliquely loaded by quoting extensively from antigay sources after each nonjudgmental statement. The material has been padded into a book by adding superficial and disjointed chapters on friendship, jealousy, sex and morality, and so on, but no coherent statement of guidance for young adults emerges.

▪ Highest Recommendation

And now for something more positive. *Changing Bodies, Changing Lives*, edited by Ruth Bell, is the most comprehensive, thorough, readable, realistic, and humane sex education book for older teens ever written. The editor was one of the group that produced *Our Bodies, Ourselves*, and she has patterned this book for teens on that landmark work. This, too, is a group effort. Hundreds of young adults all over the country shared their concerns, experiences, and questions with the many experts who wrote chapters for the book. Their words, interspersed throughout the text in anecdotes and vivid observations, give the book a relevance and immediacy that are often lacking in sex education guides written out of clinical research or, worse, out of an author's own teen memories.

The approach is completely holistic. "To us," say the authors, "being sexual and having sexual feelings is part of who we are, and part of what we bring into loving someone else." This whole-person orientation is reflected in the organization of the material. The book begins traditionally, with a description of the physical changes of adolescence and the feelings teens have about those changes. Then it moves on to new ground to discuss changes in relationships with parents and friends, exploring sex with yourself, exploring sex with someone else, sex against your will, emotional health care (including drugs and alcohol), and physical health care (including birth control, pregnancy, and sexually transmitted diseases). Each topic is grounded in reality by pithy quotations from the interviews with teens, and the authors are careful to present a variety of viewpoints and opinions.

The lengthiness of *Changing Bodies* allows topics to be treated in depth, and a number of ideas and insights emerge that have rarely or never been explored before in sex ed books. A few examples: the section on birth control includes not only methodology but a crucial discussion of the psychological reasons for the reluctance of many teens to use contraception. The emotional aspects of abortion, too, are aired, and the description of the methods used to end a pregnancy covers not only techniques but also the probable sensations of the woman undergoing each operation. The choice of a same-sex partner is included as an option throughout the book and as a natural part of the chapter on "Exploring sex with someone else." The book offers a new perspective on rape in the concept of "acquaintance rape" and puts sexually transmitted diseases in a new light by expanding this category to include such nonstigmatized ills as hepatitis. The freshness of this approach is apparent all through the book.

The authors have been careful to see that the moral and emotional dimensions of sexuality are not divorced from the physiology and they present a variety of opinions, usually in the young people's own words. The authors are especially aware of the need to bolster the young person who feels unready for sexual activity in spite of peer pressure to participate. Like Alex Comfort, they make no pretense at impartiality about birth-control methods and emphatically favor a combination of condom and foam or—preferably—mutual masturbation to orgasm.

The text is inviting. Each subject is given perspective and depth with conversations, stories, and touchingly beautiful poems from the young people themselves. The diagrams are clear and instructive, but there are also amusing posters and delightful snapshots of teens going about their lives.

Changing Bodies, Changing Lives is a superb sex education book, the culmination of all that is good in the genre. Why then, is there any need for other books? Why not hand this one out to every young person at puberty and let it go at that? Because, for one reason, although all teenagers are capable of sex, they are not all capable of reading this book. A simpler, thinner guide is necessary for those who are less than literate. Then, too, there are ultraconservative parents who find the book's open recognition of adolescent sexual activity threatening, even though their own values of abstinence are included as one possible option. A more muted book is their preference. And further, *Changing Bodies, Changing Lives* is not a first book for new adolescents. A more cautious, reassuring primer is needed as an introdution to puberty before they are ready for this book's total revelation. Last, we need to recognize that even this fine sex information book will become dated after a while and need to be replaced with some new Champion Sex Guide.

■ Sex Books for Special Needs

One way in which the old model of the sex manual is changing is in reaching out to specialized audiences that have not been addressed before. An important reader whose need for information and reassurance has previously been ignored is the adolescent homosexual. With the single exception of *Changing Bodies, Changing Lives*, the guides have been unanimous in what they had to say about the subject. A few homosexual incidents, they comforted, were nothing to worry about—lots of people do that occasionally when they're young and it doesn't mean you're going to grow up to be homosexual. This statement is always followed by supportive words for gay rights and disclaimers for the stereotypes, but for the young person who not only suspects, but *knows*, that he or she is gay, the damage has been done. His or her sexual preference has been described as a condition to be dreaded, a disease to be suspected from the symptoms. The assumption is always that the author is talking to a straight person—"you"—as contrasted with gays—"them." The experts now estimate that ten percent of the population may have mostly, or entirely, same-sex preference. Since we also now know that this identity is established at least as early as age six or seven, this means that ten percent of the teenage population is being excluded from the sexual guidance and reassurance they so desperately need.

Or were, until the 1979 publication of *A Way of Love, a Way of Life: A Young Person's Introduction to What It Means to Be Gay*, by Frances Hanckel and John Cunningham. This sensitive book offers compassionate support to young people who are struggling to clarify their sexual identity and can be read with benefit by both hetero- and homosexuals. Both authors are gay activists; Hanckel has been a hospital administrator and research technician, and Cunningham is a young adult librarian. Together they bring a diversity of understanding and sensitivity to this insider's view of gayness for young adults. They tackle such crucial problems as how to tell if you are or are not gay, how to "come out" to parents and friends and how to meet other gay people. A history of homosexuality stresses the homophile nature of ancient Greek civilization and gives perspective to our own society's attitudes. The book demystifies the legal and medical problems special to gays and urges young people to seek help if they need it—lists of sources of information, counseling, and gay-pride organizations tell where. The chapter on sexual activity is especially striking in its complete freedom from gender identification: "Sexual activity is basically the same for everyone," say Hanckel and Cunningham, and they go on to prove it by describing the range of human possibilities in the sex act, regardless of whether the partners are of the same or the opposite sex. Throughout the book the photographs and anecdotes from homosexual and lesbian friends, particularly a stereotype-destroying section called "A Dozen Gay Lives," make the book come alive.

One criticism only: since the book was written in 1979, AIDS is not mentioned, and casual sex with multiple partners is given more acceptance than might now be the case. Some cautionary words might be appropriate in a new edition. Otherwise this excellent book fills a gap in all library collections, even, or especially, in places where the ten percent have not yet felt free to become visible.

An additional introduction to gay life for teens is *Young, Gay and Proud!* by the editors of Alyson Press. Although libraries may find it problematic because of its use of four-letter words for sexual activities, it does spell out the precautions that are necessary to reduce the risk of AIDS.

Another book written with special needs in mind is *Sex Education for Physically Handicapped Youth*, by C. Edmund Hopper and William A. Allen. It is heartening that such a book exists at all, but it is too bad that it isn't better. The sexual information is minimally adequate, but the style is heavy and stilted. The best parts of the book are the sections that specifically relate to problems of the handicapped—developing a good self-concept, meeting other handicapped youths, learning about genetics and the implications for passing on a defect, getting around town with the help of ramps and railings, contacting helping agencies and referral services for counseling and employment.

But when it comes to actual sex education, Hopper and Allen are markedly uncomfortable. This shows up in a coyness of vocabulary, an unwillingness to give things their proper names: "sexual parts" for vulva, "pass water" for urinate, "stretching of a part of her genitals" for breaking the hymen. Nowhere—not in the description of intercourse or masturbation or in the index or glossary—is the clitoris named. Gender roles are described in terms of stereotypes. Sexual molestation is discussed in the chapter on homosexuality; elaborate precautions and warnings about public toilets appear in the chapter on VD; and masturbation is given only uneasy approval: "If you never start the habit, you'll never miss it." These flaws would be enough to disqualify a book addressed to the general public, but handicapped teenagers are so in need of recognition as whole and sexual persons that this guide can be used until a better one comes along.

▪ Fifties Dating Guides for the Eighties

One result of this decade's pendulum swing back to more conventional values and social behavior is the revival of dating. This peculiarly American courtship ritual had nearly died out in the freer sexual climate of the sixties and seventies. When it rose from the dead in the early eighties, the know-how had been lost, and a flood of dating-etiquette books appeared to remind teens of the rules. These harked back with almost eerie faithfulness to the pattern that had been laid down by Evelyn Duvall in 1950.

Although most of these are "little" paperbacks that quickly come and go, one hardcover title of this type is *The Teen Guide to Dating*, by Elaine Landau. In an age of New Wave rock, pregnant twelve-year-olds, and epidemic AIDS this author natters on about hay rides and "fast guys" and "ladies' choice" dances; acknowledges homosexuality only in one sentence (wrong reasons for having sex: "to prove that you are not a homosexual"); and draws a Disney-sanitized picture of dating that would have been unrealistic even thirty years ago.

A far more contemporary interpretation of the form is *The Teen Dating Guide*, by Marjabelle Young Stewart. The author touches all the familiar bases: how to start, what to do on a first (and second) date, how to give parties, how to cope with parents, what to say on a date, how to break up. She brings up the subject of sex briefly but refers readers to *Changing Bodies, Changing Lives* and *The Facts of Love* for more in-depth advice. Stewart takes into account the new egalitarianism in gender roles. Girls are told that sharing expenses is an obligation and that it is fine to call a boy for a date (but not too often). Young men are instructed to get used to asking about a girl's interests and opinions instead of talking about themselves all evening, and they are assured that it's perfectly OK for a girl to be better at some things than they are.

A number of other paperbacks of this type deal with the lighter aspects of boy-girl relations. Often they are spin-offs from the popular teen-romance series: *The Sweet Dreams Love Book*, by Deidre S. Laiken and Alan J. Schneider, for instance, or *Sweet Dreams How to Talk to Boys*, by Catherine Winters. Almost invariably they are addressed to girls, even when they are written by experts on the boys' point of view, like Peter Filichia, who speaks to young women in *A Boy's-Eye View of Girls*. A title that shows psychological insight beyond the average standard for these books is *Romance! Can You Survive It? A Guide to Sticky Dating Situations*, by Meg Schneider. These and other paperbacks of their kind are usually sensible, appealing, and useful to adolescents learning new social skills. But they are not a substitute for sound sex education. For that we still have to rely on the good old sex information guides that we have evaluated in this chapter.

■ BIBLIOGRAPHY

(Note: This is a list of books mentioned in this chapter; inclusion does not necessarily mean recommendation. For Core Collection List see Appendix.)

Bell, Ruth, et al. *Changing Bodies, Changing Lives: A Book for Teens on Sex and Relationships*. New York: Random House, 1980.

Betancourt, Jeanne. *Am I Normal? An Illustrated Guide to Your Changing Body*. New York: Avon Flare, 1983.

———. *Dear Diary: An Illustrated Guide to Your Changing Body*. New York: Avon Flare, 1983.

Carlson, Dale. *Loving Sex for Both Sexes*. New York: Watts, 1979.

Comfort, Alex, and Jane Comfort. *The Facts of Love: Loving, Living, and Growing Up*. New York: Crown, 1979; New York: Ballantine, 1980.

Eagan, Andrea Boroff. *Por Que Me Siento Tan Mal Si Estos Son los Mejores Años de Mi Vida?* Philadelphia: Lippincott, 1979.

———. *Why Am I So Miserable If These Are the Best Years of My Life? A Survival Guide for the Young Woman*. Philadelphia: Lippincott, 1976; rev. ed., New York: Avon, 1979.

Filichia, Peter. *A Boy's-Eye View of Girls*. New York: Scholastic, 1983.

Gale, Jay. *A Young Man's Guide to Sex*. New York: Holt, Rinehart and Winston, 1984.

Gordon, Sol. *Facts About Sex for Today's Youth*, rev. ed. Fayetteville, N.Y.: Ed-U, 1978, 1985.

———. *The Teenage Survival Book*. New York: Times Books; rev. ed. of *You*, 1981.

Hamilton, Eleanor. *Sex, with Love: A Guide for Young People*. Boston: Beacon, 1978.

Hanckel, Frances, and John Cunningham. *A Way of Love, a Way of Life: A Young Person's Introduction to What It Means to Be Gay*. New York: Lothrop, Lee and Shepard, 1979.

Hopper, C. Edmund, and William A. Allen. *Sex Education for Physically Handicapped Youth*. Springfield, Ill.: Thomas, 1980.

Johnson, Eric W. *Love and Sex in Plain Language*, 4th rev. ed. New York: Harper and Row, 1985.

———. *Sex: Telling It Straight*, rev. ed. Philadelphia: Lippincott, 1979.

Kaplan, Helen Singer. *Making Sense of Sex: The New Facts About Sex and Love for Young People*. New York: Simon and Schuster, 1979.

Kelly, Gary F. *Learning About Sex: The Contemporary Guide for Young Adults*. Woodbury, N.Y.: Barron's Educational Series, 1976; rev. ed., 1977.

Laiken, Deidre S., and Alan J. Schneider. *The Sweet Dreams Love Book: Understanding Your Feelings*. New York: Bantam, 1983.

Landau, Elaine. *The Teen Guide to Dating*. New York: Messner, 1980.

Langone, John. *Like, Love, Lust: A View of Sex and Sexuality*. Boston: Little, Brown, 1980.

McCoy, Kathy. *The Teenage Body Book Guide to Dating*. New York: Simon and Schuster, 1983.

———. *The Teenage Body Book Guide to Sexuality*. New York: Simon and Schuster, 1983.

———. *The Teenage Survival Guide: Coping with Problems in Everyday Life*. New York: Simon and Schuster, 1981.

———, and Charles Wibbelsman. *The Teenage Body Book.* New York: Simon and Schuster, 1978.

Madaras, Lynda, with Area Madaras. *What's Happening to My Body? A Growing Up Guide for Mothers and Daughters.* New York: Newmarket, 1983.

Madaras, Lynda, with Dane Saavedra. *The What's Happening to My Body? Book for Boys: A Growing Up Guide for Parents and Sons.* New York: Newmarket, 1984.

Mintz, Thomas, and Lorelie Miller Mintz. *Threshold: Straightforward Answers to Teenagers' Questions About Sex.* New York: Walker, 1978.

Pomeroy, Wardell B. *Boys and Sex*, rev. ed. New York: Delacorte, 1981.

———. *Girls and Sex*, rev. ed. New York: Delacorte, 1981.

Rosenberg, Ellen. *Growing Up Feeling Good.* New York: Beaufort, 1983.

Schneider, Meg. *Romance! Can You Survive It? A Guide to Sticky Dating Situations.* New York: Dell, 1984.

Simon, Nissa. *Don't Worry, You're Normal: A Teenager's Guide to Self-Health.* New York: Crowell, 1982.

Stewart, Marjabelle Young. *The Teen Dating Guide.* New York: Signet Vista, 1984.

Westheimer, Ruth, and Nathan Kravetz. *First Love: A Young People's Guide to Sexual Information.* New York: Warner, 1985.

Winters, Catherine. *Sweet Dreams How to Talk to Boys and Other Important People.* New York: Bantam, 1983.

Young, Gay and Proud!, 2nd ed. Boston: Alyson, 1985.

Chapter 10

Young Adult Fiction as Sex Education

"God, don't you hate those books for teenagers where they *have* to get married and she drops out of school and they live over a garage and he works in some used car lot. And there's always some scene where some girl who had an abortion comes to visit and she's gone insane and becomes a Bowery bum, just in case you didn't get the point," says Leda bitterly in *Beginner's Love*, by Norma Klein.

> Every other book I've read since I was *ten* is like that. The girl's a moron, the guy's a moron, they never heard of birth control. What I love are the scenes where the father takes the guy aside and says, "Son, if you marry Betsy, you'll have to give up your football scholarship to Oklahoma State." They're *always* going to some godforsaken place like Oklahoma State! And the guy says, "But, Dad, I love her!" . . . And then there's a scene where the mother says, "Dear, you haven't let him take advantage of you? You know what boys are like." Quote, unquote. . . . God, I think writers must be really dumb! Or else they're living in the Stone Age.

Leda's resentment is only marginally related to literary quality here. What is really bothering her, now as she faces an abortion decision of her own, is that she realizes that all those young adult novels she has read so faithfully have been lying about reality. She has been cheated. What she thought she had learned from fiction turns out to be no help at all in coping with life.

Of course, Klein—who is one of the most sexually outspoken young adult novelists—has tongue in cheek to some extent in this passage. The intent is satiric, and the description is accurate only for books written before the last decade. But Leda's feeling of betrayal *is* accurate.

Story is the essence of fiction, and story by its very nature must present the actions of a particular set of characters in a particular set of circumstances. Sometimes these may be quite atypical. A novelist's intention is not primarily to provide a universal model for behavior but simply to tell a good tale.

Yet people in their teens have not had enough experience with life to be able to tell when a "realistic" story reflects the norm and when it sails off on flights of individuality. Whether the writers like it or not, young adult fiction inevitably has a didactic function. Adolescents thirsty for clues on how to behave, talk, dress, read it for guidance. They identify strongly with the characters and often measure themselves against them. Fiction provides reality checks for the reader's self-image, an answer to the nagging worry, "Am I normal?" Teenagers take comfort and reassurance in learning that they are not the only ones who are embarrassed, uncertain, or scared. They look for role models. The authors of young adult novels may decline the responsibility of being teachers as well as storytellers, but teenagers will nevertheless continue to embrace their favorite "realistic" books—and even romances—as pictures of the world the way it's supposed to be.

The implications for sexuality education are obvious. As Pamela Pollack wrote in the *SIECUS Report*, May 1977:

> Potentially, children's fiction dealing with sexual themes can answer the same questions as nonfiction on the topic, and do so in a more immediate and involving way. Thus it presents a great opportunity not only to provide young people with scientific facts about sex, but also to deal with the emotional and attitudinal concerns that young people have about their own sexuality—and to do it in a form more palatable than some instructional materials, reaching many children who would not turn to formal (nonfiction) sex education books.

Or as young adult author Lois Ruby wrote in *Top of the News*, Winter 1980:

> In books for young adults we can teach about family planning, contraception, abortion, homosexuality, VD, through fictional characters, in a nonthreatening way. We can teach young people our own biases, which isn't necessarily bad to do. For example, we can

> show that sex without affection or respect is empty and not much more enjoyable than getting one's kicks going up and down on a merry-go-round pony.

Fiction, she says, can be very good at providing "behavior models, or at least rotten examples." Another of fiction's strengths is in communicating the integrated, holistic view of sexuality. The principles of good relationships are far more easily absorbed in the form of boy-meets-girl than as a dry list in a sex ed book. Emotions and sensations are best explained in story—including the answer to that urgent question, "What does It feel like?" Values, too—the struggle to define them and then the struggle to act on them—have long been the meat of fiction. And—as writers have known since paper was invented—young people will read stories about sex eagerly.

This last point is the problem. Explicit, even if educational, sex in young adult fiction is alarming to many people. Sex education in the form of a novel is subject to public attack and censorship attempts to a degree that most sex manuals, with their aura of clinical respectability, have never been (until recently). The trouble is, sex in a story is erotic. And as we have already seen, to combine sex education with titillation is the ultimate Forbidden. But to require books that teach the techniques and emotions of sex *not* to be arousing is as paradoxical and nonsensical as to prohibit cookbooks from inspiring hunger. Nothing shows the sex-negativity of our culture more clearly than this artificial divorce between sexual learning and sexual feeling. If sex is healthy and good, why should it not be all right for young people to learn about it by reading a pleasantly sexy story?

■ A Perfect Sex Education Novel

The answer to that question is revealed in the intensity of negative parental reaction to Judy Blume's novel *Forever*—and in the intensity of positive reaction it inspires in young people. It often seems that the better the quality of sexual learning in a young adult novel the more controversial it will be. *Forever* has been called the perfect sex education book by its proponents, although that was undoubtedly not the author's intent. Except for

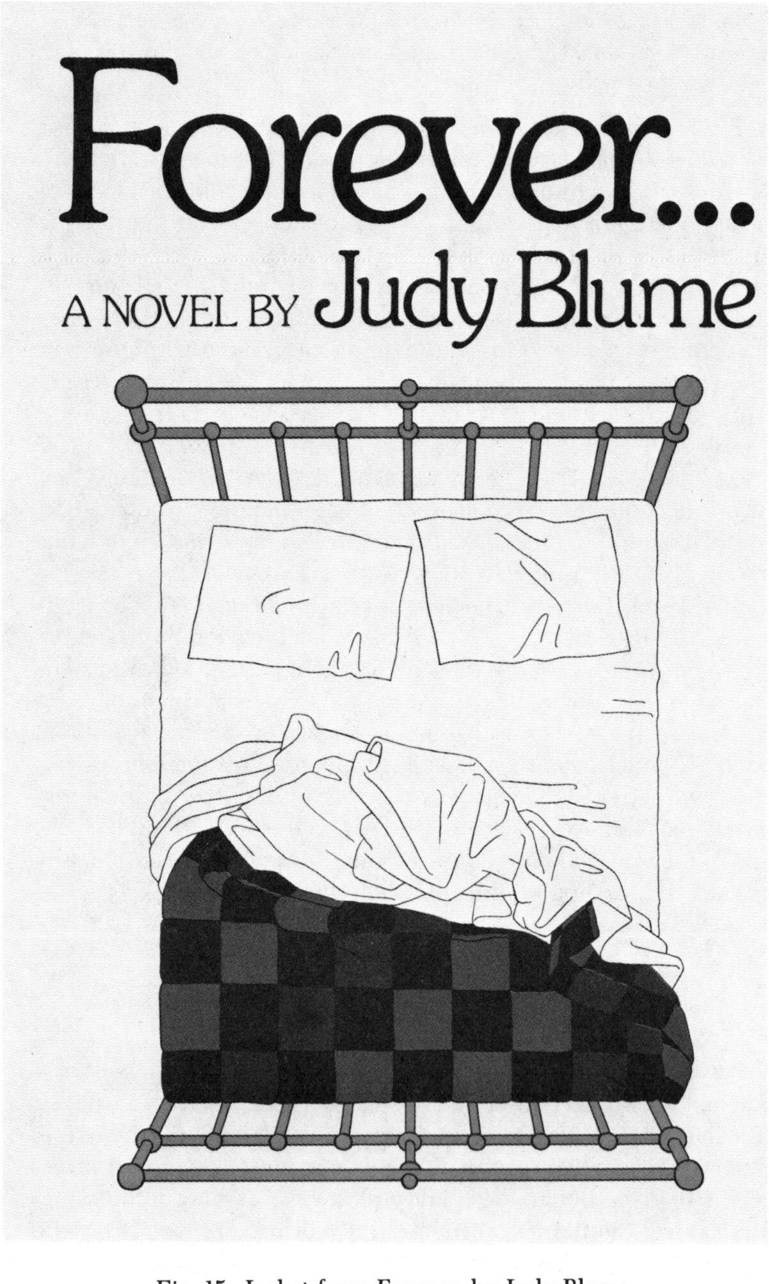

Fig. 15. Jacket from *Forever*, by Judy Blume.

the fact that it is so well-written, it might even be regarded as a case history designed to illustrate the principles of good sexual hygiene and relationship.

With delicacy and wit Blume tells the story of two nice normal kids in love for the first time. *Forever* is a romance in the sense that it is a love story, but it is not romanticized. Rather it is reality beyond reality, an ideal model for sexual unfolding if, for once, everything went exactly the way it should. Katherine and Michael are almost eighteen, intelligent and healthy, and their families are liberal, educated, financially comfortable. Katherine's family is especially attractive; her mother is a slim, witty children's librarian, her father is a handsome, tennis-playing pharmacist, and her younger sister is adorable and talented. They all get along superbly. The parents are still in love and show it; Katherine is fond of her little sister and vice versa. Everyone exudes mental health and good communication skills, even under stress. And, as Eleanor Hamilton advised in *Sex with Love*, Katherine's parents prefer that she bring her dates home to privacy and safety in the den rather than neck in parked cars.

At the beginning of the story Katherine and her best friend, Erica, are aware if not yet experienced. They know the basic facts and are even up to sophisticated jokes: when Katherine teases Erica that she is so short she'd only come up to Michael's bellybutton, Erica retorts, "He might like that!" Katherine's mother has told her how things used to be—how there were Nice Girls and Bad Girls—but they agree that these attitudes belong to the past. Katherine happily accepts her own parents' sexuality—she hears them making love sometimes—and they provide her with a loving example of a good relationship. This example is a form of sex education more valuable than the "little talks" they try dutifully to deliver when it becomes obvious that Katherine and Michael are deeply involved. By showing that these near-perfect parents still are inarticulate about sex instruction with their own daughter, Blume seems to be acknowledging that such education is more comfortably done by others and that a young person's sex life should be private. Katherine's mother later brings her a newspaper clipping that gives a list of "get ready" questions (ironically, just after she has already lost her virginity), but it is Katherine's lawyer grandmother who discreetly sends her some fact-filled pamphlets and encourages her to go to Planned Parenthood for contraception. When Katherine makes the appointment, however, she doesn't tell her grandmother because "I want it to be my own experience." She has been taught responsibility in this, as other things, by parents who care but don't clutch. For example, Katherine has no curfew but is supposed to let her parents know when she gets home.

Michael, too, is responsible and self-respecting, although he is more sensitive than practical Katherine and therefore more vulnerable. In the end it is he who is abandoned. This switch of traditional roles is one of the features (in addition to its literary quality) that distinguishes *Forever* from stereotyped formula romances. Michael is not the typical teenage dreamboat: he is tall and thin, has red hair and a mole on his cheek, wears glasses. (His habit of taking them off before he kisses is an endearing touch.) Michael is aggressive in his pursuit of Katherine. He desires her passionately, and Blume makes the physical evidence of this very clear. Yet he is considerate enough to let Katherine set the pace of their lovemaking. He might implore, but he never pressures. "Are you still a virgin?" he asks on their first date, so that he will know how cautiously to proceed. "It's nothing to be ashamed of," he reassures her—and the reader.

Katherine is a virgin by choice, although she has had opportunities. The year before she had rejected a boy who pressured her too heavily: "Sex was all he was ever interested in, which is why we broke up—because he threatened that if I wouldn't sleep with him he'd find somebody who would. . . . I told him if that was all he cared about he should go right ahead." Yet with the right boy she comes sensually alive, giving the lie to the sex education myth of the cool adolescent female. At first sight of Michael she thinks immediately of touching the mole on his cheek. On their first date at the movies she says to herself, "All I could think about was later," and when later comes and Michael uses his tongue when he kisses her she admits, "I wanted him to." But Katherine is not ready for intercourse, not because of any moral reluctance but because she needs time to be "mentally ready" for complete intimacy. Michael respects her requirement to go slowly.

Blume chronicles the progression of their lovemaking in a series of surprisingly (some would say shockingly) graphic scenes. But these scenes have a quality of innocent wonder that removes any taint of coarseness. Only after Michael and Katherine have been dating for five weeks do they proceed beyond kissing to above-the-waist touching, lying on a firelit rug in the den. Katherine stops Michael from going any further because another couple is in the house, but later she wonders if she might have allowed more intimacy if they had been alone. After several more dates, during which they play and talk and get to know each other better, they again have an opportunity for intimacy. They have just made up from a misunderstanding and have reached a new level of honesty. This time Katherine allows more and promises "the whole thing" soon. Both of them expect that "soon" has come when they plan a skiing weekend with Michael's sister and brother-in-law, but Katherine gets her period and so they sleep together in innocent near-nudity, but without heavy petting. The next night they learn to satisfy each other without intercourse, and by the time the weekend is over they have spoken as well as acted their love.

A few weeks later Michael gets the key to his sister's apartment, where they can be alone. By now they are comfortable with each other's sexual needs and know how to give satisfaction easily. The next night Katherine is ready at last for intercourse. But their first attempt is a fiasco—Michael climaxes before entering her. He is embarrassed, but she is matter-of-fact, and the difficulty is overcome after they have gone out for hamburgers and come back ready to try again. The defloration scene is instructively explicit:

> This time I tried to relax and think of nothing—nothing but how my body felt—and then Ralph was pushing against me and I whispered, "Are you in . . . are we doing it?"
>
> "Not yet," Michael said, pushing harder. "I don't want to hurt you."
>
> "Don't worry . . . just do it!"
>
> "I'm trying, Kath . . . but it's very tight in there."
>
> "What should I do?"
>
> "Can you spread your legs some more . . . and maybe raise them a little?"
>
> "Like this?"
>
> "That's better . . . much better."
>
> I could feel him halfway inside me and then Michael whispered, "Kath. . . ."
>
> "What?"
>
> "I think I'm going to come again."
>
> I felt a big thrust, followed by a quick sharp pain that made me suck in my breath. "Oh . . . oh," Michael cried, but I didn't come. I

wasn't even close. "I'm sorry," he said, "I couldn't hold off." He stopped moving. "It wasn't any good for you, was it?"

"Everybody says the first time is no good for a virgin. I'm not disappointed." But I was. I'd wanted it to be perfect.

It takes them several weeks to get their dynamics synchronized, and Katherine has begun to wonder "if things would ever work out right between us." But finally it does, and in another instructive scene Katherine takes an active part in achieving her own orgasm. From this point the story moves through other plot complications toward a conclusion. In one last sexual scene Katherine has become so much at ease that she initiates lovemaking and takes the position on top. These scenes in their variety and realism are excellent answers to the burning curiosity of young people about the emotions and sensations of intercourse. They provide healthy models for physical love that otherwise exist in fiction only in adult versions, which often are too sophisticated or even violent or pornographic.

The relationship of Katherine and Michael is emotional and mental as well as physical. They are truly in love, within the limits of their age. The most striking feature of their partnering is how open and plain-speaking they are together. Between them is no pretense, no coyness, artifice, strategy. They really try to tell each other what they think honestly, even when they quarrel. Many sex educators have defined the essence of an ethical sexual relationship as good communication, and young readers can learn the beauty of this skill from watching Katherine and Michael. Both are interested in knowing the other's thoughts and feelings, although they do not have many deep thoughts to share. Their lovemaking develops naturally from their growing closeness. As Katherine says, "I can't imagine what the first time would be like with someone you didn't love," and "The better you know a person the more you can love him." Michael, she thinks tenderly, is not only her lover but her best friend in the world.

The sexual learning in *Forever* is not limited to the techniques of intercourse itself. Katherine is an excellent contraceptor, and her experiences show the reader how to manage the tricky social and emotional aspects of birth control—a dimension that is often lacking in the lists of devices and techniques that appear in nonfiction sex education. One of the most difficult moments for a teenage (or adult) female is, on the brink of intercourse, to persuade a reluctant male to use a condom. This Katherine does very well, just before their first coupling. She insists, even though Michael is momentarily annoyed at having to get up and retrieve the rubber in his wallet. The incident is a strong example for girls who might otherwise choose the risk of pregnancy over the risk of social embarrassment.

When it becomes apparent that they are going to continue to be sexually involved, Katherine takes herself off to Planned Parenthood for birth-control counseling. This chapter is quite detailed, a walk-through that dispels the mystery and apprehension about what such a session might be like. The emphasis is on what happens and how Katherine feels about it, rather than the clinical details of what she is taught there. The friendly counselor, the description of what to expect from a pelvic examination, the pride and dignity Katherine feels afterward for taking responsibility for her own body—all these are invaluable learnings for all adolescents, whether they need the information now or later.

Katherine's friends Erica and Sybil handle the matter differently. Erica finds her virginity a worry. She is eager to lose it before going off to college and doesn't think she necessarily has to be in love to do it. But it is her mother who takes the initiative in providing her with contraception, whisking her off in alarm to the gynecologist for the Pill when her sleep-around cousin Sybil turns up pregnant. By the end of the book Erica has had second thoughts and tells Katherine, "I don't want to fuck just for the hell of it. I want it to be special, like you and Michael. So I'm going to wait." Sybil, on the other hand, is a negative example. As Blume lays flat out in the inflammatory first sentence of the book, she "has been laid by at least six different guys" and is too casual about the whole thing even to bother to consider an abortion, choosing to bear the baby "for the experience." This appalls Erica and Katherine, who agree that *they* would have had an abortion "in a minute." It is clear which conduct meets with Blume's approval on all these issues.

Another area of learning for girls that is unique to *Forever* is the whole matter of sensitivity about male genital psychology and physiology. Inexperienced young women have no way of knowing the degree of pride and affection with which men regard their penises. Michael calls his Ralph. Nor are young girls told which parts of the male anatomy are especially delicate.

Michael stops Katherine from playfully splashing shaving lotion on his testicles because he knows from previous experience that it stings. Nor do girls learn from sex education books techniques for satisfying a young man without giving in to unwanted intercourse. Michael shows Katherine just what to do. Later she learns the dynamics of an erection, his need for a rest after coitus, how to be kind about an episode of impotence.

Other sex education subjects that the story explores briefly are jealousy, venereal disease, and homosexuality. At a party Katherine has a brief flurry of jealousy but finds that it can be dispelled by talking honestly about her feelings. Although venereal disease is not a problem for these faithful lovers, they are very much aware of it (Michael has had gonorrhea) and joke half-seriously about it. Blume's attitude toward homosexuality is not so clear. Artie, Michael's good friend and Erica's boyfriend, is evidently impotent, or at least not attracted physically to girls. Whether this is because of his nonsexual emotional problems or because he actually has homosexual tendencies is never explained. At any rate he tries to hang himself because of it and is sent off to a mental hospital—not a comforting outcome for gay readers.

But perhaps the basic teaching of *Forever* that sets all this in context is that first love—complete love expressed mentally, spiritually, physically—is wonderful while it lasts, painful when it ends, but a valuable part of growing up. The book, from its first appearance in 1975, has been overwhelmingly popular with teens and even preteens, perhaps more so than any other work of young adult fiction except S. E. Hinton's *The Outsiders*. It is read voraciously by adolescents of all racial, ethnic, and economic backgrounds and all degrees of reading skill. Although it is a love story told from a girl's point of view, it is read also by boys—perhaps because its reputation as a "dirty" book allows them to do so without loss of masculine image.

Predictably, *Forever* has been wildly controversial with adults. Part of the blame for this lies in Blume's previous status as an author of books for ten- and eleven-year-olds—an audience that followed faithfully on to read this more sophisticated book, much to the outrage of their parents. Whether it would really do children any harm to read the explicit details of such a wholesome love affair is a question that perhaps has not been sufficiently debated.

The center of the controversy, however, lies in Blume's easy acceptance of teenage sexuality, her assumption that young people in love will sooner or later go to bed together. Katherine and Michael suffer no moral angst about having sex. Their ethical concerns—and Blume's—lie in different areas. The two of them genuinely respect and care for each other; they use birth control, communicate honestly, and remain loyal and faithful until they part. A moral relationship, by many people's definition.

But there are many others for whom the definition of immoral sex is unmarried sex, and to these people the comfortable plain speaking of *Forever* seems indecent and threatening. A typical complainant was the mother of a Downey, California, twelve-year-old, who told the Library Advisory Board, "In my view this is an instructional book for teenagers on how to have an affair. It gives no indication that it is wrong or even unwise behavior." Many others of the hundreds of complaints and attacks reported in the *Intellectual Freedom Newsletter* have not been so moderate or so accurate in their criticism. "We need to let the school system know that sin is sin and we're not going to put up with it anymore," said the Rev. George Crossley, of the Movement for Moral Decency in Orlando, Florida, on launching a campaign to rid the local schools of books by Judy Blume. Some Scranton, Pennsylvania, parents called the book "filth," "garbage," and "pornography" and complained that it contained four-letter words and talked about masturbation, birth control, and disobedience to parents. (Interestingly enough, *Forever* is often accused of having masturbation scenes, although the subject is actually never mentioned in its pages.) Another parent claimed that *Forever* expressed the idea that promiscuity is the best cure for teenage problems. Perhaps the very vehemence of the protest is evidence of the power of fiction to teach values. As the California mother of a ten-year-old girl said in demanding that *Forever* be removed from the public library: "These are things *we* want to tell her, not Judy Blume."

▪ Romances as "Rotten Examples"

More to the liking of such parents are the romance paperback series that flood the market with "squeaky clean" love stories. Scholastic's Wildfire was the first in the field, in 1979, followed by Bantam's Sweet Dreams and Putnam's Pacers. These little books are written to formula, and while they work well as light entertainment, they leave a great deal to be desired as sex education. The guidelines issued to prospective Wildfire authors, for example, were quoted by Pamela Pollack in *School Library Journal,* November 1981: "No books will deal with sexual matters like abortion, unmarried pregnancy, affairs . . . in fact [there is to be] no sexual involvement between the couple except kissing and feelings of attraction." Most romances allow the girl to feel euphemistic "shivers" or "quivers" when the boy touches her, but the boy himself is allowed by the writer nothing more physical than light kissing. And it is almost always he who calls a heroic halt to the embrace.

Such unrealistic writing leaves young virgins unprepared for the steamy realities of necking sessions with real boys or even any of the more subtle give-and-take of male-female social relationships. Indeed, there is a strong current of opinion among experts that a separation between romantic thinking and sex education may be a crucial factor in adolescent pregnancy. Peter Scales, in the April 1981 issue of *Medical Aspects of Human Sexuality,* wrote: "Teenage girls in particular believe that planned sex is unacceptable morally but if one is swept off one's feet by spontaneity sex is acceptable. The feeling of being out of control of the situation is a close cousin to an outright denial that one is having sex. . . . Research has shown that young people who feel guilty about their sexuality are most apt to fail to use contraception, not to refrain from sexual intercourse." Instead of promoting the preservation of virginity, the teen romances probably contribute more to its loss than realistic novels like *Forever,* in which girls are shown how to be in charge of their own sexuality.

▪ The Male Perspective

Most love stories in young adult literature, whether realistic or romantic, are told from the girl's point of view. Novels that dealt with the sexual problems of young males were rare until recently. An early exception was Judy Blume's 1971 book *Then Again, Maybe I Won't.* In this story the thirteen-year-old protagonist is mortified by sudden erections and worries about nocturnal emissions—two concerns that almost never appear in the work of other writers in spite of their universal importance to young boys.

The emotional significance of first ejaculation, too, is generally ignored, even though it is a landmark event for boys in marking their transition to potency.

Novels that view sexual learning through the eyes of teenage boys have tended to feature older protagonists and therefore to focus on a more advanced set of anxieties. The time is usually the summer before college, and the theme is most often, to put it crudely, getting laid. Crudeness is the difficulty here for the writer, because the folklore of sexology decrees that while girls are primarily interested in relationship, boys are primarily interested in impersonal physical sex. It is a tricky stylistic problem for authors to give the impression of genital preoccupation without resorting to a parade of overwhelmingly graphic images. Then, too, teachers and librarians, who make up the large part of the market for hardcover young adult fiction, are predominantly female and in the past have looked askance at novels that attempted to be realistic about the thoughts of sex-starved adolescent boys. The tendency to perceive girls as collections of interesting body parts, while attributable to high hormone levels, is not easily understood or forgiven by women. The few novels that covered this ground in the past have reaped virulent scorn from female critics: Kin Platt's *The Terrible Love Life of Dudley Cornflower*, for instance, or Don Bredes's *Hard Feelings*.

So it has been only during the last few years that male-oriented love stories have begun to appear in any number, perhaps as a reaction to the sheer quantity of sexless and sugary romances, or perhaps because only now can it be generally admitted that young men have anxieties and sensitivities that they don't dare to voice in a society where men are expected to be assertive and capable at all times. Years ago Holden Caulfield admitted plaintively that sometimes he couldn't even find what he was looking for when he was touching a girl, but nobody was listening then. Realistic novels for young men provide valuable and necessary learning about not only the physical facts but also the relational aspects of sex.

Three examples will serve to show the patterns: *Hey, Kid! Does She Love Me?*, by Harry Mazer; *A Very Touchy Subject*, by Todd Strasser; and *A Matter of Finding the Right Girl*, by Peter Filichia. In the first book a mother complains bluntly to her seventeen-year-old son, Danny, "The minute you get near a girl you lose your brains. Sometimes I think you boys have your brains in your pants." In the second book Scott Tauscher writes, "In case you're wondering why I decided to write a book, all I can tell you is that I'm seventeen years old and for the last three years I've probably spent an average of 47% of each day thinking about sex." And in the third Mike Petrino moans, "It's hard enough to find someone who'll do it with you, let alone someone you can love."

Each of these protagonists is seventeen going on eighteen, which makes for a very different situation than, say, a thirteen- or fourteen-year-old with sex on his mind. Each feels that everyone else is Doing It and that he is the last male virgin left in the western world. Each feels driven by his hormones and is embarrassed and guilty at his compulsion to sneak peeks and cop feels. In a postfeminist age sensitive young men know better, but they still feel like it. Each has a sexually experienced best friend who eggs him on in his quest for a willing female body and disparages his search for a congenial female person. None of the three has anyone he can really talk it over with. As Scott says, "If you're a guy and you talk to other guys about sex, they either don't know the answers or they just BS you to death. And forget about parents and teachers. This may make a lot of adults mad, but frankly I think you'd have to be an absolute nerd to sit down and discuss the intimate aspects of your life with your biology teacher or someone." So they muddle through, groping in an obscuring fog of lust toward a glimmering of understanding of love and relationships.

The dynamics of this universal masculine problem are most clearly laid out in Peter Filichia's *A Matter of Finding the Right Girl.* Mike and his best friend, Wally, had made a Vow—a solemn promise that by the time each was eighteen "he would get it or die trying." Now Wally has already achieved the objective, but for Mike, two weeks before his birthday, it is T minus 335 hours and counting. He has set his calculator watch for the countdown, and as the minutes and hours tick by his search for the right girl grows more desperate. He really likes redheaded Leslie, who works beside him at Zella's Superette. They have fun together and are good friends, and besides, he can't help noticing her nice breasts. But Leslie is going with someone else, so Mike dates Corinne (who on their third date tells him she has decided to become a nun) and then little Rochelle Twombley (whose reputation for easiness turns out to be based on one pathetic incident). At last, with only three hours, twenty-nine minutes, and thirty-five seconds left to go, he "gets it" in the back seat of his car with Susan, an angry girl who is bent on getting back at her parents for uprooting her from her beloved Wyoming. It isn't as great as he'd expected. In fact it's pretty mechanical, and Mike, in a neat switch on the usual way of the world, has the distinct impression he's been used. For a while he worries that he might even be gay, until his Uncle David, who *is* gay, reassures him: "My guess is that you're going to feel a lot better about making love when you make love with someone you love." It looks like this is going to turn out to be gloriously true when Leslie breaks up with her boyfriend and she and Mike discover that their friendship has laid the basis for some very satisfactory passionate caring.

A Very Touchy Subject, by Todd Strasser, is a bit slicker, but the conflict is the same. "Sex alone isn't a good enough reason to be interested in someone," says Scott Tauscher, sounding like a sex ed manual. "You should enjoy being with her, you should like and admire and respect her, you should feel some kind of emotional caring that's different from your desire to jump in bed with her." Scott is sophisticated enough to know the right attitudes, but it's hard for him to remember them when his longtime girlfriend, wealthy Alix, continually refuses to have sex, for no special reason (it seems to him) except that she wants to exercise the right to refuse. In this vacuum he finds himself reluctantly attracted to his fifteen-year-old neighbor Paula, mostly because he knows she has a lover and therefore (by male teenage logic) is available for sex. But Paula is a waif, and Scott finds himself unwillingly drawn into helping her deal with her alcoholic mother and abusive boyfriend. When his romance with Alix dies of malnutrition, he finds that he has become Paula's friend and has grown past his desire to exploit her for sex (although he makes her promise never to tell his buddies that he has passed up the Golden Opportunity).

Hey, Kid! Does She Love Me?, by Harry Mazer, is more sentimental—a touching story of a young man's unrequited grand passion for an older (but not much older) woman. Jeff Orloff more than anything wants to become a film director. Two years before, when he was a sophomore and she was a senior, he was smitten with Mary Silver's acting talent but never got up the nerve to speak to her. Now she is back in town—with a baby—

and living at the boardinghouse run by his best friend's mother. Jeff plots and schemes to get near her and eventually does break through her prickly defensiveness to win her trust and that of her baby, Hannah. But all his romantic daydreams come to nothing against Mary's cool determination to stay just friends. Distressed at her abandonment of her acting career, he persuades her to try for a scholarship to a weekend acting workshop. Mary wins, and Jeff offers to care for Hannah, privately planning to hand the baby over to his mother. But his parents have arranged to be out of town that weekend, and Jeff finds himself singlehandedly (in one of the funniest passages in young adult fiction) taking care of a squalling, diaper-filling, utterly charming baby girl for four endless days. Fantasies of Mary falling into his arms (and bed) with gratitude sustain him. Eventually he gets pretty good at the job of baby-tending and begins to feel a new emotion of tenderness for the bossy little creature in his care.

And he begins to understand the life-changing demands that women accept when they decide to bear a child. "Maybe it's a good thing men don't get pregnant. We're too selfish to have babies. I am, anyway," he muses, in a striking monolog. "Now, in a just world, pregnant women—pardon me, pregnant persons—would have time off for good behavior, check out of the scene when it got to be too much."

Finally Mary returns, aglow with new plans and opportunities, and although grateful, she makes it plain that they are still no more than friends. Jeff's fantasies die hard. For a while, even after she has left town to live with a young theater troupe, he clings to hope. Only after he has punctuated the end of the romance by getting drunk, wrecking his friend's truck, and spending a night in jail is he able to get on with his life and let his passion for Mary be transformed into the same tenderness he feels for Hannah.

The theme of a young man's adoration for an older woman recurs frequently in young adult literature. Examples are M. E. Kerr's *If I Love You, Am I Trapped Forever?* and Barbara Wersba's *The Carnival in My Mind* and *The Country of the Heart*. (This last, a desperately romantic story about the affair of a teenage boy and a dying poet in her forties, is probably more appealing to girls—or older women.) Such a theme naturally often leads into Oedipal complications, as in *Dark but Full of*

Diamonds, by Katie Letcher Lyle, in which a boy loves an older woman who wants to marry his father, or *Father Figure*, by Richard Peck, in which a son is in love with his father's girlfriend.

In other versions of this theme a young man is initiated sexually by an older, more sophisticated, or more experienced girl—a common male teenage fantasy. *Hard Love*, by Cynthia Grant, and *Center Line*, by Joyce Sweeney, deal realistically with the complications of such a relationship. In *The Disappearance*, by Rosa Guy, the seductress is more sinister. The situation appears often in the works of Norma Klein: *It's OK if You Don't Love Me*, *Give and Take*, and especially *Beginner's Love*.

This last is a close second to *Forever* in the explicitness and variety of sexual detail, but from the male perspective. For instance, the defloration scene is from the other side of the bed:

> Finally, I even put my hand inside her. She didn't seem to mind. In fact, about a minute after I did that, she whispered, "Why don't we. . . ."
>
> Okay, so I did a classic thing. I absolutely couldn't help it. I entered her and it felt so great, just the *idea* that we were really doing it, plus the feeling, just everything, that I came. There's no way on earth I could've held off. When I was finished, I lay there on top of her, embarrassed.

Although the author is a woman, the book is convincing in its depiction of this and other male sexual traumas, such as erections at inconvenient moments. Masturbation is part of the story in the commonplace way that is appropriate. Joel, the protagonist, struggles with the typical sexual conflict of young men in the 1980s, the unacceptable split between sexual desire and relationship:

> I always feel there's something slightly hypocritical going on between us and I don't know if it's my fault or what. It's like there are four of us. First, just Leda and me, two regular people who sometimes get along and sometimes don't. . . . But then there are our bodies, which basically just want to fuck. I hate to put it that crudely, but it's true. Leda once said she hated some book she read where a man cheated on his wife or girl friend and said, as an excuse, "It wasn't me, it was him," meaning his cock. I admit that's kind of a dodge, but I also know what he means.

Beginner's Love is unique in being the only young adult novel in which oral sex is part of the young lovers' repertoire. It also has the only sympathetic portrayal of a young man's feelings of guilt and exclusion during and after his girlfriend's abortion.

The role of young men in the pregnancy epidemic and how they might feel about it has not been adequately explored, either in nonfiction or fiction. Only Jeannette Eyerly, in *He's My Baby, Now*, and Lois Ruby, in *What Do You Do in Quicksand?* have shown young fathers with some affection for their babies. But male fictional concerns for possible offspring are usually limited to the condom-in-the-wallet syndrome. Impotence is another alarming subject in which fiction might offer adolescent boys some comfort and guidance, but only occasionally does it appear in stories. The incident in *Running Loose*, by Chris Crutcher, is almost unique, except for Michael's brief impotence in *Forever*.

It should not be thought that all young adult novels from the male perspective present sex as problematic and anxiety-laden. A number of excellent books put the subject in proportion as a natural and comfortable part of other growing and learning. The young men in these books are, in the area of sex, healthy and affectionate young animals just doing what comes naturally. In *Center Line*, by Joyce Sweeney, five brothers leave home to escape their murderous father. Adventures with girls are a normal part of their experiences on the road. Like all young men away from home for the first time, they look for sexual opportunities a lot, but not to the exclusion of other more important matters. Terry Davis is the master at writing sexual scenes of joyful lightness, and his beautiful novels *Vision Quest* and *Mysterious Ways* have many lovely descriptions of the horseplay of young lovers.

■ Preggers Novels

Although the social role of young men in pregnancy has been slighted in fiction, the plight of the gravid adolescent female has been a literary staple since long before Faust got Gretchen with child. The "preggers novel" is so common in young adult fiction as to be almost a subgenre. The form has a venerable history, going back to early fate-worse-than-death efforts like *Mr. and Mrs. Bo Jo Jones*, by Ann Head, in which everybody's life is ruined when the young couple try to make a go of a forced marriage.

The heroines of later books in the seventies, probably warned off from a wedding by the Jones's experience, were more likely to terminate their pregnancies, at great physical and emotional cost. Abortion in these stories was uniformly pictured as painful, bloody, and psychologically damaging. See, for instance, *Bonnie Jo, Go Home*, by Jeannette Eyerly, or *My Darling, My Hamburger*, by Paul Zindel. After the legalization of abortion in 1973 the subject was less dramatic and therefore appeared less frequently. But when it did, as in *Beginner's Love*, it was still given an aura of gloom. Almost never in young adult fiction is the termination of an unwanted pregnancy treated as a logical, safe, and relatively comfortable experience. The young mothers-to-be in current adolescent fiction consider abortion as one of their options but seldom actually choose it—probably because at that point the story would be over.

Instead they spend most of the pages of the book procrastinating and agonizing over options and usually end up giving birth. *Lauren*, by Harriett Luger, is a realistic and educational book of this type. A young girl struggles with the hard choices her pregnancy imposes. She rejects her parents' pressure to abort and runs away to a shabby part of town, where she is taken in by two young mothers on welfare. Their gritty poverty and their frustration at the conflicting demands of babies and unfinished adolescence are touchingly and realistically portrayed. Eventually Lauren returns home and decides to give up her child to a barren young couple who have befriended her.

Others merely float with the situation and passively accept whatever institutional help is offered. The cheerful slut who has a baby during senior year is a stock minor character. Blossom Elfman has written several witty and sympathetic books out of her own experience as a teacher in a California "pregnant school" that explore the institutional mindset: *The Girls of Huntington House*, *A House for Jonnie O*, and *The Butterfly Girl*. Everywhere in young adult literature pregnancy is tinged with tragedy, and if a girl has intercourse it is almost guaranteed that she will conceive before too many more chapters. "Sex is the crime, pregnancy is the punishment," says Leda in *Beginner's Love*.

A refreshing exception to all this bungling and jaw-clenching is

Unbirthday, by A. M. Stephensen, the story of a young couple who are responsible and intelligent about their sex lives. Louisa and Charlie are high-school seniors who have a strong and loving relationship. They have always used condoms, even postponing that first time when it was so hard to wait until they could get protection. But Louisa eventually gets pregnant anyway. Even with this they keep their heads, although they are scared and troubled. They talk the problem through and then find confidential help at the Women's Center at a nearby college. A young counselor helps Louisa weigh her options and is honest about the emotional difficulties of a decision for abortion. When she decides to trust her own instinct for self-preservation and to terminate the pregnancy, Charlie stands by her and insists on paying his half. The details of the abortion are vividly described, from Louisa's point of view, but in a way that demystifies the procedure and makes it less frightening. There are no complications and no real regrets, and in the end she is sure she made the right decision.

The message is unabashedly proabortion, although there is respect for those individuals who feel strongly that to interfere in a pregnancy means ending a human life. The "pro-life" movement, however, gets some harsh words from the young feminist counselor. As a source of information the book is excellent, communicating facts, as well as feelings and emotions, better than many nonfiction titles on the same subject. But Louisa never tells her parents, and that, plus the fact that the characters talk like real adolescents, has made the book controversial. Even more problematic for some people, it shows with intelligence and wit that wholesome, responsible teenage sex doesn't necessarily mean ruined lives.

Unbirthday is unique in one more way: the characters go to books and libraries for help in solving their problems—but with varying degrees of success. The couple's original contraceptive decision is based on Louisa's library research:

> The basic information was pretty easy to find, but the details . . . took a lot of digging. . . . Unless the Tollefson Falls Public Library had some secret forbidden files you had to ask for, which I wasn't about to since my mother and the librarian had been friends since grade school, the closest thing they had to what I needed was a book on investing in condominiums. Finding information about pregnancy wasn't much easier. . . . There was . . . an

> ancient book in which a famous advice columnist gave "teens" the "inside scoop" about sex. Charlie and I had run into that one on one of our research missions, and we'd nearly gotten ourselves kicked out of the library for laughing uncontrollably at poor Dear Dora's attitude that anything more serious than French kissing was an act of wickedness and depravity.

Novels have been no help either:

> There was only one book I could remember where a girl got an abortion. It was so badly botched she ended up puking blood all over the upholstery of her boyfriend's car on the way home, and when she got into her house and puked more blood on the rug before collapsing on the floor, her exceptionally swift parents suddenly realized what was going on and virtually disowned her.

Later, Louisa's faith in the helpfulness of the printed word is justified when the counselor lends her some pamphlets on abortion and her own treasured copy of *Our Bodies, Ourselves.*

▪ Preventing Pregnancy

Contraception is a crucial adolescent learning that could be effectively taught in fiction. Techniques and devices could be described in action, fear of an internal exam and a diaphragm fitting could be allayed, and, most important, characters that young readers like and admire could be shown using birth control as an indispensable part of lovemaking. Contraception could be made to seem necessary for social acceptance, and its omission could be ridiculed. But this powerful potential influence is to a large extent not being utilized.

There are a few exceptions, of course. Katherine's visit to Planned Parenthood we have already discussed. Leda, in Norma Klein's *Beginner's Love,* has a diaphragm, but, alas, gets pregnant anyway because she forgets to wear it every time—not an encouraging example for teens considering this method. Only rarely do parents help their daughters get contraception: fathers in both *Beginner's Love* and Klein's *Love Is One of the Choices,* Erica's mother in *Forever.* More often the parental literary role toward birth control is discovery and outrage, followed by a stormy scene. Gail, in Richard Peck's *Are You in the*

House Alone? has responsibly gotten herself a prescription for the Pill but suffers for it when her mother finds the packet.

Unfortunately, novelists seem to find something inherently comical about the condom—the birth-control method most recommended for young teens by sex counselors. In fiction it is found in drawers or pockets by appalled moms or impedes the romantic progress of a love scene with awkward difficulties of application. Even more often it is carried in wallets (a practice frowned on by experts) so that boys can impress their buddies and themselves with their impending sexual initiation. The literary possibilities of contraceptive foam, understandably enough, seem to be almost zero.

▪ Growing Up Gay

Homosexuality, like pregnancy, is a theme that appears extensively and for the most part negatively in adolescent fiction. For a number of years it was an unspoken tradition that if a teenage boy had a homosexual experience in a novel, be it explicit, fleeting, or rumored, there would be a violent death in the next to the last chapter. The bludgeon murder of a psychotic gay schoolmaster in James Kirkwood's *Good Times, Bad Times*, the graphic gunshot suicide of a young homosexual in Paul Covert's *Cages*, the car crashes in Lynn Hall's *Sticks and Stones* and Sandra Scoppettone's *Trying Hard to Hear You*, the heart attack of an older gay who befriends a lonely young boy in Isabelle Holland's *The Man Without a Face*, even the death of the dachshund in John Donovan's *I'll Get There, It Better Be Worth the Trip*—all this mayhem conveyed the message that while writers might be allowed to create a sympathetic homosexual character, somebody just better be punished for it before the end of the book. Articles in the library and educational press and protests from gay organizations brought the pattern to the attention of writers and publishers and it eventually faded away, but not without a satirical in-joke salute by Sandra Scoppettone in the title of her lesbian novel *Happy Endings Are All Alike*.

The homophile inclinations of girls have fared better in young adult fiction. Writers seem to perceive far more clearly when the lovers are female that a passing homosexual experience or even a homosexual love affair during the formative adolescent years does not necessarily mean that the participants must define themselves as gay. Deborah Hautzig, in *Hey Dollface!* has shown with sensitivity and understanding that a close friendship between two girls can be expressed physically, and Rosa Guy has also dealt with the same theme in *Ruby*. The lovers in *Happy Endings Are All Alike* act out their passion on a blanket in the woods; when the affair is over, one of them has decided that she is gay, the other is still unsure. No one dies for the "crime," but literary tradition is upheld when one of the girls is brutally raped. An entire boarding school rises up in horror when a lesbian is uncovered in their midst in the old-fashioned story *The Last of Eden*, by Stephanie Tolan. A tender love affair between two girls ends in disclosure and public shame in Nancy Garden's *Annie on My Mind*, both for the teenagers and the older lesbian couple in whose house they are discovered. In general, however, lesbian characters and tendencies have never inspired the fear and loathing that in the past has been the lot of gay males in adolescent fiction. The young protagonist in *Tunes for a Small Harmonica*, by Barbara Wersba, cheerfully experiments with kissing another girl to see if she herself might be lesbian, and in *Breaking Up*, by Norma Klein, a teenager receives the news of her mother's love affair with a woman with only casual interest.

A different kind of gay novel, one in which the homosexual preferences of the protagonist are already established, has until recently been confined to underground status. These books, as contrasted with mainstream young adult fiction, are told from the point of view of a gay teenager, and while they show the difficulties sympathetically, they do not assume that homosexual identity is a problem to be punished or solved or explained away. The prototype is *Rubyfruit Jungle*, by Rita Mae Brown, which follows the comic sexual adventures of an extroverted young lesbian. *Patience and Sarah*, by Isabel Miller, is a love story based on historical fact. Later books of this type tend to be more or less autobiographical: *The Best Little Boy in the World*, by John Reid, or *Reflections of a Rock Lobster: A Story About Growing Up Gay*, by Aaron Fricke. *Independence Day*, by B. A. Ecker, shows a young boy's forbidden yearnings for his unsuspecting best friend, and *Counter Play*, by Anne Snyder and Louis Pellitier, also deals with the difficulties of gay-straight friendship. Aidan Chambers's *Dance on My Grave* tells of a young man's grief when his lover is killed.

▪ Drama vs. Education

Other sexual matters appear in the pages of young adult fiction in direct proportion not to their educational importance but to their dramatic possibilities and their literary acceptability. Masturbation, as an almost universal practice and the primary sexual outlet for adolescents, should be part of the internal dialog of any protagonist, if novels accurately reflected the teenage mentality. Actually, it appears only briefly in a few of the "boys' books" mentioned earlier. Although it has been heartily endorsed by sex educators at least since the 1968 publication of *Boys and Sex*, the old Victorian taboos still make this one of the most combustible subjects for young adult novelists. Robert Cormier wrote a stunningly sensual chapter for *The Chocolate War* in which the vicious Archie masturbates to climax while he achieves the idea for a diabolic revenge. But on the advice of his editor, Cormier took it out of the final version. Female masturbation is even more forbidden. Three sentences in Judy Blume's *Deenie* have been almost as controversial as the chapters and chapters of explicit sexual action in *Forever*. A young girl says innocently: "As soon as I got into bed I started touching myself. I have this special place and when I rub it I get a very nice feeling. I don't know what it's called or if anyone else has it but when I have trouble falling asleep, touching my special place helps a lot."

Menstruation is another universal experience (at least for half of the population) that almost never shows up in adolescent fiction. When it does, it is most often used as a plot device to postpone something, usually sexual intimacy, as in *Forever*, or *The Year of Sweet Senior Insanity*, by Sonia Levitin. Only two books deal sensitively with the anxieties of young girls awaiting their first period: *Are You There God? It's Me, Margaret*, by Judy Blume, and *Saturday the Twelfth of October*, by Norma Fox Mazer.

Venereal disease, too, has been avoided in fiction like the plague. Granted, it is an untidy and unpleasant subject but not without a certain inherent drama. When gonorrhea and other sexually transmitted diseases are rampant partly because so many teenagers either do not recognize the symptoms or are ashamed to seek treatment, it would seem that more characters in fiction would reflect that reality and that more writers would feel a responsibility to educate their young readers about it. To date only *Forever's* Michael has been afflicted—and that was *last* summer, before the book began—and the heroine of *To Take a Dare*, by Crescent Dragonwagon and Paul Zindel, who becomes sterile from untreated gonorrhea when her abusive father throws away her antibiotic capsules.

Crushes have always been a fact of adolescent sexual awakening, and they occur often in junior novels. Examples of feminine adoration from afar are to be found in *The Handsome Man*, by Elissa Haden Guest; *Tunes for a Small Harmonica*, by Barbara Wersba: and *Crush*, by Jane Futcher. Novels sometimes carry this fantasy on into wish-fulfillment: the Parisian-garret romance of a schoolgirl and a forty-year-old artist in *A Matter of Feeling*, by Janine Boissard; the affair of the young boy and the dying poet in *The Country of the Heart*; the desperate crush of a high-school senior for a young woman doctor and its unlikely outcome in marriage in the subplot of *Beginner's Love*; the shy girl who replaces her English teacher's wife in *Love Is One of the Choices*, by Norma Klein.

But the actual sexual exploitation of adolescents by adults is another matter entirely. Incest, while statistically more and more common, occurs in young adult novels rarely and then only in the form of seduction attempts by a stepfather or uncle or mother's boyfriend. Two exceptions are *Abby, My Love*, by Hadley Irwin, and *A Solitary Secret*, by Patricia Hermes, in both of which a young girl confesses that her father has been sexually abusing her for years. Brother-sister incest, which is probably far more common than anyone wants to acknowledge, has never been the subject of a junior novel, although the turgid and heavy-breathing potboilers of V. C. Andrews that fixate on that topic (*Flowers in the Attic*, *Petals on the Wind*, and so on) are an underground cult with teenage girls. Prostitution formerly appeared in young adult literature only in a sad little scene in *Catcher in the Rye*, until the recruiting of pubescent girls for commercial sex became such a national scandal that it was recognized in *Steffie Can't Come Out to Play*, by Fran Arrick, and *Making It*, by Barbara Corcoran. Violent rape has been explored adequately in at least three novels: Scoppettone's *Happy Endings Are All Alike*, Peck's *Are You in the House Alone?* and *Did You Hear What Happened to Andrea?* by Gloria Miklowitz. However, the far more frequent and subtle problem of acquaintance rape has not been fictionalized.

Adolescent resentment of the sexual activity of single parents is often an important part of the plots of fiction, although this subject is almost totally lacking in nonfiction sex education. The usual situation is the dating or remarriage of a divorced parent, and the protagonist's resistance to accepting the implied parental sexual activity. Norma Klein broke ground for this kind of story with her critically acclaimed but highly controversial book *Mom, the Wolfman and Me*, in which an independent mother lets her boyfriend sleep over and contemplates having his child without marrying him. Especially good examples are *The Divorce Express*, by Paula Danziger, and its sequel, *It's an Aardvark-Eat-Turtle World*. In these books Phoebe and Rosie are best friends until their parents become live-in lovers. The theme of unconscious parental-child sexual rivalry is skillfully carried to its extreme in *Surrogate Sister*, by Eve Bunting, a tale about an earth-mother who shames her daughter by bearing a child for money.

There are even novels that show young women choosing to enjoy a good relationship with a boyfriend without sex. They differ from the dishonest virgins (and writers) of the paperback romances in confronting their sexuality openly rather than denying it altogether. One of the best books of this type is the beautiful love story *Very Far Away from Anywhere Else*, by Ursula LeGuin, which tells of a pair of gifted young people who care for each other very much, but because of more urgent and immediate life goals postpone the emotional involvement that would come with sex. A second young-love story by this science-fiction author, *The Beginning Place*, uses the same theme in a fantasy setting—the young couple must defeat a strange misshapen creature who in some respects is a metaphor for desire. In *Up in Seth's Room*, by Norma Fox Mazer, a girl struggles successfully against the sexual needs of her older and more experienced boyfriend. And in *The Year of Sweet Senior Insanity*, by Sonia Levitin, the narrator is prevented from sleeping with her boyfriend by an untimely menstrual period but later finds she is glad to have been stopped.

Other stories revolve around aspects of love other than sex, although a physical relationship may be implied in the background. *Someone to Love*, by Norma Fox Mazer, is a subtle picture of the joys and sorrows of a short-lived cohabitation, and by anatomizing a bad relationship it teaches a great deal about good ones. *The Day the Senior Class Got Married*, by Gloria

Miklowitz, shows a young engaged couple learning about the hard economic realities of married life in a social-studies class, an experience that persuades the young bride-to-be that breaking off a wedding is less traumatic than a lifetime with the wrong man. But most love stories are simply lighthearted romps like Marjorie Sharmat's *How to Meet a Gorgeous Guy* and *How to Meet a Gorgeous Girl.*

Novelists, after all, are tellers of tales. And sex is only a small part of the raw material with which they weave stories of the trials and pleasures of growing up. They do not admit to being in the business of sex education—even if sometimes they are.

■ BIBLIOGRAPHY

(Note: This is a list of books mentioned in this chapter; inclusion does not necessarily mean recommendation. For Core Collection List see Appendix.)

Andrews, V. C. *Flowers in the Attic.* New York: Simon and Schuster, 1979; New York: Pocket Books, 1982.

———. *Petals on the Wind.* New York: Simon and Schuster, 1980; New York: Pocket Books, 1982.

Arrick, Fran. *Steffie Can't Come Out to Play.* Scarsdale, N.Y.: Bradbury, 1978; New York: Dell, 1979.

Blume, Judy. *Are You There God? It's Me, Margaret.* Scarsdale, N.Y.: Bradbury, 1970; New York: Dell, 1974.

———. *Deenie.* Scarsdale, N.Y.: Bradbury, 1973; New York: Dell, 1974.

———. *Forever.* Scarsdale, N.Y.: Bradbury, 1975; New York: Pocket Books, 1976.

———. *Then Again, Maybe I Won't.* Scarsdale, N.Y.: Bradbury, 1971; New York: Dell, 1974.

Boissard, Janine. *A Matter of Feeling.* Boston: Little, Brown, 1980.

Bredes, Don. *Hard Feelings.* New York: Atheneum, 1977.

Brown, Rita Mae. *Rubyfruit Jungle.* Houston: Daughters, 1973; New York: Bantam, 1977.

Bunting, Eve. *Surrogate Sister.* New York: Lippincott, 1984.

Chambers, Aidan. *Dance on My Grave.* New York: Harper and Row, 1982.

Corcoran, Barbara. *Making It*. Boston: Little, Brown, 1981; New York: Archway, 1985.

Cormier, Robert. *The Chocolate War*. New York: Pantheon, 1974; New York: Dell, 1975.

Covert, Paul. *Cages*. New York: Liveright, 1971.

Crutcher, Chris. *Running Loose*. New York: Greenwillow, 1983.

Danziger, Paula. *The Divorce Express*. New York: Delacorte, 1982; New York: Dell, 1983.

———. *It's an Aardvark-Eat-Turtle World*. New York: Delacorte, 1985.

Davis, Terry. *Mysterious Ways*. New York: Viking, 1984.

———. *Vision Quest*. New York: Viking, 1979.

Donovan, John. *I'll Get There, It Better Be Worth the Trip*. New York: Harper and Row, 1969.

Dragonwagon, Crescent, and Paul Zindel. *To Take A Dare*. New York: Harper and Row, 1982; New York: Bantam, 1984.

Ecker, B. A. *Independence Day*. New York: Avon, 1983.

Elfman, Blossom. *The Butterfly Girl*. Boston: Houghton-Mifflin, 1980.

———. *The Girls of Huntington House*. Boston: Houghton-Mifflin, 1972; New York: Bantam, 1973.

———. *A House for Jonnie O*. Boston: Houghton-Mifflin, 1977; New York: Bantam, 1978.

Eyerly, Jeannette. *Bonnie Jo, Go Home*. Philadelphia: Lippincott, 1972.

———. *He's My Baby, Now*. New York: Archway, 1978.

Filichia, Peter. *A Matter of Finding the Right Girl*. New York: Fawcett Juniper, 1985.

Fricke, Aaron. *Reflections of a Rock Lobster: A Story About Growing Up Gay*. Boston: Alyson, 1981.

Futcher, Jane. *Crush*. Boston: Little, Brown, 1981; New York: Avon, 1984.

Garden, Nancy. *Annie on My Mind*. New York: Farrar, Straus, Giroux, 1982.

Grant, Cynthia D. *Hard Love*. New York: Atheneum, 1983; New York: Ballantine, 1984.

Guest, Elissa Haden. *The Handsome Man*. New York: Four Winds, 1980.

Guy, Rosa. *The Disappearance*. New York: Delacorte, 1979; New York: Dell, 1981.

———. *Ruby*. New York: Viking, 1976; New York: Bantam, 1979.
Hall, Lynn. *Sticks and Stones*. New York: Follett, 1977.
Hautzig, Deborah. *Hey Dollface!* New York: Greenwillow, 1978.
Head, Ann. *Mr. and Mrs. Bo Jo Jones*. New York: Putnam, 1967; New York: New American Library, 1973.
Hermes, Patricia. *A Solitary Secret*. New York: Harcourt Brace, 1985.
Hinton, S. E. *The Outsiders*. New York: Viking, 1967; New York: Dell, 1969.
Holland, Isabelle. *The Man Without a Face*. New York: Lippincott, 1972.
Irwin, Hadley. *Abby, My Love*. New York: Atheneum, 1985.
Kerr, M. E. *If I Love You, Am I Trapped Forever?* New York: Harper, 1973; New York: Dell, 1974.
Kirkwood, James. *Good Times, Bad Times*. New York: Fawcett, 1978.
Klein, Norma. *Beginner's Love*. New York: Dutton, 1983; New York: Fawcett Juniper, 1984.
———. *Breaking Up*. New York: Pantheon, 1980; New York: Avon, 1981.
———. *Give and Take*. New York: Viking, 1985.
———. *It's OK if You Don't Love Me*. New York: Dial, 1977; New York: Fawcett, 1978.
———. *Love Is One of the Choices*. New York: Dial, 1978; New York: Fawcett Juniper, 1982.
———. *Mom, the Wolfman and Me*. New York: Pantheon, 1972; New York: Avon, 1982.
LeGuin, Ursula K. *The Beginning Place*. New York: Harper and Row, 1980: New York: Bantam, 1981.
———. *Very Far Away from Anywhere Else*. New York: Atheneum, 1976; New York: Bantam, 1978.
Levitin, Sonia. *The Year of Sweet Senior Insanity*. New York: Atheneum, 1982; New York: Ballantine, 1983.
Luger, Harriett. *Lauren*. New York: Viking, 1979; New York: Dell, 1981.
Lyle, Katie Letcher. *Dark but Full of Diamonds*. New York: Coward, 1981.
Mazer, Harry. *Hey, Kid! Does She Love Me?* New York: Crowell, 1985.

Mazer, Norma Fox. *Saturday the Twelfth of October.* New York: Delacorte, 1975; New York: Dell, 1976.

———. *Someone to Love.* New York: Delacorte, 1983; New York: Dell Laurel-Leaf, 1985.

———. *Up in Seth's Room.* New York: Delacorte, 1979; New York: Dell, 1981.

Miklowitz, Gloria D. *The Day the Senior Class Got Married.* New York: Delacorte, 1983; New York: Dell, 1985.

———. *Did You Hear What Happened to Andrea?* New York: Delacorte, 1979; New York: Dell, 1981.

Miller, Isabel. *Patience and Sarah.* New York: Fawcett Crest, 1973.

Peck, Richard. *Are You in the House Alone?* New York: Viking, 1976; New York: Dell, 1977.

———. *Father Figure.* New York: Viking, 1978; New York: New American Library, 1979.

Platt, Kin. *The Terrible Love Life of Dudley Cornflower.* Scarsdale, N.Y.: Bradbury, 1976.

Reid, John. *The Best Little Boy in the World.* New York: Ballantine, 1976.

Ruby, Lois. *What Do You Do in Quicksand?* New York: Viking, 1979; New York: Fawcett Juniper, 1981.

Salinger, J. D. *Catcher in the Rye.* Boston: Little, Brown, 1951; New York: Bantam, 1964.

Scoppettone, Sandra. *Happy Endings Are All Alike.* New York: Harper and Row, 1978; New York: Dell, 1981.

———. *Trying Hard to Hear You.* New York: Harper and Row, 1974.

Sharmat, Marjorie. *How to Meet a Gorgeous Girl.* New York: Delacorte, 1984.

———. *How to Meet a Gorgeous Guy.* New York: Delacorte, 1983.

Snyder, Anne, and Louis Pellitier. *Counter Play.* New York: New American Library, 1981.

Stephensen, A. M. *Unbirthday.* New York: Avon, 1982.

Strasser, Todd. *A Very Touchy Subject.* New York: Delacorte, 1985.

Sweeney, Joyce. *Center Line.* New York: Delacorte, 1984; New York: Dell, 1985.

Tolan, Stephanie. *The Last of Eden.* New York: Warne, 1980.

Wersba, Barbara. *The Carnival in My Mind*. New York: Harper and Row, 1982.
———. *The Country of the Heart*. New York: Atheneum, 1975.
———. *Tunes for a Small Harmonica*. New York: Harper and Row, 1976.
Zindel, Paul. *My Darling, My Hamburger*. New York: Harper and Row, 1969; New York: Bantam, 1978.

Chapter 11

Religious Sex Prevention Guides

While secular sex education has always looked to medical science and the current attitudes of society for authority, religious sex education has always claimed to be based on the word of God—or a particular interpretation of the word of God. What the Lord has to say about it, according to religious sex guides, from flaming fundamentalist tract to reasoned liberal discussion, can be summed up in one sentence: Thou shalt not have sexual intercourse before marriage. Impressing young people with this prohibition is the primary motivation behind all religious sex and dating guides for adolescents. Some of the more conservative books consist of nothing more than long essays on the theme, as if the entire complex content of human sexuality could be encapsulated in one dictum. As the Victorians felt that they had done their whole educational duty if young people could be warned away from masturbation, so religious sex educators seem to feel about preventing premarital sex.

Although they are unanimous about theme and intent, the various religious presses cover a broad range of styles in sex education books. On the far right are crudely printed hellfire-and-brimstone tracts. A bit less threatening are the paperback dating guides written for young born-again Christians, which are studded with references to Bible chapter and verse; this category ranges from books that lean heavily on warnings about the temptations of the Devil to gentler texts that focus on the loving personhood of Jesus Christ for guidance in relationship. A third style, intended for a broader audience, are the books written from a conservative Christian perspective but without the specific religiosity of the fundamentalist guides. Liberal Christian sex education books for private reading are often accepted into the mainstream and lose their identity as religious instruction (although most liberal Christian denominations produce extensive sex education study materials for youth groups and these do tend to be restricted to religious bookstores). Catholic and Jewish sexuality guides reflect the ethical and spiritual concerns and the styles of their respective traditions. Mormons have made a specialty of "Christian fiction."

To the secular world of publishing these books are invisible. The presses that produce religious literature are outside of the New York book establishment. They are more commonly located in towns in the Midwest or Southern California, rather than in the large cities of the Northeast. Their books are seldom reviewed in standard sources, distributed through major outlets, or bought by school or public libraries, but nevertheless they sell extraordinarily well. *Just Like Ice Cream*, by Lissa Halls Johnson, for example, an obscure title from Ronald N. Haynes Publishers, racked up sixty thousand volumes in sales in its first thirteen months. (For comparison, *The Chocolate War*, by Robert Cormier, one of the most widely read young adult novels ever written, sold twenty-two thousand hardcover copies in ten years.)

Religious publishing has its own distribution channels. The sales outlets are the thousands and thousands of Christian bookstores that can be found in small towns and suburbs everywhere in America. The bookstores vary in character as much as their wares. At one end of the spectrum are the musty storefronts with racks of lurid tracts. Far more numerous are the attractive, clean, and well-lighted conservative Christian bookstores that specialize in glossy paperbacks from large fundamentalist publishers like Fleming H. Revell and Zondervan. National chains of bookstores are owned by some large religious publishing houses, such as Cokesbury and Augsburg, and their stock tends to reflect the preferences of their denominational affiliates: liberal Methodist for Cokesbury, conservative Lutheran for Augsburg. Liberal Christian books can also sometimes be found in secular stores. Catholic sex education manuals are sold only in Catholic bookstores and parochial schools, and Jewish books are distributed through synagogues and scholarly libraries. Local congregations, parochial schools, and church libraries are also a large market for fundamentalist presses.

Conservative religious sex education must be sought out in bookstores because it is seldom found on the shelves of public libraries. Librarians, who by and large are liberals themselves, often are repelled—when they are aware of these books at all—by the heavy proselytizing in print of the born-again philosophy. But even when they are making sincere efforts to build balanced collections that represent all points of view, there are sound reasons why many of the fundamentalist religious sex and dating books are not valid choices for library purchase. Some are badly produced—shoddy paper, careless printing, amateurish illustrations. Errors or distortions of facts about sexual functioning are not uncommon. Even worse is a tendency to "prove" trends by quoting outdated statistics or research. Slang that is elderly enough to alienate even a conservative readership is a disqualifier, as is an unhealthy emphasis on guilt or the Devil.

Although religious writers may feel that what they have to say on sexual ethics is eternal and unchanging, in some sensitive subject areas it is mandatory that they be aware of shifts in current medical and social thinking. A tricky problem appears here. In judging these books for suitability it is important that librarians or teachers distinguish carefully between secular fact and religious opinion. For instance, to say that masturbation is sinful is a matter of religious belief, but to imply that it causes physical harm is a factual error. And to claim that the practice causes crippling guilt is probably true in the case of a person who believes that it is sinful. A further example: for a writer who believes in a literal interpretation of the Bible it is an article of belief that God forbids homosexuality. Yet for that writer to accuse homosexuals of sin because they *choose* not to be heterosexual flies in the face of the recent finding that sexual gender preference is unalterably established early in life. And for that same writer to equate child molestation and homosexuality would be entirely wrong and a cause for rejecting the book. But an author who maintains that God decrees that woman's place is in the home is entitled to his religious opinion, and that statement ought not to disqualify the book, no matter how repugnant it might be to a feminist librarian making the purchase decision.

Deny as they may that *their* sexual ethics shift with the winds of popular culture, authors of religious sex education books find that they, too, must update their works from time to time if they want to stay in print. They lag behind in making the necessary adjustments, but adjust they do, eventually. Although they keep up with the times, it takes them longer than secularists, a group whose own writings (as we have repeatedly shown) are by no means always au courant with sexual behavior. Yet however old-fashioned these books may seem, there are reasons why they should be considered seriously for inclusion in library and school collections.

First is the legitimate demand by fundamentalists and other conservative religious groups that their views be represented. Librarians are missing the point when they insist that this is already being done because secular sex guides give support to abstinence as one of many possible sexual choices. Such moral relativism is repugnant to the far right. The ethic embraced by most conservative leaders is that abstinence until marriage is the *only* morally valid option, and only books that restrict themselves to this approach are acceptable to them.

A second reason for some judicious selection of religious sex education is the obvious need, in the light of teen pregnancy statistics, for materials that intelligently reinforce a commitment to abstinence or at least postponement of first intercourse. If religious convictions can be utilized to this end (but without invoking the fear and guilt that lead to denial and sexual irresponsibility), then this source of persuasion should not be ignored.

All of the books evaluated in this chapter (except the one Jewish guide) have been gleaned from the current stock of Christian bookstores. It should be emphasized that lacking a comprehensive in-print list of religious publishing, these represent a geographically limited selection. Many titles are so old that they would long ago have been dropped from secular publishers' catalogs and from library shelves. But because they are still being offered for sale, it has seemed relevant to evaluate them as current purchasing decisions rather than in historical perspective.

▪ Scorched Pages

The first example, found in a dim inner-city shop, dates from 1943. *Courtship and the Dangers of Petting*, by John R. Rice, reeks of sulfur and brimstone. It is one of over a hundred lurid tracts written by this prolific Baptist pamphleteer on subjects ranging from "The Double Curse of Booze" to "Speaking in

Tongues." In its hellfire-scorched pages he points the finger of scorn at modern immorality:

> On every bathing beach, in every darkened movie theater, on front porch swings, even on the dance floor and (most deadly of all) in automobiles far from chaperons, young people make free with each others' bodies; hug, kiss and fondle each other. They pet when there is no pretense of actual love nor holy intention to marry. They do it promiscuously, as shamelessly as the mating of promiscuous barnyard animals. . . . Then in countless millions of cases they take the next step, one that naturally follows, and commit the scarlet sin, adultery.

Sex desire, once aroused, is irresistible, Rice warns. He illustrates: "A young woman attended a dance with her sweetheart to whom she was engaged to be married. After dancing several times with a high school friend whom she did not love, she and he both became deeply aroused, and they were led into the scarlet sin." Rice reinforces his warnings with Bible verses, including a long, lingering examination of the more sensual passages of the Song of Solomon. Fortunately, this heavy-breathing style has been supplanted by a more sophisticated tone in most contemporary sex guides, even from the far right.

▪ The Bible as Sex Education

By far the greatest number of sex and dating guides to be found in Christian bookstores are the books addressed to young people who already have a commitment to fundamentalist ideas, those who are "born again." These writers rely heavily on biblical verses to give weight to their pronouncements, but here they encounter a difficulty. Nowhere in the Bible is there a clear prohibition of premarital sex. Indeed, Scripture is far less concerned with sex as a source of sin than are the authors of religious sex instruction. Only one of the Ten Commandments, which lay down the basic rules for an ethical life, is about sex. The Seventh Commandment forbids adultery, which is strictly defined as "voluntary sexual intercourse between a married person and a partner other than the lawful husband or wife" (*American Heritage Dictionary*, 1975). Jesus himself, although he had a great deal to say about loving care for one's fellow beings, is silent on the subject of sex between unmarried young people. He did, however, on at least two occasions set an example of forgiveness toward older women who were involved in sexual hanky-panky (John 8:3–18 and John 4:17–19).

The historical fact is probably that in the biblical patriarchal society, where young girls were strictly closeted within the family until an early marriage, premarital sex was so rare as to be not worth mentioning in the rules. The "sexual licentiousness" that appears in later books of the New Testament as an item in lists of forbidden behavior refers, according to biblical scholars, to adultery or contact with prostitutes. Excerpts from these lists are favorite quotes for religious sex educators to demonstrate the sinfulness of premarital sex.

Without plain instruction from Jesus Christian dating guides must fall back on the words of Paul, a man who gave only reluctant approval even to legitimate physical love within marriage. But when quoting from Paul's letters the authors sometimes distort meaning to make it say what they want it to say. For example, a passage frequently cited is 2 Timothy 2:22: "So shun youthful passions and aim at righteousness, faith, love, and peace, along with those who call upon the Lord from a pure heart." But the "passions" named here are not sexual but "impatience with status quo, aversion to rule and routine" and other youthful enthusiasms, according to such a respected authority as the *Interpreter's Bible* (Nashville, Tenn.: Abingdon, 1952).

Another technique is to misinterpret Old Testament stories out of historical context to fit current sexual ideas. For example, the story of Onan was often told in older books to prove God's horror of masturbation. But a close reading of the passage shows quite plainly that the sin was not self-abuse when Onan "spilled his seed upon the ground" but a refusal to fulfill his obligation to conceive a child with his dead brother's wife, a child who would symbolically be his brother's and not his own.

In the broader implications of recorded Judeo-Christian thought, however, it is quite clear that a loving monogamous relationship between two human beings is the ideal sexual context and that uncaring behavior that treats other people as objects for self-gratification will eventually put one out of step with God and humanity. When religious sex educators speak from this more positive perspective they have far more credibility than when they attempt to put words in God's mouth about the Scarlet Sin.

▪ Born-Again Books

Certain ideas and topics appear in all of the following books aimed at a young fundamentalist readership. First, of course, is the dominant theme that sex is to be postponed until marriage and that virginity is a gift to bestow on one's new spouse. God has planned it this way and the Bible specifically forbids sex outside marriage, they say. Sex, they imply, is always followed by guilt and other bad things, such as pregnancy. A growing relationship is stopped in its tracks when the couple begins to have sex and usually dies away shortly afterward. Abortion, when it is mentioned at all, is classified as murder. Going steady is comfortable but dangerous. Any caresses or thoughts that arouse sexual desire are off-limits, even between engaged couples.

Dating a non-Christian is energetically discouraged. Boys are always the initiators and aggressors and girls the victims—tales of predatory males and seduced and abandoned females abound. Long outdated "problems," such as the evils of flirting, the conduct of engaged couples, and whether to kiss on the first date, are revived. There is almost no information on the physical facts of sex—no diagrams of sexual organs, no discussion of coitus, menstruation, nocturnal emissions, conception, orgasm. Nor is birth control or sexually transmitted diseases mentioned—since the readers are not going to go to bed with anybody, these subjects are evidently irrelevant.

An extreme example of the sex prevention manual addressed to young born-agains is *A Handbook on Christian Dating*, by Greg Laurie. The author presupposes a readership whose every waking moment is devoted to "witnessing for the Lord." In answer to the question "What do Christians do on dates?" he says: "A Christian's ideas of fun are serving the Lord, getting into the Word, and praying. . . . Pray together before you even do anything. Get in that car and seek the Lord together. . . . Read the Bible together. Go to Church together. Go on and enjoy the Lord together. . . . One of the best things to do together is to witness." Dating the unsaved is dangerous because "old Beelzebubble starts nailing you." Readers are assured that God will find them the perfect mate, and in the meantime energy spent worrying about dating could better be used to witness and wait on the Lord. The author is the young pastor of Calvary Chapel of Riverside, California, where he presides over a congregation the majority of whose members are between fifteen and twenty-five. He is also a talented cartoonist and has produced Christian comic books. *A Handbook on Christian Dating* is adorned with his drawings in the manner of the sixties (the "Jesus People" style of the text also recalls that era). Although the book is appropriate only for those within this Christian sect, there is something attractive in its youthful tone and the earnest sweetness of its total dedication.

Another book with a young perspective is *A Love Story*, by Tim Stafford. It is better written and more friendly than many books of this type, possibly because Stafford is young, an editor of *Campus Life*, and author of a column in that magazine on "Love, Sex and the Whole Person." He makes at least token recognition of plurality: "Right now a half-dozen ideas about how to handle our sexuality are with us. Each one seems to work for at least some people. . . . I believe that when you add up all the columns, Jesus' ideas on sex come out ahead of anyone else's." Chapters on "Why Wait," "How Far Do We Go?," "Masturbation," "Singleness," "Homosexuality," and "Going Out" are built around Stafford's responses to poignant letters from teens troubled by their sexual urges. His answers, often reinforced by anecdotes from his own experience as a single man, are honest and practical within the framework of an absolute commitment to chastity outside of marriage. The pros and cons of masturbation warrant fourteen pages of discussion, although he concludes the matter is not an important ethical concern for God: "If it's a sin, it's one the Bible deals with less than gossip, overeating, and kicking the cat." Neither is homosexuality a serious sin; according to the Bible, "envy and gossip are in the same class," if the person with homosexual tendencies resists acting them out and prays to God to be changed. Stafford's final chapter is a passionate paean to "marriage, the Christian focus of sex, as a metaphor for the relationship of God to His people." Although this book is firmly rooted in the conservative Christian belief system, it is appropriate for public libraries serving evangelical populations because of the practical help it offers young people struggling to control their sexual desires.

Yet one more book with a young style—at least compared with the others of this type—is *Dating: Guidelines from the Bible*, by Scott Kirby. The focus is a detailed examination of dating rituals and etiquette from a fundamentalist Christian orientation. Discussion questions at the end of each chapter explore Bible passages the author considers relevant.

More appropriate for general library purchase is *Christian Ways to Date, Go Steady, and Break Up*, by John Butler, a young editor at Standard Publishing. He takes a positive, practical approach to all problems of human interaction involved in dating and reflects a careful concern for other people: "All the wrong reasons for dating involve exploitation." Although he gives practical advice on how to maintain chastity on a date, he doesn't emphasize it out of all proportion. The style is warm and aware, and the cartoon illustrations are amusing. The section on breaking up humanely is especially good. The book is addressed to evangelical Christians, but there is much in it that could be useful to other young adults.

When Can I Say, "I Love You"?, by Max and Vivian Rice, is strongly focused toward marriage, although the authors recommend that young people should not be in a hurry to find a partner. Instead, they should work on the fundamentals of sacrificial Christian love, practicing in their own families. True love in a lasting marriage can be found only with the guidance of the Holy Spirit, they maintain. The Rices, who are the directors of a South Carolina Christian camp called Look-Up-Lodge, write in a restrained and relatively literate style, and their book should be reassuring to young people who have a Christian commitment.

Looking for Love in All the Wrong Places is also written by a Christian camp director. Joe White is president of Kanakuk-Kanakomo Kamps and lives in Missouri. Cartoon illustrations give his book a lighthearted look, but the text is weighted down with heavy-handed proselytizing and lugubrious anecdotes proving the evils of sex and drugs. These stories are often drawn from the author's previous life as a sinner before he was saved. Each chapter ends with a set of questions for thought and discussion, such as "At what point does sex become sin?"

Many other books of this kind range from elderly to ludicrous.

The Dating Game, by Herbert J. Miles, is drawn from the author's twenty-three years of experience as a teacher of college-level marriage and family courses and as a columnist for several Southern newspapers. His vocabulary creaks ("courtship" is used throughout, despite the title), and his anecdotes and bits of advice are antiquated. A girl who has had sex is called "a bird with a broken pinion"; the Kinsey study is labeled "an insult to American women."

You Me He, by Texas evangelist Sammy Tippit as told to Jerry Jenkins, tips its hand with the subtitle: "Sex Really Isn't a Dirty Word." A couple who park or go to an empty apartment are told they are committing spiritual suicide. Dates should pray together when they first get into the car, dedicate the date to God, and flee the Devil.

Questions Teenagers Ask About Dating and Sex is drawn from Barry Wood's ministry to youth. Each chapter answers a question. Sample queries are: "Is French kissing a sin?" "Can sexy clothes be a 'turn-on' that displeases God?" "Is thinking about sex a sin?" "Should I stop dating a non-virgin?" The book ends with a glossary, which includes the terms chastity belt, fondle, fornication, lasciviousness, lust, temptations, and an indictment of masturbation as emotionally damaging as well as sinful.

Another example of the sex-as-sin school of thought is *How to Be Happy Though Young*, by Darien B. Cooper. The author, a graduate of Carson Newman College in Jefferson City, Tennessee, developed the book from her "sought-after lecture series for groups of teenagers in the Atlanta area." Teens are not only to beware of any sexual feelings or actions before marriage but are also to watch for other lures of the Devil, such as alcohol, cigarettes, marijuana, and dating non-Christians. Cartoon illustrations show teens coping with temptation.

A chapter is devoted to exposing the evil effects of listening to rock and country music. "Our enemy, Satan, uses unhealthy music to weaken Christians. Much like drugs, rock music's pulsating, hard-driving beat can, over a period of time, affect one's will, making him vulnerable to satanic influence." Cooper deplores the personal lives and beliefs of the Eagles, the Beatles, the Rolling Stones, Frank Zappa, the Beach Boys' Brian Wilson, Elton John, and Peter Frampton. "Anyone listening to hard-rock groups or singers such as Kiss, Santana, Black Sabbath, Eagles, Rolling Stones, or Alice Cooper, is, in my opinion, placing himself in very dangerous company." Their lyrics should be carefully examined. "Be on guard against songs which approve sexual promiscuity, crime, revolution, peace at any price, disarmament, fear of death, atheism or anti-Christianity, internationalism, committing suicide, occultic practices, defeatism, or a pessimistic outlook on life."

A particularly bad abuse of scriptural authority characterizes *Update: A New Approach to Christian Dating*, by Fred Hartley. The book bristles with chapter and verse out of context, and the author sometimes even goes so far as to put bracketed words into the quote to make it fit his intentions—as in I Peter 5:5–9: "Likewise you that are younger be subject to the elders," an instruction to the junior members of a Christian congregation to respect the older leaders of the group. Hartley changes it to "Likewise you that are younger [children] be subject to the elders [parents]" and uses the passage to prove "advice from parents gives us protection from the temptations of the devil." In Hartley's mind the words "sin" and "passion" are interchangeable with the word "sex," and so he is able to find many places in Scripture that seem, out of context, to support his arguments. "These are the last days," he proclaims,

> "and wickedness is being multiplied. In the high schools and colleges across the globe sex is making slaves of men and women. Television, newsstands, and movie theaters are filled with impurities. Never has wickedness been so worldwide. The end is coming soon and Satan knows it. He has vomited demons of filth upon the earth, and many of our brothers and sisters who are now in love with Jesus will lose their affections because they will refuse to date God's way.

Young Christians should beware not only of dating non-Christians but should also not date or even "fellowship" with immoral Christians—"those who consistently don't call upon the Lord." Sex poisons everything, according to Hartley's stories from his own pastoral counseling, in which he advises young people to break up with a partner with whom they are tempted to be erotically involved. They should dump the offending party and will feel much better afterward. Because, as he says, "it is amazing to watch boy-girl relationships fall apart when lust enters in. As soon as sex is resorted to, things begin to decay." Even "praying with someone of the opposite sex should generally be limited to a group situation" lest uncontrollable intimacy result.

▪ BROADER BOOKS FOR CONSERVATIVES

Another type of religious sex education is written out of conservative Christian conviction but does not necessarily assume that readers share that doctrinal commitment. Although Jesus, God, and the Church are occasionally invoked, these authors do not depend on biblical quotations to back up their arguments but rely instead on generally accepted conservative attitudes. They are more likely to acknowledge the possibilities of venereal disease and unwanted pregnancy and so to give at least minimal mention to basic sexual physiology and birth control—although the information they provide on these subjects is often inaccurate and incomplete. Drawings of the sexual organs are never included, nor are glossaries of sexual terms or even indexes. It should not be assumed that because the intended audience is broader, the authors' ideas are, too. The same narrow obsession with the preservation of virginity dominates their thinking.

Honest Answers About Dating and Sex isn't. The author, Gwen Pamenter Aseltine, bases many of her statements on books, articles, and studies from the late fifties and sixties and so reaches conclusions that are no longer valid. For instance, she cites a 1961 study by Lester Kirkendall to prove that physical intimacy has the effect of driving an unmarried couple apart. But two major factors in Dr. Kirkendall's study were loss of respect by the male and the necessity for secrecy—neither of which is a serious problem today. Aseltine is not hopeful at all for the prospects of sexual pleasure for girls. She repeatedly stresses the difficulties of learning to reach orgasm and sternly tells girls that it is "unrealistic" for women to expect the same degree of satisfaction in intercourse as their husbands.

Each minichapter is built around a question from a young person, questions presumably gleaned from the author's experience teaching classes in Marriage and the Family at "a state university." But no matter what the query, the answer eventually is worked around to premarital chastity. The style is condescending in the extreme: "The next time you feel that you are having difficulty with your erotic impulses, take a cold shower—then go out and do something nice for someone else."

The tone of *Preparing for Adolescence*, by James Dobson, is also suffocatingly preachy. The book, which was originally offered for sale in the format of cassette tapes, is aimed at thirteen-year-olds—extremely naive thirteen-year-olds. It would be hard to find a young person pliant and uninformed enough to sit through—much less read—these dull and overbearing lectures without rebelling. Beginning with a long section on self-esteem, Dobson moves on to the dangers of conformity (drugs, alcohol, and sex), the changes of puberty, misconceptions about love, and a long "rap session" in which four older teens describe their own young adolescent feelings. At one point the group is joined by the tape technician, who shares a story about how God healed his addiction to drugs. His attempts at the vernacular of the drug culture are not even close: "My friend's big sister was a big 'loader,' and she used to make us roll up lids for her. . . ."

In a chapter on the physical manifestations of adolescence Dobson is so intent on emphasizing that puberty is nothing to fear that he creates the opposite effect ("Menstruation is not an awful event for girls to dread. . . . You will not bleed to death, I promise you. . . . Sex is not dirty and it is not evil. . . . Sex is not a dirty thing at all . . ."). Young people who commit the sin of premarital intercourse are told that they may be endangering their eternal salvation. Not the least of the unpleasant features of *Preparing for Adolescence* is a long, excruciatingly detailed, sad story about the death of the author's little dog when he himself was thirteen. The dubious justification for including this painful tale is to demonstrate the intensity of adolescent emotions. Dr. Dobson is Associate Clinical Professor of Pediatrics at the University of Southern California School of Medicine and serves on the attending staff for Children's Hospital of Los Angeles. He is the author of a number of books on medicine and psychology that are respected in their fields. *Preparing for Adolescence* is not one of them.

A pair of much more moderate books are *Sex, Love, or Infatuation: How Can I Really Know?* and *Sex, Dating and Love—77 Questions Most Often Asked*, by Ray E. Short. The author, a Methodist minister and professor of sociology at the University of Wisconsin, lectures frequently to high-school and college students; *Sex, Dating and Love* is arranged around their questions. *Sex, Love, or Infatuation* is a long and detailed examination of the characteristics of lasting "real love" as contrasted with the more transitory state of being "in love." To help young people diagnose their own relationships he provides fourteen clues (What is the major attraction? How did it start? How does it affect your personality? What does distance do? Are you jealous?). Each of these he analyzes at some length. Short has a penchant for checklists and charts; others are "The nine known facts about sex before marriage," "The road to arousal" (from full repression to sexual intercourse), "A checklist of arguments for and against premarital sexual intercourse" (twenty-five for, thirty-four against), and a "Profile of the typical traits of unwed live-in couples in the United States and their relationships."

To Short's credit he does footnote and document statements based on statistics and studies, and most of his sources are reputable and reasonably recent. However, sometimes his conclusions are more extreme than the data would seem to warrant. He also has an occasional tendency to reach for outdated research to prove a foregone assumption. For instance, he bases the claim that "those who have premarital sex tend to have less happy marriages" on information from a book published in 1953.

Unlike any other author of this kind of sex guide, he recognizes the plurality of religion in America ("Check it out with your priest, minister, or rabbi"), admits that venereal disease can be cured, and discusses herpes as well as syphilis and gonorrhea. He gives at least minimal birth-control information but seems to have the peculiar idea that to be effective condoms should be tested "for tiny holes" underwater before use. On homosexuality he has very little to say, only reassuring a boy that masturbation will not make him gay and telling a girl who has been "pawed" by another girl to "avoid her; it could get complicated." He discusses cohabitation at great length in both books, concluding that it has a bad effect whether or not the couple eventually marry. Most of the arguments in the two books are devoted, of course, to persuading young people to postpone sex until marriage. Short presents the conservative position with reason and respect for young people; his books are satisfactory choices for libraries and even schools that wish to include this point of view in their collections.

Another acceptable book representing the conservative outlook is *The Great Date Wait and Other Hazards*, by William L. Coleman. Written in the form of letters from a father to his own teenagers, it is illustrated with charming photographs of young teens. Each page-long devotional focuses on one aspect of building self-esteem and developing relationships and ends with a short Bible verse and three discussion questions. The tone is realistic, practical, and sympathetic. Coleman's theme is that teens should get on with living abundant, useful lives without putting too much emphasis on dating as a source of happiness and self-worth.

The Dating Maze, by Brent D. Earles, has a similar format. One or two pages of discussion are focused on a problem or technique of dating, ending with a line from the Bible (often wrenched out of context) and a "Beatitude" composed by the author to drive home the message ("Happy are those who don't find their excitement in the bottom of a bottle or can, for their thrills don't make them wake up feeling like a loser the next morning."). Earles works hard to sound jazzy and contemporary, but misses by fifteen years. His advice includes not only warnings about sexual temptation and dating nonbelievers, but also diatribes against alcohol and dancing (which he terms "sexual slithering"). Only the most naive teens would not be offended by his condescending style.

The Stork is Dead, by Charlie W. Shedd, is probably the best-known book of this type, both because it has been around for awhile (original edition 1968) and because its author is widely visible as a columnist (*Teen* magazine and "Strictly for Dads"), lecturer, radio personality, and, with his wife, Martha, promoter of the Fun Marriage Forums. The revised edition of 1982 makes almost no changes from the 1968 version, but, interestingly enough, in the light of the new conservatism the book seems less dated now than it did in 1975. Shedd's style is brisk and colloquial, and the short chapters built around poignant letters from teens have punch and energy. Only occasionally is there a false note in the contemporary tone ("This girl in our school wears clothes that really turn a fellow on . . .").

The chapters on "Lines Guys Use" and "Why Girls Give In" are particularly realistic. Shedd gives limited approval to abortion when the health of the baby or the mother is endangered but recommends that a pregnant girl bear her child and then give it up for adoption. Surprisingly, he describes masturbation as a "gift of God." He accepts that some teens are going to have sex no matter what and urges them to use birth control—although he doesn't give any particulars. Other unusual passages are a list of "Twelve Ways to Handle Your Parents" and an explanation of why Protestants believe in contraception (without the expected diatribe against interfaith marriages).

Shedd's friendly, nondidactic style and general good sense would make this a highly useful title to represent the conservative outlook, if it were not for two serious lapses. The first is a discussion following the question "Can a Nymphomaniac Be Cured?" in which Shedd gives credence to this long-discredited idea. The second is a chapter in which he classifies mutual masturbation, oral sex, incest, and homosexuality as "sordid things to consider." It is a pity that these two errors in judgment were not corrected in the new edition. With them, the book can be given only a marginal recommendation.

▪ Religious Fiction

Although the fundamentalist presses have made a few clumsy attempts to tap the power of fiction for their own purposes, the Mormons are the only denomination that has produced readable and well-written religious novels in any quantity. These usually serve the purpose of explaining the beliefs of the Church of Latter Day Saints in a historical setting or show young people living by those beliefs in contemporary society. Some are good enough to transcend the didactic intent.

An outstanding example is *What Now, McBride?*, by Gary Lee Davis. The hardcover production is excellent: handsome jacket, catchy title, good binding, attractive and readable page. More than that, the story moves along briskly, the scenes are well paced, the characters are believable, and best of all, the dialogue is genuinely funny.

The author is a professional comedian, among other things, and a master of the fast wisecrack. There is none of that smug mustiness that usually taints these books. Even when the lead character explains why he is against abortion, the reasoning is low-key. One almost wishes he would explain Mormon doctrine—but he doesn't. The story stays away from religious apologetics and concentrates on the romance of Paula Cohen and Nephi McBride.

She is a UCLA student in theater arts and he is a young carpenter who is a devout Mormon and one of the most charismatic characters ever to appear in YA fiction. They meet when her comparative-religion class takes a tour of the gigantic Mormon Temple in Westwood Village. Paula is Jewish, although atheistic, and a talented budding actress and singer. Nephi and Paula fall in love to the tune of some wonderful repartee and have an idyllic courtship, during which Paula discovers that Nephi is strong but gentle and understanding, idealistic but not above practical jokes, knows influential people everywhere but will spend a whole afternoon helping a clumsy, underdog kid. The question of sex never arises. Only when it is too late do they face the difficulties of their future together. His church decrees conversion of intended spouses and devotion of women to home and babies, Nephi explains in despair. Then Paula discovers an additional complication—she is pregnant by her last lover. She breaks off the romance and disappears. Nephi searches desperately for her and is reviled by her strident, stringy-haired, feminist roommates. At last he finds her at the home of his aunt, barefoot and pregnant and fully converted to his faith. They get married, and as a wedding present he stages a scene in the foyer of Mann's Chinese Theater so that she can put her handprints in wet cement, be asked for her autograph by the wedding guests, and sign herself in concrete as "Mrs. Nephi McBride."

So skillfully is this plot developed that only later does the reader realize that this girl has given up her ethnic heritage, her beliefs, her potential career, her name, and her very identity in exchange for marriage to a very attractive man. Whether the sacrifice is worth the reward is a social and religious, but not a literary, judgment.

The fascinating subject of polygamy is explored in a number of Mormon novels, such as *The Principle*, by Kathryn Smoot Caldwell, and *A Woman of Destiny*, by Orson Scott Card. Other Mormon young adult novels with some bearing on sex education are *Summer Fire*, by Douglas Thayer, and *Today, Tomorrow, and Four Weeks from Tuesday*, by Carol Lynn Pearson.

But other conservative evangelical publishers are much less skillful with fiction. The bestselling paperback *Just Like Ice Cream*, by Lissa Halls Johnson, is as simplistic in its message as a Victorian cautionary tale. The cover makes it appear to be a teen romance, but actually it is the standard predictable preggers story: innocent girl seduced by glib young man, painful and unpleasant sex, agonized pregnancy, bloody delivery, and a brave but mournful decision to give the baby up for adoption. A subplot concerns the girl's conversion to fundamentalist Christianity.

The "Christian" novels of John Benton surpass in sordid detail any of the realistic secular YA novels that are so vehemently opposed by conservatives. The cover of each book of the "New Hope" series shows a fully clad but provocatively posed young woman, and the titles are feminine names. *Carmen* is typical. A young girl runs away from her brutal, alcoholic father to a life as a junkie and prostitute. There is no explicit sex or four-letter words, only hints and suggestions for the imagination to fill in. But there *are* lingering, loving descriptions of the joys of shooting up with heroin; there are enthusiastic scenes of beatings, muggings, knife fights, razor slashings.

Carmen is uncomfortable whenever she runs out of dope, but turning a few tricks is always a convenient and easy way to make the price of a fix. The life of the hooker is made to seem attractive and exciting, with hard drugs the ecstatic reward for a night's work. (The marijuana scene is more overblown than the ludicrous classic antidope film *Reefer Madness.*) In the very last chapter Carmen gets saved by David Wilkerson's Teen Challenge, but this is tame stuff compared with what went before. Carmen and all the rest of John Benton's ladies are close relatives of the heroines of the obscene "needle novels" that are passed from hand to hand by inner-city teenagers. This is dangerous, poisonous stuff and not at all justified by the fake religious conversion stuck on at the end.

▪ Catholic Sex Manuals

Most Catholic sex education books are meant to be used in an institutional setting. Official hierarchical approval is indicated by the presence of the Nihil Obstat and the Imprimatur on the reverse of the title page. However, these are followed by a formal disclaimer: "The Nihil Obstat and the Imprimatur are a declaration that a book or a pamphlet is considered to be free from doctrinal or moral error. It is not implied that those who have granted the Nihil Obstat and Imprimatur agree with the contents, opinions or statements expressed." This apprehensive attitude is further revealed by careful instructions for the circumstances under which young people may be exposed to the contents of such books. For instance, *Sexuality and Dating: A Christian Perspective* carries the explicit directive "intended for use in conjunction with the Student Guide for Personal Reflection, under the supervision of a teacher employing the approach outlined in the Teaching Manual, and with the written permission of the students' parents."

Since these books are burdened with such heavy cautions, it might be expected that they would cleave rigidly to the Vatican's directives on sexual matters. Surprisingly, this is not always the case. Although the position on abortion and premarital sex is undeviating, there is room for examination of personal conscience concerning masturbation, contraception, and even homosexuality. Gone, too, is the traditional teaching that sex is only for purposes of procreation. And, although Protestant sex guides often warn against dating Catholics, the reverse doesn't seem to be true.

Sexuality and Dating: A Christian Perspective, by Richard Reichert, emphasizes the goodness of sex when used as God intended, to express full humanity. The first chapter stresses "the importance of getting the facts about the biology of the human reproductive system" but doesn't provide any information on the subject other than to tell students "this course is a useful forum for asking serious questions and for getting some straightforward answers."

Intelligent chapters on sex-role stereotyping and the real differences and similarities between men and women lead into a discussion of the "dating game" and the one cardinal rule for playing: "Respect the person you are dating." Although recent liberation movements have achieved some praiseworthy results in overcoming injustice, the author says, the momentum has carried things too far, so that young adults should not fall into the trap of presuming that current sexual attitudes and practices are normal. "Undoubtedly the most horrendous side effect of these movements has been the legalization of abortion." Almost as bad has been the increasing number of divorces.

"Within marriage as viewed by Jesus, sexual intercourse is a prayer, a sacrament—and fun." But other sexual expressions: "rape, adultery, prostitution, nonmarital intercourse (even when the couple is in love), mutual or solitary masturbation, genital sexual relationships between homosexuals or lesbians—all these must at the minimum be judged as less than fully human. . . ." But are these actions sinful? This is a much more complex question in Catholic theology. Masturbation is "sinful in principle" but "rarely involves serious personal guilt" and should be discussed with a priest. Homosexuality, since its practitioners have not chosen to be as they are, is not in itself a sin. "The Church does not approve of homosexual acts, but it reserves moral judgment to the individual and God." This statement is followed by the very unusual (for religious sex manuals) acknowledgment that the reader may be an incipient gay. "If it happens over the period of the next few years that you discover you have a homosexual orientation, get good advice from someone who can help you to feel good about yourself." But nonmarital sexual intercourse is "immoral, period" and "seriously sinful." Petting, too, is in principle "considered immoral for unmarried persons" because it might tempt them to sin further.

Contraceptives are discussed in the context of "how would you decide if you were a parent today and you had a daughter your age?" Brief mention is made of the Pill ("medically risky"), the IUD ("kills newly-conceived babies"), the diaphragm ("more for someone who is planning to be sexually active"), and foam ("not considered a highly reliable contraceptive"). Condoms get tentative approval as "the best method, other than abstinence, for preventing the spread of VD." But the morality of contraceptive use is left an open question.

A final chapter points out that celibates are "special people in God's eyes." Reichert's style is much more liberal than this analysis of content would seem to indicate. The book is attractively illustrated with photographs of teenagers and excerpts from the comic strip "Cathy."

Sex, Sexuality & You, by Nancy Hennessy Cooney with Anne Bingham, is not nearly as slick and handsome, but it has far more information. Cooney is Youth Ministry Consultant for the Archdiocese of Milwaukee and a member of the U.S. Catholic Conference's Committee on Family and Human Sexuality. She provides sound and adequate text and drawings on the physiology of sex and reproduction (making this the only religious sex education book to name the clitoris). Sex roles are discussed in the context of the mutuality of family living. The concept of "skin hunger" is useful in learning to deal with sexuality, the author explains, but masturbation is a wrong way to relieve this need because "sexual expression ideally should take place in the context of a loving relationship with one's spouse."

Contraceptive methods are divided into those that do and do not have official approval of the Catholic Church. *But*, "many couples, including Catholics, have turned to manufactured or surgical methods of birth control because these methods generally are more effective than biological methods. . . . Whichever decision is reached, it's important that the couple take responsibility for their decision. The Church wants each person to have an informed conscience and act according to it."

Cooney explains that the Church's attitude toward homosexuals—since it is now understood that "the condition is not a choice"—is changing. "The Church desires that Catholic homosexuals remain in touch with the Church and obtain help from the . . . community," although "the Church does not approve of homosexual acts." A reader who suspects such tendencies should find a person to talk to who can "help you feel good about yourself."

The teaching on abortion is less flexible: "it is wrong because it destroys innocent human life." However, Cooney, unlike many prolife activists, is willing to bear responsibility for the consequences of enforcing her beliefs: "If we oppose abortion, we also must make a commitment to the children who will be born to women who otherwise might have had abortions."

She concludes with a celebratory statement: "Sexuality is not limited to genital expression. It's literally 'all that we are, and all that we offer.' Intercourse, and everything else we do, can reveal to us the presence of God and the deeper meaning of life."

Celebration is the name of the game, man, with a flower-child guide that bloomed only four years after Vatican II but is still on sale in Catholic bookstores. Entitled simply (in the manner of the era) *Sex Sex Sex*, it was written by Marcena and Trevor Wyatt Moore and published jointly in 1969 by the Catholic Ave Maria Press and the Protestant Pilgrim Press of the United Church. It bears no Imprimatur. Reading (or digging) this little volume brings on an acute attack of nostalgia for the good old days of laidback psychedelic peace and joy. The words wander freely over, up, and around the page, interwoven with splashes of color, outsized exclamations, and amusing bits of Victorian (copyright-free) etchings.

But even this super-hip proclamation, if read closely, is making a case for the traditional sexual arrangements:

> Like not all sexual love consists of horizontal exercises au contraire cheri it's freely giving one's self to the other rather than perpetual panting pursuit of internal combustion that makes love sexcessful . . . like dig before the pillow comes the person special creature beloved by God person someone not something beloved by God can you do less? person The cool cats are persons usually hip enough to forego [sic] sex until they have committed themselves to each other a lot of rap about commitment? It may be an old fashioned word but so is Sex and without committed love the whole scene gets distorted as hell like baby, no matter how high the fever may rise, when it breaks, two uncommitted persons may find themselves just used, lonely people, utter strangers like nowhere commitment means love that wills intensely the greatest good of the one loved & Marriage r.s.v.p. (after more or less relevant & costly ceremonies) is generally regarded as the state of life most suitable for fulfillment of mutual commitments. . . .

▪ A Liberal Jewish Perspective

Historically the Jewish tradition has depended for guidance on the careful reasoning of scholars bringing thoughtful and prayerful analysis to bear on the torah (the body of Jewish literature and oral tradition as a whole, containing the laws, teachings, and divine knowledge of the religion). *Love, Sex and Marriage: A Jewish View*, by Rabbi Roland B. Gittelsohn, is grounded firmly in that tradition. The 1980 edition of this work is a combined revision of the author's *Consecrated unto Me* (1965) and *Sex and Marriage* (1976) and is intended as a textbook for older teens.

Rabbi Gittelsohn is a master of the rabbinical style. Even the fictional cases for discussion that appear at the end of each chapter reveal his warmth and concern. With simple dignity and a scrupulous care for fairness he lays out the evidence on both sides of every question. Speaking from the reform, or liberal, Jewish position, he explains that a deep appreciation of the validity of tradition need not preclude flexibility for modern circumstances. "Most of the ethical insights of Judaism are at least as valid today as when they were first conceived by our ancestors. In some areas, however, because we have knowledge which was unavailable to them, it becomes necessary for us to revise or even discard their judgments."

Beginning with a positive approach, he extolls the excellence of Jewish family life. He praises the beauty of the Jewish marriage rite and the enduring nature of real love. "Jews are likely to have more stable marriages than others," he claims—a verifiable fact. Historically this has been because "Jewish survival depends on the kind of home they establish."

In this setting, which presupposes a solid marriage, dating is seen in perspective as the prelude to family life. He discusses its etiquette (including the safe use of the car, a topic often not given enough importance). The discussion moves naturally to questions of physical intimacy. Quoting from Eleanor Hamilton's *Sex Before Marriage*, Rabbi Gittelsohn gives a qualified approval to petting to orgasm if both partners love and respect each other.

But the ethical issue of premarital sex is not so easily settled. Fair as always, the rabbi says, "Today we must offer young people more alternatives; we must give them both sides of such controversial questions as the advisability of premarital intercourse, then trust them to arrive at their own decisions." This he does, beginning with the honest admission that "nowhere in either the Bible or the Talmud is there an explicit prohibition of intercourse before marriage," because in biblical times couples were betrothed in mid-teens and married a year later. He realizes that postponed maturation has created a problem of sexual expression in our society. "To tell a young person that it is wrong to feel what nature itself impels one to feel is to create an almost intolerable problem."

He urges young people to make an active choice, not to drift into conduct that may be harmful. "The only person on God's earth who has a right to decide that question is *you*." But he makes no secret of where his own sympathies lie: enjoying sex on a purely physical level may make it impossible to experience it later on a spiritual plane, he says, and "studies show" that those who have had premarital sex are more likely to have extramarital sex. For those who nevertheless choose not to wait he stresses the moral imperative of birth control. But finding himself unable to present the arguments in favor of premarital sex with any impartiality, he turns that chapter over to colleague Judith Fales.

Family planning and contraception within marriage are appropriate ways to shape the ideal family. But in the long view "the modern Jew confronts a most painful dilemma between a knowledge that the human population of this earth must be curbed if disaster is to be averted, and an insistence that it is important—for us and for humankind in general—that we Jews survive."

Other controversial matters are also put into historical and ethical perspective. "The spirit of liberalism of genuinely traditional Judaism . . . allows abortion where the physical or mental health of a mother would otherwise be threatened," although "there are some Orthodox rabbis . . . whose views on abortion are scarcely distinguishable from the Catholic position." Discussing homosexuality, he contrasts the ancient Jewish traditional harshness toward such practices with modern liberal acceptance. The attitudes toward masturbation, too, have changed since ancient times; Rabbi Gittelsohn gives unhesitating approval to the practice. On the subject of VD, however, he is out of date, basing his discussion on statistics collected between 1960 and 1974 and making no mention of recent developments like herpes or AIDS.

The subjugation of women in a patriarchal society has long been a vulnerable point in Jewish ethical thought. The rabbi admits freely that "the ancients were regrettably less sensitive to sexual equality than we are today." However, to be fair he points out their "astonishing sensitivity to the fact that women possessed active sexual needs." Although Judaism has historically not considered women equal, this tradition has treated women better than other cultures at the same time, he proves, and has been willing to grow and change in its attitudes toward women.

With characteristic moderation and far-sightedness he sums up his argument: "Human progress and creativity seem to accompany a measure of restriction on sexual activity." Although *Love, Sex and Marriage* is long and sober, it deserves respect and a place in every library collection that serves a population that includes Jewish teenagers.

▪ The Invisible Liberal Christians

As we have seen, liberal Christian books are not usually perceived as religious sex education. This is because their basic premise—that sexual morality can be defined as respect for the personhood of others—is the same as that of secular sex education. Many well-known sex educators could, in the broader sense, be termed Christian writers. Eric Johnson, for instance, is a devoted Quaker. But his works are never found in "Christian" bookstores.

One writer whose work does occasionally appear in Cokesbury as well as secular stores is Richard Hettlinger. An Episcopalian minister, he is professor of religion at Kenyon College in Ohio. While thus technically a liberal Christian, Hettlinger's social attitudes are conservative. *Growing Up with Sex* in its 1980 edition is an intelligent and thoughtful presentation of this position. Hettlinger adopts the traditional stance that sexual intercourse should be reserved for couples who have made a life commitment to each other. Although he says, "I do not think intercourse before marriage is degrading or terribly sinful, provided it expresses concern and respect between two people," he also says, "A girl who will go to bed with a boy on the first date is pretty universally regarded as a tramp: in fact, she is emotionally sick." The solution he recommends is mutual petting to orgasm.

Nor does he shrink from taking definite stands on other sticky matters. Masturbation is "God's provision of a temporary substitute for the full joys of sexual intercourse," and "now that abortion is legal in the United States it is inevitable and proper that a couple consider it if an unwanted pregnancy occurs." A married couple, that is.

The chapter on homosexuality is more ambiguous. Although he has expunged some offensive references to "faeries and queens" and "the gaudy attractions of the gay life" that appeared in the 1971 edition and although he supports the right of homosexuals to live without unfair social and legal discrimination, his acceptance of gayness is less than wholehearted. "If you eventually grow up homosexual, don't be ashamed of what you are but make your sexual relationships as rich and mature as you can."

His coverage of basic physiology, birth control, and STD is adequate but not outstanding. A chapter on teenage marriage and a glossary of sexual terms (from which a section of the alphabet is inexplicably missing) complete the book.

■ BIBLIOGRAPHY

(Note: This is a list of books mentioned in this chapter; inclusion does not necessarily mean recommendation. For Core Collection List see Appendix.)

Aseltine, Gwen Pamenter. *Honest Answers About Dating and Sex: A Book for Teenagers.* Old Tappan, N.J.: Revell, 1982.

Benton, John. *Carmen.* Old Tappan, N.J.: Revell, 1970.

Butler, John. *Christian Ways to Date, Go Steady, and Break Up.* Cincinnati: Standard, 1978.

Caldwell, Kathryn Smoot. *The Principle.* Sandy, Utah: Randall, 1983.

Card, Orson Scott. *A Woman of Destiny.* New York: Berkley, 1984.

Coleman, William L. *The Great Date Wait and Other Hazards.* Minneapolis: Bethany, 1982.

Cooney, Nancy Hennessy, with Anne Bingham. *Sex, Sexuality & You: A Handbook for Growing Christians.* Dubuque, Iowa: Brown, 1980.

Cooper, Darien B. *How to Be Happy Though Young.* Old Tappan, N.J.: Revell, 1979.

Davis, Gary Lee. *What Now, McBride?* Orem, Utah: Raymont, 1982.

Dobson, James. *Preparing for Adolescence.* Ventura, Calif.: Vision House, 1978.

Earles, Brent D. *The Dating Maze.* Grand Rapids, Mich.: Baker, 1984.

Gittelsohn, Roland B. *Love, Sex and Marriage: A Jewish View,* new ed. New York: Union of American Hebrew Congregations, 1980.

Hartley, Fred. *Update: A New Approach to Christian Dating.* Old Tappan, N.J.: Revell, 1977, 1982.

Hettlinger, Richard P. *Growing Up with Sex: A Guide for the Early Teens,* new rev. ed. New York: Continuum, 1980.

Johnson, Lissa Halls. *Just Like Ice Cream.* Palm Springs, Calif.: Haynes, 1982.

Kirby, Scott. *Dating: Guidelines from the Bible.* Grand Rapids, Mich.: Baker, 1979.

Laurie, Greg. *A Handbook on Christian Dating.* Riverside, Calif.: Harvest, 1978.

Miles, Herbert J. *The Dating Game*. Grand Rapids, Mich.: Zondervan, 1975.

Moore, Marcena, and Trevor Wyatt Moore. *Sex Sex Sex*. Notre Dame, Ind.: Ave Maria, and Philadelphia: Pilgrim, 1969.

Pearson, Carol Lynn. *Today, Tomorrow, and Four Weeks from Tuesday*. Salt Lake City: Bookcraft, 1983.

Reichert, Richard. *Sexuality and Dating: A Christian Perspective*. Winona, Minn.: St. Mary's Press, Christian Brothers, 1981.

Rice, John R. *Courtship and The Dangers of Petting*. Murfreesboro, Tenn.: Sword of the Lord, 1943.

Rice, Max, and Vivian Rice. *When Can I Say, "I Love You"?* Chicago: Moody, 1977.

Shedd, Charlie W. *The Stork Is Dead*. Waco, Texas: Word, 1968. Rev. ed., 1982.

Short, Ray E. *Sex, Dating and Love—77 Questions Most Often Asked*. Minneapolis: Augsburg, 1984.

———. *Sex, Love, or Infatuation: How Can I Really Know?* Minneapolis: Augsburg, 1978.

Stafford, Tim. *A Love Story: Questions and Answers on Sex*. Grand Rapids, Mich.: Zondervan, 1977.

Thayer, Douglas. *Summer Fire*. Midvale, Utah: Orion, 1983.

Tippit, Sammy, as told to Jerry Jenkins. *You Me He*. Wheaton, Ill.: Victor, 1978.

White, Joe. *Looking for Love in All the Wrong Places*. Wheaton, Ill.: Tyndale, 1982.

Wood, Barry. *Questions Teenagers Ask About Dating and Sex*. Old Tappan, N.J.: Revell, 1981.

Chapter 12

Sex Guide Spin-offs

As certain aspects of teen sexuality become more and more complex and controversial, it becomes less and less possible to discuss them adequately in a few paragraphs or even a chapter of a general sex manual. The subjects of STD, contraception, abortion, rape, menstruation, gay identity, and—most especially—teen pregnancy and parenting have now accumulated enough data and opinions to justify whole books for young people. Clearly these are spin-offs from the sex guide genre. Although most of these books are obviously addressed to teens, the intended audience of others is not so apparent. Some are relevant to the general population as well as young adults, and a few have only one chapter that focuses on adolescent needs within the larger context of the subject. But all of them, however subtly or indirectly, reveal their origins by the didactic intent to influence behavior and bring it within the range of the socially accepted norm. (A few books have been included in this chapter that do *not* fit this definition of the spin-off because they contain important and useful information that has not yet been filtered through the sex guide mentality.)

▪ Loathsome Diseases

The VD book is the oldest kind of special-topic sex guide derivative. Early in the seventies, when educators began to realize that gonorrhea was becoming a serious teenage epidemic, dozens of books appeared that described symptoms of that and other loathsome diseases in technicolor and encouraged infected adolescents to have the courage to tell their contacts and to go for treatment. Among these titles were *VD: Facts You Should Know*, by Andre Blanzaco; *The V. D. Story*, by Stewart M. Brooks; *What About VD?*, by Phyllis S. Busch; *VD: The ABC's*, by John W. Grover; *VD: The Silent Epidemic*, by Margaret Hyde; *How to Avoid Social Diseases: A Practical Handbook*, by Leslie Nicholas; *VD: A Doctor's Answers*, by Suzanne M. Sgroi; *The Love Bugs: A Natural History of the VDs*, by Richard Stiller; *VD: The Love Epidemic*, by Mari Stein; *The VD Book*, by Joseph Chiappa; *V.D.*, by Eric Johnson; and *Facts About VD for Today's Youth*, by Sol Gordon. All of these, while useful for their time, are now outdated. For one thing, they saw the problem in terms of syphilis and gonorrhea, with a few other random diseases thrown in around the edges to fill up the pages.

We now know that the picture is far more complex and that symptomology and treatment are not nearly so clear-cut. Chlamydial infections, which often have no symptoms at all, are probably the diseases that affect the most people—4.5 to 10 million reported cases annually.[1] Or it may be herpes, which the Centers for Disease Control estimate now afflicts 20 million Americans, with half a million new cases reported every year.[2] Compared with this, gonorrhea with 1 to 3 million and syphilis with 70,000 fade to insignificance.[3] But the most frightening sexually transmitted disease is undoubtedly AIDS, from which no one has ever recovered since it first appeared in 1981. Although the numbers are as yet small, research scientists estimate that in five years, if it continues at its current rate of growth, AIDS will strike 1.6 million people.[4]

All of this is especially pertinent to young adults—seventy-five percent of STD occurs among people fifteen to twenty-four,[5] and the age group with the highest rate of increase is eleven to fourteen.[6] Unfortunately, the ongoing radical changes in the nature and understanding of socially transmitted disease mean that books on the subject date quickly. Only one of the many that have been written for young teens is still valid: Sol Gordon's *Facts About STD* (1983). This is a revision of *Facts About VD for Today's Youth*, first published in 1973 and updated in 1979. In spite of its slimness, it gives simple but adequate coverage of the major illnesses and clear guidance for prevention and treatment. (Although there is never any answer at the phone number given as the California VD Hotline.) Like Gordon's *Facts About Sex*, it is practical for reluctant or unskilled readers and young adolescents.

Although at the present time there are no STD books aimed exclusively at older teens, there are at least three books on the adult level that meet adolescent needs perfectly well. As Dr. Hans Neumann says, "If you're old enough to be sexually active, you're old enough to have the straight story." His *Guide to the New Sexually Transmitted Diseases* is a readable, friendly, and authoritative source of complete information. His discussion of AIDS is slightly behind the times, and he proposes a rather eccentric theory that cortisone use may be related to the etiology of the disease. Otherwise the book is an excellent source both for reference and general reading.

STD: A Commonsense Guide to Sexually Transmitted Diseases, by Maria Corsaro and Carole Korzeniowsky, is a sensible, clearly presented alphabetical arrangement of information on the various STDs. However, AIDS is left out entirely, which is surprising considering the 1982 publication date from Holt, Rinehart, and Winston—until a closer examination reveals that the original book was issued by St. Martin's in 1980.

A third adult STD guide is *Healthy Sex and Keeping It That Way: A Complete Guide to Sexual Infections*, by Richard Lumiere and Stephani Cook. This is the most medically detailed of the three although it is so skillfully organized and written that this is no deterrent for a reasonably literate layperson. The authors are not above an occasional outbreak of humor to relieve the grim topic. On pubic lice, for instance: "It is hard to mistake a case of crabs for anything else, even if you've messed yourself up with too much scratching: you can *see* the little suckers, and they look like . . . crabs."

The book is divided into three sections. The first covers some basic information, providing things like body maps and symptom charts, and includes an excellent discussion on how to break the news tactfully to sexual partners after the fact. The second section describes the infections and their treatment with great thoroughness and correctness, even including some gruesome color pictures. The third section has chapters addressed to the special information needs of women, men, gay men, and teenagers and gives sources of medical help (including that same nonanswered California Hotline). Like Dr. Neumann's book, *Healthy Sex* can be used both as a reference resource at time of need and for preventive browsing. One or both titles belong in any library serving your adults in their mid- or late teens.

▪ Woman Talk

Books on feminist sex education topics, unlike STD books, have aged very little in the last few years. This is probably because the major developments in current social thinking on these subjects took place in the seventies at the height of the women's movement. Many of the best books on menstruation, rape, abortion, and contraception (although this last is not an exclusively feminine subject) were written in the second half of that decade and are still completely valid.

Menstruation is a subject that should be explained to girls in some detail before their first period. Since the average age of first menses in the U.S. is 12.9 years,[7] books designed to prepare girls for this event should be addressed to eleven- or even ten-year-olds. *Period*, by JoAnn Gardner-Loulan, Bonnie Lopez, and Marcia Quackenbush, is one of the few books that seems to recognize this obvious fact. The tone is comforting and cheerful, with lots of words from girls themselves, and the story is told in amusingly amateurish cartoon drawings by Quackenbush. There is much emphasis on feelings, although physiology is not slighted. A valuable feature is the reassuring section on the pelvic exam. The book's theme is that menstruation, while sometimes uncomfortable, is a part of becoming a self-sufficient adult woman in tune with the rhythms of life and so should be something to be proud of.

Other volumes on menstruation are disconcertingly reminiscent of those little talks by gym teachers. *The Girls Guide to Menstruation*, by Ellen Voelckers, and *Menstruation*, by Hilary C. Maddux, are sober and informative but a bit dull. The standard source of instruction on the menses, of course, has always been the pamphlets provided free by manufacturers of sanitary napkins, such as *It's a Woman's World* and *Accent on You* from Tampax. These are adequate for a brief introduction to the facts, although the writers are understandably more interested in selling lots of the product than in helping young women feel good about their bodies.

Rape information is a grim but necessary part of sex instruction for girls (and even boys). Margaret Hyde's *Speak Out on Rape!* was one of the first books on the subject written for adolescent readers. It is a well-researched and usually objective presentation of the social problem; Hyde only occasionally expresses a righteous anger as she points out the urgency for change in the attitudes of police, the courts, and the medical establishment, as well as male society's perception of women. Many of the changes she calls for have now begun to be implemented. Her descriptions of callous police and doctors are no longer widely accurate and might have an inhibiting effect on the willingness of young victims to seek help and publicly accuse their attackers. For these two reasons the book seems a bit less useful than it once was.

More helpful to potential rape victims (and all women *are*) is the more personal approach of *Rape: Preventing It; Coping with the Legal, Medical, and Emotional Aftermath*, by Janet Bode, and *Rape: What Would You Do If . . . ?* by Dianna Daniels Booher. Bode, who has also written a book for adult women on the subject, begins by saying that the threat of rape "shapes and restricts all women's lives." She demolishes the myth of "Godzilla and Little Red Riding Hood" as the typical encounter between rapist and victim and paints a more statistically realistic picture of the nature of sexual attacks (sixty percent of teenage victims know their assailants, for instance). She describes the stages of emotional reaction to rape, including long-range effects, and discusses the reality of getting medical and legal help. She is realistic but not discouragingly negative about the possibility of occasional less-than-sympathetic treatment and equally honest in explaining what to expect in court. Safety precautions can prevent at least some stranger rape, she says and lists some, although acquaintance rape and incest are more difficult to anticipate. Bode writes in an interesting conversational style and often couches her points in personal accounts and anecdotes.

Booher is equally personal and readable. She begins her presentation from the opposite end, stressing prevention rather than reaction. She lists many specific dangerous situations—at home, on the street, or in social settings—and discusses the safest responses to them. On the basis of recent research she characterizes rapists as belonging to seven types and describes the kind of resistance most likely to be effective with each pattern. If a girl should be raped in spite of all precautions, Booher strongly encourages her to go immediately for medical help and to report the crime to the police. She is honest about the unpleasantness of court procedures but firm about the absolute necessity to prosecute.

There are no books specifically for teenagers on abortion, in spite of the fact that half of adolescent pregnancies end this way.[8] However, *A Woman's Guide to Safe Abortion*, by Maria Corsaro and Carole Korzeniowsky, is easy to read and clear and informative about clinic procedures. It is written for women who have already decided to abort and offers no help to those who are still trying to make up their minds. There is a good chapter on choosing a personally appropriate method of contraception to prevent another pregnancy.

For background and understanding of political aspects of this extremely controversial issue public libraries should have at least *Abortion and the Politics of Motherhood*, by Kristin Luker; *The Ambivalence of Abortion*, by Linda Bird Francke; and *Abortion and the Conscience of the Nation*, by Ronald Reagan.

Good contraception, of course, precludes abortion. The importance of getting accurate birth-control information into teenagers' heads can hardly be exaggerated. As we have seen, most sex guides make a point of providing at least a once-over of methods and techniques. Two books for adolescents have centered on the topic.

What Are You Using? A Birth Control Guide for Teenagers, by Andrea Balis, is small but concise, informed, and thorough. After an introductory rundown on reproductive biology and the history of contraception Balis devotes one chapter to each of the currently approved methods, describing not only techniques of use but also potential problems. Each section is followed by short taped dialogs in which a group of teens discuss their contraceptive fears and successes and the funny, awkward, and sexy things that can happen in the process. These discussions are delightful—and undeniably real—in their innocent candor about the problems of the new sexual etiquette.

The most complete source of contraceptive information specifically for teens is the 1981 edition of *Sex and Birth Control: A Guide for the Young*, by E. James Lieberman and Ellen Peck. The authors set the stage with a chapter on research into teen sexuality, focusing on the basic study done by John Kantner and Melvin Zelnik in 1971 and 1976 at Johns Hopkins University. They then proceed in an authoritative but friendly style to summarize the facts about each of the accepted birth-control methods, beginning with a strong argument for abstinence. A chapter on VD concentrates on gonorrhea and syphilis, but a table summarizes a variety of other sexually transmitted diseases (with the omission of AIDS). The discussion of abortion is strongly prochoice, although it acknowledges the controversy. Chapters on the need for sex education, sexual morality, and population control round out the book. An appendix lists an amateurish selection of books and some national organizations, clinics, and hotlines (most of which are no longer in service). In spite of this minor shortcoming, this is an excellent and dependable guide.

It seems like a giant compared to the pygmy efforts of Peter Mayle and Arthur Robins in *Congratulations! You're Not Pregnant: An Illustrated Guide to Birth Control.* This ridiculous book, like Mayle's other works, comes in a large picture-book format. Most of each page is taken up with huge, brightly colored drawings of the adventures of Mr. Penis and Ms. Vagina (the ultimate nonholistic approach). "It's impossible to generalize too much about such a personal act," say the authors—and then go on to disprove that thesis. Mayle seems more intrigued with showing how cute he can be than with presenting accurate information. There are a number of serious errors: douching is described as "better than nothing," crabs "won't nest in clean surroundings," NSU is "almost entirely a male problem," and in the rhythm method ovulation is indicated by a *drop* in temperature. Male worries about penis size are equated with female worries about vagina length (breast size would be a far more accurate comparison). He spends what for this sketchy treatment is an inordinate number of pages on performance anxieties and the difficulty of breaking the hymen. Although it must be admitted that some parts of the book *are* funny (Mr. Penis looking cross-eyed at his "nose" sheathed in a pink condom and tied with a red bow), it should not be taken seriously as sex education.

▪ The Pregnancy Epidemic

The problems of adolescent pregnancy are too drastic and too far-reaching to allow room for fooling around. The numbers alone are appalling: more than one million girls a year become pregnant. But the long-range consequences of adolescent child-bearing are even worse. This age group has the highest rate of both infant and maternal mortality. Teen mothers tend to drop out of school and thus lack job skills and must be supported at public expense. Their chances of lifelong poverty are substantially increased. Their children fall behind measurably in social and cognitive skills and are more likely later to become teen parents themselves.[9] And the suicide rate for adolescent mothers is seven times that of the general population.[10]

Although there has been much hand-wringing and nationwide concern about this social phenomenon, no clear understanding of the causes or guidelines for action have yet been developed, although many people are trying. There has, naturally, been an explosion of books and articles attempting to interpret and offering guidance. A number of these have been written for the young women themselves (although almost none, regrettably, for the actual or potential fathers). Pregnancy books for adolescents fall into three categories: help with decision-making, collections of real or fictionalized case histories, and practical advice for prenatal and baby care and marriage.

▪ HARD CHOICES

A simple book of the first type is *Kids Having Kids: The Unwed Teenage Parent*, by Janet Bode. The typeface and format seem to indicate a young junior-high-school audience. Bode briefly puts the problem in historical, international, and statistical perspective and then offers an overview (with many anecdotes) of choices and sources of help.

Several other books do a far better job of this task. *What to Do if You or Someone You Know Is Under 18 and Pregnant*, by Arlene Kramer Richards and Irene Willis, is one of the best recent books of counsel for pregnant teens. The range is comprehensive: conception and contraception, abortion, pregnancy, adoption, marriage, infant care. A chapter called "Where to Get Help" consists of forty-one pages of resources: abortion clinics, adolescent medicine clinics, adoption agencies, counseling and information services (including the public library), and an excellent bibliography of both fiction and nonfiction. The authors are knowledgeable; Richards is a psychoanalyst and Willis has been a secondary-school teacher, counselor, and administrator for twenty-five years. Together they have written several other books for young adults on social problems. Their approach is careful and thorough, and the long list of experts who were interviewed for the book is impressive. Their style is simple but not condescending, with a well-defined format. Most chapters open with anecdotes so lively that it is almost a disappointment not to find out what happened next to the characters.

Mom, I'm Pregnant: A Personal Guide for Teenagers, by Reni L. Witt and Jeannine Masterson Michael, is also excellent—complete, authoritative, readable. It lays out the choices clearly and gives calm step-by-step guidance for the girl whose pregnancy has thrown her into a terrified muddle. "The decision you make about the outcome of your pregnancy may be the most difficult one you have ever had to face," the authors level. "Yet the problem of what to do can be broken down into small pieces." In five basic steps they show how to weigh alternatives and accept the consequences of choice.

Coauthor Jeannine Masterson Michael counsels pregnant teens at Eastern Women's Center, a gynecological health-care facility in New York City, and her years of experience are evident as she leads the reader skillfully past the first stages of denial to seek help and take action. Michael knows all the myths and excuses and secret reasons. She gives careful unflinching explanations of the pregnancy test, the pelvic exam, the difficult task of telling boyfriend and parents, and the primary decision of whether to continue or end the pregnancy.

Chapters on abortion, marriage, adoption, and foster care are detailed and realistic, presenting facts but also helping the girl deal with feelings about each choice. A final section outlines prenatal care and birth and works through the negative feelings many young women have about contraception. An invaluable feature of the book is the exhaustive sixty-seven-page list of hotlines and agencies in the United States and Canada. The excellent bibliography includes both articles and books (unfortunately, books addressed to teens are not listed separately).

The tone throughout is friendly but tough, and many brief quotations from girls add anecdotal interest. The underlying theme, as the authors explain in "A Special Word for Parents," is "achieving self-knowledge and independence, as well as accepting responsibility"—a vision of hope for the young women who can gain self-respect and strength from these hard decisions well made.

An inexpensive source of data for pregnancy decision-making is the paperback *Your Choice*, by Caryl Hansen. To help clarify options and urgencies the author gives a timetable for the pregnancy with each trimester clearly marked for write-in deadlines. Each choice—abortion, single-parenting, adoption, marriage—is considered thoroughly. There are also valuable chapters for the unwed father and for the couple's parents. The information is sensibly and fully presented, but the small print and dense page as well as the somewhat formal style make the book more appropriate for educated women in their late teens and early twenties.

Young Parents, by Jane Claypool Miner (who has also written teen historical romances), is for early adolescents or older teens who don't read well. Miner comes down hard in favor of abortion while acknowledging that some girls may find this option morally unacceptable. She is strongly in favor of the right to legal choice, telling young women that "those ads that begin, 'Pregnant? Need help?' are actually agencies that will give a girl a place to stay during pregnancy and arrange for adoption later. Girls who are considering abortion should avoid those ads or right-to-life organizations."

A discussion of adoption presents this as a sensible choice, even for mothers of toddlers who may find that under the stress of child care they are beginning to neglect or abuse their little ones. Some young marriages, good and bad, illustrate the third possibility. The latter half of the book takes a hard look at the reality of raising a child alone: the exhausting and repetitive work, the constant attention needed by a helpless and demanding baby or toddler, the necessity to put the baby's needs first, the loneliness and isolation from other young people. "Parenting is a twenty-year commitment," she says seriously. But "being a mother is challenging work and the payoff—successful, happy children—is worth it for most young women." Many teens explain their desire for pregnancy in rosy, romantic terms of wanting a baby so that they can have "someone to love me." This realistic, readable book should throw cold water on those poignant fantasies of babies as cuddly dolls.

Handbook for Pregnant Teenagers, by Linda Roggow and Carolyn Owens, is a much slighter work but is appropriate for girls whose religious convictions rule out abortion as an option. In an opening scene a young girl agonizes about her decision to abort and finally cancels her appointment because "abortion means taking a human life." From there the book goes on to consider thoughtfully the alternatives of marriage, adoption, or raising the baby alone. The orientation is middle-class, and many of the factors for decision-making are financial. With the exception of the final chapter, "Faith Helps," there is little specific religiosity. The authors often make points in the form of reasonably believable anecdotes or quotations. Although there are a few general remarks about the advisability of good prenatal care, there is no description of birth, the pelvic exam, attitudes or feelings about past or future sex, or any other physical matters. The only form of contraception mentioned is repentance and prayer. An appendix lists "Crisis Pregnancy Centers" that offer counseling for those who do not wish to consider abortion. A page of "Suggestions for Further Reading" lists other relevant books from evangelical publishers. In general this is a sound book for the readership for which it is intended, although it certainly should not be the only book on the subject in the library collection.

In former years secretive confinement and adoption was the most common solution for an unwanted pregnancy. Nowadays, regrettably, only eight percent of unmarried teens choose to relinquish their babies. Most attempt to go the hard road of raising the child alone. A helpful discussion of the adoption choice—and the only book on this subject written for adolescent mothers—is *Pregnant Too Soon: Adoption Is an Option*, by Jeanne Warren Lindsay. The author, who coordinates a teen-mother program for a school district in southern California, has worked with hundreds of young women. Their stories fill these pages in between the wise counsel and fact-filled discussions of the legal and psychological complexities of adoption.

▪ Pregnant Testimonials

Scary stories, as we have seen, are a time-honored device for frightening teenagers away from sexual behavior that is not condoned by society. A writer doesn't have to search too hard to find scary stories about adolescent pregnancy and childbearing. A number of books have used this technique, with varying degrees of integrity.

"Mom . . . I'm Pregnant," by Bev O'Brien, is a religious tear-

jerker, written by a mother, ostensibly for other mothers. But some girls with a born-again Christian orientation may find this story of a close mother-daughter relationship inspirational. (Care should be taken not to confuse this book with the Witt and Michael volume of the same title reviewed above.) When nineteen-year-old Sandy turned up pregnant, her mother, Bev, was numb with shock that her good Christian daughter could ever do anything that would lead to such a result. She needed to work through her own anger and grief before she could help her daughter. During the pregnancy Bev and Sandy come to terms with the shame and guilt and make the decision to allow the baby to be adopted, although this causes them both great pain.

A highly emotional book, this has little information to offer and what there is centers on legal matters—the rules of adoption, the laws on discrimination against pregnant women, the statutes concerning paternity (a distasteful chapter describes their attempt to punish the young non-Christian father by taking him to court).

In the last two chapters Bev ponders whether she, or any mother, should give her daughter detailed birth-control information. She dismisses this idea on the grounds that no contraceptive method is foolproof, and (ironically) "she may construe this to mean that we expect her to experiment with sex." Sexual values, if not clinical facts, should be taught in the home, she maintains, difficult as it may be for parents to speak of such things. Unfortunately, her short, unselective bibliography gives little help.

In *Only Human: Teenage Pregnancy and Parenthood* Marion Howard makes use of interlaced fictional stories of three young couples to make points about early pregnancy and marriage. The narrator's voice interrupts the action from time to time to inject facts and instructions. The stories, which resolve the problem in three different ways, trace the lives of the six young people from the discovery of pregnancy through the first year of the baby's life.

Deep Blue Funk and Other Stories: Portraits of Teenage Parents is also told by a narrator, but these stories are achingly true. Daniel Frank spent two years hanging out at Our Place, a community center run by the social-service agency Family Focus, in a black enclave of the middle-class Chicago suburb of Evanston. There Dan, who is white and Jewish, learned to fit in. He tutored pregnant black teenagers for their GED exams and listened to them talk about their lives. These stories are vividly detailed scenes and conversations from that time, showing young women who are themselves children struggling to care for the babies they had so blithely conceived—for in this community pregnancy is a mark of status for a teenager. The young fathers, too, get their say in this book. One of the most touching scenes is a rap at a meeting of the Fathers' Group, in which they express their hurt at being excluded from the tight circle of baby, mother, and grandmother; their bewilderment at the weight of new responsibilities; and their struggles for respect as fathers and men in a society that rejects them at every turn.

It Won't Happen to Me: Teenagers Talk About Pregnancy, by Paula McGuire, covers a broader geographic and socioeconomic spectrum, but the message is just as painful. The book is a collection of interviews with young women, fifteen to nineteen, who have dealt with their unintentional pregnancies in a variety of ways. To round out the picture the author has included interviews with a high-school counselor for pregnant girls, a social worker with Planned Parenthood and her physician husband, and two adoption caseworkers.

At first the rambling monologues seem monotonous—McGuire does not have the knack of giving style and shape to a taped transcription. Then insights and understandings begin to emerge from the sheer mass of data. These girls have been caught in a vicious double bind: peer pressure to end their virginity, and then peer disapproval when they became pregnant. Planning for sexual activity with contraception is definitely not cool, they say, and besides—. Then follows a list of bizarre misconceptions about every common form of birth control. Sex must be a romantic accident, and very few of these girls find it pleasurable at all. At the end it becomes clear that these girls are victims of social forces, of their boyfriends, and, ultimately, of their own lack of self-esteem.

A more positive picture emerges from the testimonies in *The One Girl in Ten: A Self-Portrait of the Teen-Age Mother*, by Sallie Foster. The young women who speak in this book seem less passive, more thoughtful and in control of their own lives, perhaps because they were interviewed several years after the births of their children. Sallie Foster was for many years a social worker with the Los Angeles County Department of Social Services, specializing in helping pregnant girls and young mothers.

The seventy-seven girls she interviewed for this book had all given birth to their first child while they were still of school age. Most were from middle-class families living in East Los Angeles. The ethnic mix is an accurate representation of that area: over half Anglo, twenty-five percent Mexican-American, ten percent black. The girls seem eager to talk about their experiences, and while their words often illuminate feelings and insights about adolescent childbearing, the sample is too small and too localized to be statistically important and too large to come alive as individual stories with any impact.

▪ And Baby Makes Two

Even if the young father is willing to marry her, the odds are weighted heavily that the girl will end up raising the child alone sooner or later. When both partners are under eighteen, fifty percent of marriages end in divorce in four years or less.[11] The difficulties in assuming two new roles—spouse and parent—before the developmental tasks of adolescence are done are overwhelming.

A book that offers help with this tough job is *Teenage Marriage: Coping with Reality*. Author Jeanne Warren Lindsay speaks from experience she has gained in her eleven years of counseling teenagers as school-district coordinator of a teen-mother program in California. For this book she undertook a national survey to measure the attitudes toward marriage of three thousand teenagers, including extensive interviews with fifty-five young people who were married before they were twenty. Anecdotes and long quotes from these young husbands and wives make the book almost unbearably poignant.

Lindsay is able to focus with unrelenting accuracy on the areas in which young marriages founder. Money, predictably, is the primary problem—young high-school dropouts have few job skills. Living with in-laws is another source of stress. (Two thirds of Lindsay's interviewees moved in with parents, even though only one in twenty thought this was a good idea.) Emotional immaturity, lack of communication skills, conflicts about sharing housework, jealousy—all cause their share of troubles, and Lind-

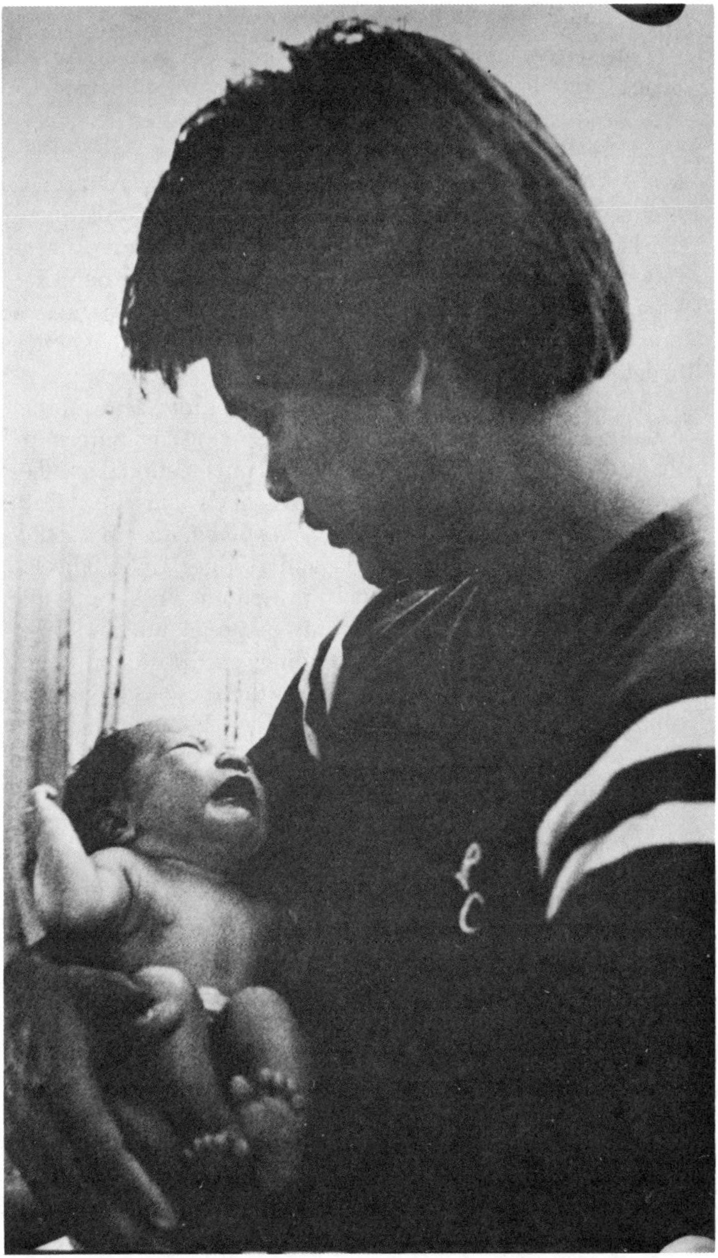

Fig. 16. Young father. From *Teenage Marriage*, by Jeanne Warren Lindsay.

say and her interviewees offer insights and practical suggestions for coping.

One serious and common problem in young marriages is battering, and in a chapter called "People Are Not for Hitting" Lindsay insists that such behavior should never be tolerated or excused. But there are happy stories here, too, tales of courage and love and perseverance that help to make a warm, lasting union. An appendix includes a good bibliography, a quiz scorecard for predicting potential success of a marriage, and a marriage-attitude test. Lindsay has seen too much to be in favor of teen marriage, but she is still in favor of good marriage, and her book will help young adults move toward that goal, whether now or later.

Books focusing on prenatal care for adolescent mothers are usually designed to be used in a class or discussion group. Two that are easy to read and cheerfully conversational are *Teenage Pregnancy: A New Beginning*, by Linda Barr and Catherine Monserrat, and *Teen Pregnancy: The Challenges We Faced, the Choices We Made*, by Donna and Rodger Ewy. The latter is simply written and attractively presented, with many pictures and cartoons. Both cover anatomy of pregnancy and birth, diet and exercise, delivery, breastfeeding, and postnatal contraception. Although the original format of these books (spiral binding, oblong shape) signals "textbook," *Teen Pregnancy* (Ewy) also appears as a small paperback suitable for library purchase.

Although there are innumerable books on caring for new babies and toddlers, almost none of them addresses the special problems of the very young and inexperienced single mother. A third book from Jeanne Warren Lindsay, *Teens Parenting: The Challenge of Babies and Toddlers*, is realistic in its comprehensive discussion of the day-to-day business of coping happily with a baby while also coping with school, limited money, and shared living quarters. Quotes from sixty-one young mothers substantiate and flesh out Lindsay's down-to-earth advice on everything from what to expect from a newborn to how to limit a three-year-old's television viewing. Lindsay links the emotional and physical needs of the young moms inextricably with the baby's welfare, and the final chapter, "Your Future—Your Child's Future," leans hard on the importance of continuing education.

▪ Some Special Needs

Adolescence can be a difficult time for young people who are gay. These are the years in which they must confront and accept their own preference for same-sex partners, face the implications of that fact for their futures, and decide whether to tell the world. Coming out to parents can be particularly traumatic. The brief autobiographical essays in *One Teenager in Ten: Writings by Gay and Lesbian Youth* center on these transitions. Editor Ann Heron collected these twenty-eight stories by mail, in response to a request printed in the back of a previous book.

Behind a shield of adolescent bravado, pain and loneliness bleed from these pages—tales of rejection, ridicule, even arrest and confinement in mental institutions. Several grapple with feelings that God Himself has turned His back. (One essay includes a useful list of denomination-affiliated religious gay groups.) And yet through it all these young people fight to find a sense of their own self-worth. Their stories should be heartening to the one teenager in ten who is homosexual or lesbian and enlightening to those who are not.

If learning the words with which to talk about sex can be hard for most adolescents, it is even trickier for those who are deaf and communicate silently. *Signs for Sexuality*, by Susan D. Doughten, Marlyn B. Minkin, and Laurie E. Rosen, is a guide to the vocabulary they need. "Hearies" too will enjoy leafing through this pictorial dictionary. Again and again one is reminded that signing is its own language, not simply a transliteration of English. *This* language is earthy and amused in its communication about sex. Many of the signs have a sly humor: the wide-flung coat and wide-open smile of "exhibitionist," the upraised forefinger at the temple for "horny," the exaggerated ecstatic expression that is an integral part of the sign for "orgasm." Other signs carry meaning beyond the English equivalent: the lingering way in which the two hands slide apart for "divorce," the interlocked fingers that by their distance from the belly indicate degree as well as condition of "pregnancy," the variations to indicate male or female, solitary or mutual "masturbation." Many signs are unabashedly graphic in miming the action ("fellatio," "erection") or using the signer's own body to demonstrate ("nipples," "Fallopian tubes"). It is interesting to note that this language, too, shows transition in its attitudes toward homosexuals. The signs for "gay male" and "lesbian" have two versions—the preferred, neutral signs and the secondary (and presumably older) versions, which use a dampened little finger on the eyebrow or a mimed beard to communicate the respective stereotypes. In the larger sense this view from slightly outside is a fascinating commentary on the euphemisms of our verbal communication about sex.

▪ Love at Last

And finally a book about l'amour. Wisdom would seem to be the essential quality for a writer who sets out to explain this profound, disturbing, and joyful emotion to adolescents. Unfortunately, Dianna Daniels Booher has settled for research, and superficial research at that. *Love* is a simplistic and confused amalgamation of pop psychology gleaned from books by self-help gurus like Leo Buscaglia and articles from women's magazines like *Redbook*. Half-digested bits from various sources bob to the surface, giving an odd bumpy quality. Coined words from other writers ("girlspeak," "limerance") appear briefly and are never used again; provocative ideas are mentioned and then not pursued (women are inherently not as adept as men at the game of love; you can tell someone is interested in you if his pupils dilate; body language reveals trustworthiness or availability, and so on). The first chapter defines love as a game, but then that orientation is abruptly dropped in favor of several other perceptions of its nature.

The flavor is negative, and the intent seems to be to describe all the many ways love can be destructive, painful, and misleading; not until the fifth chapter do we get to healthy relationships, and even then the advice begins "revive it before it wilts." Jealousy is discussed only in the context of loss, and in this and in many other discussions and anecdotes there is something peculiarly off-target. (The description of a person with a negative mindset, for instance, veers off at the end into a picture of homocidal paranoia.) Other than this, and a general lack of unity of concept, there is nothing actually wrong with Booher's second-hand counsel, and much of it would probably be useful and interesting to young women struggling to understand what real love is all about. But the emotion that our culture defines as fundamental to happiness deserves a better press.

■ NOTES

[1]Lidia Wasowica. "Leading Venereal Disease, Chlamydia, Spreading Rapidly." *Los Angeles Times,* July 8, 1984, Section II, p. 1.

[2]Elbert D. Glover. "Herpes: Removing Fact from Fiction." *Health Education*, August/September 1984, p. 6.

[3]Hans H. Neumann with Sylvia Simmons. *Dr. Neumann's Guide to the New Sexually Transmitted Diseases*. Washington, D.C.: Acropolis, 1983.

[4]Margot Joan Fromer. *AIDS: Acquired Immune Deficiency Syndrome*. New York: Pinnacle, 1983.

[5]Evan G. Pattishall, Jr. "Health Issues in Adolescence." In Richard M. Lerner and Nancy L. Galambos, eds. *Experiencing Adolescents: A Sourcebook for Parents, Teachers, and Teens*. New York: Garland, 1984, p. 209.

[6]Sol Gordon and Judith Gordon. *Raising a Child Conservatively in a Sexually Permissive World*. New York: Simon and Schuster, 1983.

[7]Vern L. Bullough. "Age at Menarche: A Misunderstanding." *Science*, July 17, 1981.

[8]Jane Claypool Miner. *Young Parents*. New York: Messner, 1985, p. 27.

[9]Judy A. Shea. "Adolescent Sexuality." In Lerner and Galambos, p. 71.

[10]Miner, p. 136

[11]Louise Guerney and Joyce Arthur. "Adolescent Social Relationships." In Lerner and Galambos, p. 104.

■ BIBLIOGRAPHY

(Note: This is a list of books mentioned in this chapter; inclusion does not necessarily mean recommendation. For Core Collection List see Appendix.)

Accent on You. Lake Success, N.Y.: Educational Dept., Tampax Inc., 1983.

Balis, Andrea. *What Are You Using? A Birth Control Guide for Teen-Agers*. New York: Dial, 1981.
Barr, Linda, and Catherine Monserrat. *Teenage Pregnancy: A New Beginning*. Albuquerque, N.M.: New Futures, 1978.
Blanzaco, Andre, with William F. Schwartz and Julius B. Richmond. *VD: Facts You Should Know*. New York: Lothrop, Lee and Shepard, 1970.
Bode, Janet. *Kids Having Kids: The Unwed Teenage Parent*. New York: Watts, 1980.
———. *Rape: Preventing It: Coping with the Legal, Medical, and Emotional Aftermath*. New York: Watts, 1979.
Booher, Dianna Daniels. *Love*. New York: Messner, 1985.
———. *Rape: What Would You Do If . . . ?* New York: Messner, 1981.
Brooks, Stewart M. *The V. D. Story*. New York: Barnes, 1971.
Busch, Phyllis S. *What About VD?* New York: Four Winds, 1976.
Chiappa, Joseph A. *The VD Book*. New York: Holt, Rinehart and Winston, 1977.
Corsaro, Maria, and Carole Korzeniowsky. *STD: A Commonsense Guide to Sexually Transmitted Diseases*. New York: St. Martin's, 1980; New York: Holt, Rinehart and Winston, 1982.
———.*A Woman's Guide to Safe Abortion*. New York: St. Martin's, 1980; New York: Holt, Rinehart and Winston, 1983.
Doughten, Susan, Marlyn B. Minkin, and Laurie E. Rosen. *Signs for Sexuality—A Resource Manual*. Seattle: Planned Parenthood of Seattle/King County, 1978.
Ewy, Donna, and Rodger Ewy. *Teen Pregnancy: The Challenges We Faced, the Choices We Made*. Boulder, Colo.: Pruett, 1984; New York: New American Library, 1985.
Foster, Sallie. *The One Girl in Ten: A Self-Portrait of the Teen-Age Mother*. Claremont, Calif.: Arbor, 1981.
Francke, Linda Bird. *The Ambivalence of Abortion*. New York: Random House, 1978; New York: Dell, 1978.
Frank, Daniel B. *Deep Blue Funk and Other Stories*. Chicago: University of Chicago Press, 1983.
Gardner-Loulan, JoAnn, Bonnie Lopez, and Marcia Quackenbush. *Period*, rev. ed. San Francisco: Volcano, 1981.
———. *Periodo*, rev. ed. San Francisco: Volcano, 1981 (in Spanish).
Gordon, Sol. *Facts About STD*. Fayetteville, N.Y.: Ed-U, 1983.

———. *Facts About VD for Today's Youth*. Fayetteville, N.Y.: Ed-U, 1973; new ed., 1979.

Grover, John W. *VD: The ABC's*. New York: Prentice-Hall, 1971.

Hansen, Caryl. *Your Choice: A Young Woman's Guide to Making Decisions About Unmarried Pregnancy*. New York: Avon, 1980.

Heron, Ann, ed. *One Teenager in Ten: Writings by Gay and Lesbian Youth*. Boston: Alyson, 1983.

Howard, Marion. *Only Human: Teenage Pregnancy and Parenthood*. New York: Seabury, 1975; New York: Avon, 1976.

Hyde, Margaret O. *Speak Out on Rape!* New York: McGraw-Hill, 1976.

———. *VD: The Silent Epidemic*. New York: McGraw-Hill, 1973.

It's a Woman's World. Lake Success, N.Y.: Tampax Inc., n.d.

Johnson, Eric W. *V.D.: Venereal Disease and What You Should Do About It*. Philadelphia: Lippincott, 1973; rev. ed., 1978.

Lieberman, E. James, and Ellen Peck. *Sex and Birth Control: A Guide for the Young*, rev. ed. New York: Harper and Row, 1981.

Lindsay, Jeanne Warren. *Pregnant Too Soon: Adoption Is an Option*. Buena Park, Calif.: Morning Glory, 1980.

———. *Teenage Marriage: Coping with Reality*. Buena Park, Calif.: Morning Glory, 1984.

———. *Teens Parenting: The Challenge of Babies and Toddlers*. Buena Park, Calif.: Morning Glory, 1981.

Luker, Kristin. *Abortion and the Politics of Motherhood*. Berkeley: University of California Press, 1984.

Lumiere, Richard, and Stephani Cook. *Healthy Sex and Keeping It That Way: A Complete Guide to Sexual Infections*. New York: Simon and Schuster, 1983.

McGuire, Paula. *It Won't Happen to Me*. New York: Delacorte, 1983; New York: Delta, 1983.

Maddux, Hilary C. *Menstruation*. New York: Tobey, 1975.

Mayle, Peter, and Arthur Robins. *Congratulations! You're Not Pregnant: An Illustrated Guide to Birth Control*. New York: Macmillan, 1981.

Miner, Jane Claypool. *Young Parents*. New York: Messner, 1985.

Neumann, Hans H., with Sylvia Simmons. *Dr. Neumann's Guide to the New Sexually Transmitted Diseases*. Washington, D.C.: Acropolis, 1983.

Nicholas, Leslie. *How to Avoid Social Diseases: A Practical Handbook*. New York: Stein and Day, 1973.
O'Brien, Bev. "*Mom . . . I'm Pregnant.*" Wheaton, Ill.: Tyndale House, 1982.
Reagan, Ronald. *Abortion and the Conscience of the Nation*. Nashville, Tenn.: Nelson, 1984.
Richards, Arlene Kramer, and Irene Willis. *What to Do if You or Someone You Know Is Under 18 and Pregnant*. New York: Lothrop, Lee and Shepard, 1983.
Roggow, Linda, and Carolyn Owens. *Handbook for Pregnant Teenagers*. Grand Rapids, Mich.: Zondervan, 1984.
Sgroi, Suzanne M. *VD: A Doctor's Answers*. New York: Harcourt, 1974.
Stein, Mari. *VD: The Love Epidemic*. Palo Alto, Calif.: Page-Ficklin, 1973, 1977.
Stiller, Richard. *The Love Bugs: A Natural History of the VDs*. Nashville, Tenn.: Nelson, 1974.
Voelckers, Ellen. *Girls Guide to Menstruation*. New York: Rosen, 1975.
Witt, Reni L., and Jeannine Masterson Michael. *Mom, I'm Pregnant*. New York: Stein and Day, 1982.

Chapter 13

Larger Than Life, or, 16-mm Sex

by Susan B. Madden

From the earliest peep shows and "blue" movies sex has been a popular celluloid subject but never a particularly respectable one for general public viewing. Although European filmmakers were experimenting with this new medium in the field of legitimate sex education, it wasn't until the 1930s that any widespread application was seen in this country, and that was through the auspices of the military. Early recognized as a powerful propaganda tool, film was also seen as a useful method of instructing the thousands of raw recruits being called for active duty in World War II. Innumerable young men were exposed to the perils of wartime promiscuity by required viewings of lurid films graphically depicting the horrors of venereal disease. Grainy, crude, and both heavy-handed and simplistic, these harshly moral training films became the butt of veterans' jokes as well as the basis for many present-day attitudes toward sex education on film.

Thousands of GIs returning to college campuses brought the peacetime application of educating huge classes via screen. Educators, soon faced with baby-boom enrollments and increased technological improvements, quickly adopted this educational aid and brought it into classrooms at all levels. By the sixties it was basic to all curricula, and by the seventies it and television were so heavily used that critics were concerned about the quality of education. (They still are, but no longer give all the blame to media.)

In the eighties students, by constant exposure in home, school, and theater, have become highly sophisticated critics of film techniques. As a society we are visually oriented and literate in screen and film usage, but we still bring older attitudes of morality and respectability to the content of film, especially in areas of sexuality. This can be seen not only in our adoption of the heavily biased and very limited Motion Picture Association of America (MPAA) codes but also in the traditional methods and content still utilized in sex education media.

■ Media Other than Film

Considering the current state of the art in the various audiovisual media, 16-mm film is at the moment the most practical choice for use with young adults in sex education. There are several reasons for this:

Audiotapes and recordings can be highly informative but are also fairly boring. Given a choice between the top ten and "educational" tapes, the average young adult will make the obvious choice. (Before you sneer, think how often you've actually sat down and listened to a whole playback of a professional conference workshop you couldn't attend.)

Slides are either superb or awful and almost always require an accompanying booklet, projector, spare bulb, and lots of "fiddling." They're hard to catalog, store, circulate, and keep in order, and they usually cost more than they're worth.

Filmstrips can be wonderful personal-discovery items, especially those with good audiotape accompaniments (think kits). But my personal bias is that the equipment requirements, as well as the same logistic problems involved with slides, block ease of use.

Realia, such as plastic models, puppets, transparencies, dolls, and birth-control devices, are useful teaching aids and belong in all formal sex education programs. But they require instruction, planned storage and access, and funds way beyond regular library budgets. If you have strong community support, agency contracts, or special grants for planned programs, investigate these with the staff members who are to use them. Look at the Tactile Media reference in the Resource/Review section.

Video is *the* nonprint media for the eighties. The next edition of this book will probably have a full chapter devoted to it. But at this point there are several problems with this format, not the least of which is cost. Box-office or popular-fiction video is cost-effective at a range of $35 to $75 per tape, but educational or nonfiction materials are just now becoming affordable. The ballpark is still $150 to $350, and the quality doesn't yet justify such a playing field. People have a tendency to equate video with film. But size, pacing, photography, scripting, and audience are radically different. Both producers and consumers need to become better able to determine the appropriateness of a given video's application.

▪ Anticipating Controversy

Film uses sight, sound, and motion to convey verbal and nonverbal messages; it is a highly expressive, emotional, appealing, and often controversial medium. Larger-than-life images presented in vividly glowing color tend to create a lasting impact, which for many people makes film a stronger medium than the printed word. And while this may raise some intellectual-freedom specters, it certainly is a boon for sex education, especially where reading ability may not match interest or need level. It has some drawbacks—cost, projector and screen needs, and space—but these may be countered by other factors that are detailed in the next section.

As for the controversial aspects, schools and libraries operate under a broad range of policies, the most pertinent here being acquisition or selection and curriculum criteria. The Library Bill of Rights, nationally endorsed by the American Library Association and other educational bodies, covers all materials—not just books (see Appendix III). Most libraries have adopted the Freedom to Read Statement, and many are also including the Freedom to View Statement adopted by the Educational Film Library Association in 1979:

FREEDOM TO VIEW

The FREEDOM TO VIEW, along with the freedom to speak, to hear, and to read, is protected by the First Amendment to the Constitution of the United States. In a free society, there is no place for censorship of any medium of expression. Therefore, we affirm these principles:

1. It is in the public interest to provide the broadest possible access to films and other audiovisual materials because they have proven to be among the most effective means for the communication of ideas. Liberty of circulation is essential to insure the constitutional guarantee of freedom of expression.

2. It is in the public interest to provide for our audiences, films and other audiovisual materials which represent a diversity of views and expression. Selection of a work does not constitute or imply agreement with or approval of the content.

3. It is our professional responsibility to resist the constraint of labeling or pre-judging a film on the basis of the moral, religious, or political beliefs of the producer or filmmaker or on the basis of controversial content.

4. It is our professional responsibility to contest vigorously, by all lawful means, every encroachment upon the public's freedom to view.

▪ Film-Evaluation Checklist

In judging film, as in judging the printed word, there are some vital considerations to be used in selection, especially in the area of sex education. There are three basic areas of concern in film evaluation: content, technique, and utilization.

Content Criteria

Presentation

Does the film have unity of theme?

Is it dated or obsolete? Will it become so soon?

Does it creatively inform or is it just a lecture?

Is it free from stereotypes?

If sponsored, is too much time spent in advertising?

Is the dramatization, animation, and/or factual analysis appropriate?

If innovative or controversial, does the presentation aid in understanding?

Accuracy

Are there any obvious factual errors?

Does it have misleading images or information?

Are the images relevant to the subject?

Are the facts distractions rather than amplifications?

Is it too long or too short? (Does it cover too much or not enough?)

Are unusual examples presented as typical?

Usefulness

Are you glad the film was made?

Will it appeal to adolescent age groups and/or parents and/or educators?

Does it require a discussion leader, or can it stand on its own?

Does it fill a definite need?

Is it most useful as a film, or could it be presented just as well or better as a book, slides, filmstrip, video, tape, or record?

Technical Criteria

Photography

Is the film visually pleasing?

Is there good use of color or black-and-white?

Does the camerawork show quality and originality?

Are the images and camera style appropriate to the subject?

Is the handling of focus, exposure, special effects useful?

Sound

Do the actors or narrators have good voice quality, diction, and timing?

Can the sound be heard in a well-modulated and -recorded manner?

Is the use of music, special sound effects, or silence effective?

Does the narration match the visuals?

Is the narration condescending in mannerism or style?

Is the vocabulary appropriate to audience age level?

Direction

Do the settings, cast, and costumes contribute to the mood of the film?

Is the rhythm, pacing, and editing smoothly and appropriately done?

Are animation, flashbacks, and process photography, when used, effective?

Is it produced with imagination, style, originality, and humor?

Is the medium of film used effectively?

Utilization Criteria

Cinematic and Aesthetic Value

Does it show originality of treatment?

Are the elements of film, sound, image, and structure well-handled?

Are the treatment and form suitable to the thesis or content of the film?

Does it have high technical quality?

Accuracy and Quality of Information

Is the main objective clearly and concisely presented?

Does it have unity of purpose?

Are the facts accurately presented?

Is the vocabulary appropriate for the subject and audience?

Information and/or Cultural Value

Does the film stimulate interest or enjoyment?

Does the audience have to view it more than once to understand?

Does it duplicate or expand existing information?

Does it attempt to affect attitudes, build appreciation, develop new concepts or critical thinking? Does it succeed?

Program Potential

Does the film provide motivation for further discussion and participation after the showing?

Does it fill a need for a specific audience?

Does it fill a need for a broad range of audiences?

Can it be used with other components (speakers, books, and so forth)?

These may initially appear to be repetitious points, and to a large degree they are, but by design. Just as with books, one must balance content and quality with use. Restating points under different headings helps avoid costly "shelf-sitters," and with repeated use of the checklist the evaluative process becomes second nature for a critical reviewer. Of course, the cardinal rule is PREVIEW EVERY FILM FOR PURCHASE OR USE! Some nasty surprises can result from ignoring this requirement.

▪ PREVIEW FORMS

After the evaluation process the selection decision must be recorded on some sort of official form for the files. Even small informal groups may want to use a form of some kind to preserve their thinking on why a particular film was or was not chosen. These records will help in future decisions and can prove useful in the controversial area of sex education if a film draws censorship attack. The following examples offer a broad range of adaptable ideas that may be changed to suit the needs of an institution or group.

▪ YA SEX ED FILMS AND TEEN PICS

All these forms stress use and audience, and that is of paramount importance with sex education films. Unless there is a specific school, library, or community program geared to the use and discussion of these films, a difficult question must be asked. Will young adults or parents voluntarily come into the library and check out some of these carefully chosen films for personal use?

Our experience at King County Library System indicates a strong negative to such a use pattern, though we have the largest public-library film collection in the Northwest. Curious adolescents tend to be wary of exploring such intensely personal and sensitive subjects through film, which is so distinctly a group-related format. The whole rigamarole of projector and screen set-up is also a deterrent. It has been proven, however, that small preset viewing rooms reduce this factor significantly. (But books offering such vital personal information *are* designed for individual use, and they get remarkably high circulation, although much use is oddly in-house—under pillows in the reading room, stuffed

Appropriate for public libraries:

TITLE: ______________________________

COPYRIGHT: ______________ DISTRIBUTOR: ______________

AGES:	USEFUL IN:
☐ All Ages (family)	☐ Library Programming
☐ Preschool	☐ Day Care (preschools)
☐ Lower Elementary	☐ Home Situations
☐ Upper Elementary	☐ Parties / Groups
☐ YA	☐ Other ______________
☐ Other ______________	

COMMENTS:

Purchase soon ☐ Consider for purchase ☐ Forget ☐

Evaluator: ______________ Library: ______________ Date: ______________

Appropriate for community groups:

Film Preview Sheet

FILM TITLE:

TIME: PRICE, COLOR:

PRICE, B&W:

EVALUATION: Circle applicable remarks

Color:	necessary	helpful	unnecessary
Photo:	excellent	good	poor
Sound:	excellent	good	poor
Narration:	excellent	good	poor
Subject:	excellent	good	poor
Presentation:	excellent	good	poor

Group appeal: ______________________________

Value for program use: high good low

Value for purchase, PCL: high good low

Recommendation: yes no

Comment:

Reviewer: ______________ Date: ______________

Appropriate for schools:

Film Evaluation Form

Task I—Record Essential Information

Title of Film ______________________________

Color ___ B/W ___ Copyright Year _____

Producer and/or Distributor ______________________

Evaluator's Name ______________________________

School District ______________ Date of Preview ________

Task II—Collect Data

1. Does the film logically present material that has *relevance* for specific curricular concepts? Please explain:

2. Is the content of the film or its technical elements likely to become *obsolete* within the next five years? Please elaborate:

3. Are *biased* points of view presented, or does the content portray individuals or groups in *stereotyped* ways? Please cite examples:

4. What are some of the specific *photographic techniques* employed by the producer that tend to make the film effective or to detract from its quality? Please list:

5. In general, are the filmic images presented at a high enough level of *professionalism* to have adequate appeal to the intended audience? Please elaborate:

6. In general, what *editing techniques* have been used to strengthen the impact of the film? Please list:

7. Is the *soundtrack* appropriate and supportive of the visual messages? Give evidence:

8. Is the arrangement of the *teacher's guide* convenient, and is sufficient information included to facilitate the use of the film? Please explain:

9. Does the *title* give clues to the film content, and is it free of distractive or suggestive words? Please elaborate:

10. Give evidence of ways that the film *applies the principles of instructional design*:
    A. Prepares, organizes, and motivates the viewer.
    B. Uses repetition adequately.
    C. Uses aural and visual cues appropriately.
    D. Arranges for participation by the viewer.
    E. Promotes feedback on viewer responses.

Task III—Evaluate Data and Make Recommendation.

1. This film is not recommended for purchase because:

2. Check appropriate grade levels—double-check the most appropriate:

   A. Primary ___ Intermediate ___ JH ___ HS ___ College ___ Prof. ___

   B. Film is intended primarily for use with which strategy: Cognitive ___ Psychomotor ___ Affective ___

   C. Film is recommended for use in the following subject(s):

___ art	___ language arts
___ biology	___ mathematics
___ business & office	___ music
___ chemistry	___ P.E. & health
___ civics	___ physical science
___ contemp. affairs	___ physics
___ creative writing	___ reading
___ economics	___ social studies
___ English language	___ soc./psych.
___ environmental ed.	___ U.S. history
___ family liv./sex ed.	___ vocational ed.
___ geography	___ Washington history
___ guidance	___ world history
___ homemaking	___ values clarification
___ humanities	___

3. This film is recommended for use in attaining the following specific course goals or instructional outcomes.

4. Do you recommend this film for purchase? Yes ___ No ___

   Overall Rating: 1 2 3 4 5 6 7 8 9 10
   low — high

behind innocuous stacks, and tucked in the pages of mundane periodicals.)

Undoubtedly the most dynamic "sex education" in media is in the flood of feature-length films geared to adolescent appetites and interests. Much like *Forever* and other young adult fiction, the current teen movies offer behavior and conversation models as well as attitudes. If you want to sample the range of these films, watch *Risky Business, All the Right Moves, Little Darlings, Class of 1984, Over the Edge, The Breakfast Club, The Karate Kid, Fast Times at Ridgemont High, Bad Boys, Oxford Blue, Porky's I* and *II, Sixteen Candles, The Outsiders, No Small Affair, Tex, Teachers, The Sure Thing, Spring Break, Nightmare on Elm Street, Revenge of the Nerds, Valley Girls*, and whatever else is playing at the theaters in your town. Some are charming, some are appalling, but they are all box-office blockbusters with young adults. Although tremendously varied in content and impact, all have state-of-the-art technical quality and convey powerful messages of contemporary sexual manners and mores. But are these messages useful sex education, or even true?

Sarah Crichton thinks not, in a witty and perceptive article for *Ms.* magazine (June 1985), "Off the Beach Blanket and into the Bedroom":

> Teen pics, whether they're in the sleazoid "Porky's" department, the charming fantasy school. . . , or the let's-tackle-adolescent-alienation mode . . . are all, when you get down to it, about sex. Or more specifically, they're about Boys Getting Laid.
>
> Oh, the joy in the hearts of these male filmmakers. They can make their adolescent fantasies come true over and over again. It's the American Dream. Any boy can do it. . . . You can woo and make them come back for more. The wooing takes time, but the rest is gravy: no muss, no fuss; no bras to fumble with, no birth control to fret over.
>
> Like all moviegoers before them, today's teenagers are fed fantasies, only these hide the lies better. The filmmakers pepper the screen with obscenities, sprinkle them with drugs; make them seem hip, in-the-know. We know you—we know teens, they promise their audience, but the only realistic thing about teen sex in their movies is that no one uses birth control. And the movies end before anyone can see the result.

After sampling the teen pics, compare the offerings of the sex education market. What a contrast! Generally nonfiction films on teen sexuality are pedantic, slow, humorless, repetitious, technically dated, and reminiscent of those awful films of forty years ago. The manner in which they're done seems to reflect an "ought-to-know" point of view rather than a "want-to-know." The successful lessons taught by Disney, Henson, Coppola, and Spielberg are ignored for "serious" educational purposes.

▪ Some Selected Films with Annotations

Now, I don't expect patrons to queue outside libraries for any of these titles, but the following are films I've found useful despite the aforementioned reservations. These choices reflect the needs of a general public-library collection with no tie-in to a formal sex education program. Consequently there are some wonderful films that are glaringly absent here, although they are heavily touted in most of the resource materials. Such films need to be used in combination with discussion led by a trained sex education professional. Others that may have been omitted are more curriculum-oriented and so more appropriate for a school-library film collection.

Am I Normal?
1979 color live action 23 minutes New Day Films $375
Very believable young male adolescents discover facts about puberty and sexual development in a series of situation-comedy routines. Masculinity, peer pressure, and personal identity are issues identified in a humorous but valid manner. The clever tongue-in-cheek approach has been called "flip" by some critics, but this is a fun, entertaining, and quite informative film.
Audience: 10 to 14, parents, educators, youth-service providers

Better Safe Than Sorry III (A Vitascope Film)
1985 color live action 19 minutes
Filmfair Communications $400
Narration interspersed with dramatic segments covers contemporary concerns, such as date rape, incest, and molestation, with suggestions for personal safety and avoidance. Victim's guilt feelings and teen's increased responsibilities are given recogni-

tion and assurance by TV personality Stephanie Edwards.
Audience: 12 to 18, parents, educators, youth-service providers

Condom Sense
1981 color live action 25 minutes
Perennial Education $400
An extremely original and clever film that uses humor à la *Saturday Night Live* to explore the myths, rumors, and facts of choosing and using this important form of contraception and protection. (The image of a six-foot walking, talking condom causes such laughter and shock that this usually gets double playing.)
Audience: 15 to 21, parents, educators, youth-service providers

Dear Diary
1981 color live action 25 minutes New Day Films $394
A witty and educational film about female puberty from the makers of *Am I Normal?* (with a few visual puns referring to that film). In the same situation-comedy format information about body changes and maturation is presented tastefully with humor and reassurance. Issues of self-image, peer pressure, and dating/kissing awkwardness are dealt with in a creative and informative way.
Audience: 10 to 14, parents, educators, youth-service providers

Marsha and Harry
1982 color object animation 10 minutes
Focus International $225
A humorous look at the joys and tribulations of first-time intercourse as personified by Marsha and Harry, vulva and penis puppets. Fears, anxieties, and contraceptive awkwardness are addressed in this funny and informative film.
Audience: 16 to 21, parents, educators, youth-service providers

A Masturbatory Story
1978 color animation 15 minutes
Perennial Education $249
A series of still pictures highlighting the humorous and typical experiences of a young adult learning about autoerotic pleasure. Guitar backs the rhyming narration.
Audience: 14 to 21, parents, educators, youth-service providers

Fig. 17. Line-up. From the Film *Condom-Sense*.

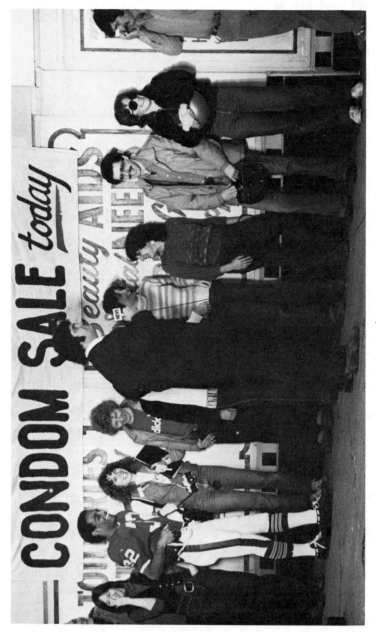

Michael, a Gay Son
1981 color live action 28 minutes Filmmakers Library $450
Michael's gay support group shares a variety of experiences involved in informing parents of homosexuality. He acts on this advice, but only his sister is supportive until a therapist intervenes.
Audience: 16 to 21, parents, educators, youth-service providers

Schoolboy Father
1982 color live action 30 minutes
Learning Corp. of America $450
Based on Jeanette Eyerly's *He's My Baby Now*, this popularly done film tells of sixteen-year-old Charles, who wants to care for the baby he helped create instead of allowing adoption.
Audience: 12 to 16, parents, educators, youth-service providers

Shatter the Silence
1981 color live action 29 minutes Phoenix Films $485
A dramatic and realistic depiction of father-daughter incest, the film shows the psychological impact on thirteen-year-old Marianne and her evolution into confused and scared womanhood. The therapy group provides other reactions to the situation, so the viewer realizes there are resources and rights for such abuse victims.
Audience: 14 to 21, crisis groups, parents, educators, youth-service providers

Teenage Father
1979 color live action 10 minutes Children's Home Society of California $350
This Academy Award-winning documentary is about the unplanned pregnancy of a fifteen-year-old girl and a seventeen-year-old boy. Emphasizing his position, scenes show parental reactions, options, and decisions.
Audience: 13 to 17, parents, educators, youth-service providers

What Can a Guy Do?
1980 color live action 15 minutes Serious Business Co. $250
Using dramatized vignettes and interviews, this film points up

the variety of attitudes and awareness levels of typical adolescent males. Rather than dwell on answers, this encourages responsible information seeking.
Audience: 12 to 16, parents, educators, youth-service providers

Mother May I?
1981 color live action 33 minutes Churchill Films $450
A tongue-in-cheek approach to adolescent sexuality issues, this story points up the parental as well as the young woman's fears, emotions, and actions when she thinks she's pregnant. A useful aid for cross-generation communication.
Audience: 12 to 18, parents, educators, youth-service providers

When Teens Get Pregnant
1982 color 19 minutes Polymorph Films $395
This candid interview documentary of five pregnant teens brings out personal experiences, attitudes, worries, and details of the issues they must face. Despite a blurry sound track, this precipitates instant discussion.
Audience: 13 to 18, parents, educators, youth-service providers

■ Resources and Reviews

Although there are excellent reviews and resource guides available, do not rely on them exclusively. For one thing, they're even more dated than book reviews. (I'm always astounded to read a new film review on a title we've had circulating for two years!) And for another, they aren't written to meet your program needs.

Even more important, remember to go back and reconsider existing films in your collection. Because of the high cost of these materials, there's a tendency to keep them forever. Weeding the 16-mm collection is just as important (if not more so) than throwing out those dated books.

Get to know the film vendors; they are marvelously knowledgeable resource people. Get on their mailing lists for catalogs. Do take advantage of preview opportunities at film programs of national, regional, and state conferences of your professional association. Talk to media specialists, and above all else watch lots of movies—nothing will make you more aware and critical. Happy viewing!

Film Distributors

Children's Home Society of California
5429 McConnell Avenue
Los Angeles, CA 90066
(213)306-4114

Churchill Films
662 North Robertson Boulevard
Los Angeles, CA 90069
(800) 334-7830, (213) 657-5110

Filmmakers Library Inc.
133 East 58 Street, Suite 703A
New York, NY 10022
(212) 355-6545

FilmFair Communications
10900 Ventura Boulevard
Studio City, CA 91604
(818) 766-9441

Focus International
1776 Broadway
New York, NY 10019
(212) 586-8612

Journal Films, Inc.
930 Pitner Avenue
Evanston, IL 60202
(800) 323-5448, (312) 328-6700

Learning Corporation of America
1350 Avenue of the Americas
New York, NY 10019
(212) 397-9330

New Day Films
Box 315
Franklin Lakes, NJ 07417
(201) 891-8240

Perennial Education Inc.
930 Pitner Avenue
Evanston, IL 60202
(800) 323-9084, (312) 328-6700

Phoenix Films
468 Park Avenue South
New York, NY 10016
(800) 221-1274, (212) 684-5910

Polymorph Films Inc.
118 South Street
Boston, MA 02111
(617) 542-2004

Serious Business Co.
1609 Jaynes Street
Berkeley, CA 94703
(415) 527-6800

Resources

Adolescence: Choices and Changes, 2nd ed. King County Library System, Young Adult Department (300 8th Avenue North, Seattle, WA 98109). 1983.
A free list of books, films, videos, and resources for young adults and concerned adults.

Audio-Visual Resources. Planned Parenthood, Southeastern Pennsylvania, The Resource Center (1220 Sansom Street, Philadelphia, PA 19107).
Subject and title arrangement of annotated films, filmstrips,

slides, videotapes, and teaching aids available for use by any interested parties. (Note: Most local or regional Planned Parenthood offices can offer similar lists. This entry is representative of the excellent resources available from this national organization. Discussion leaders and program providers are also available.)

Common Focus: An Exchange of Information About Early Adolescence. Center for Early Adolescence, University of North Carolina at Chapel Hill (Suite 223, Carr Mill Mall, Carrbora, NC 27510). Five issues per year.
Call or write to get on the mailing list of these remarkable folks for a broad variety of applicable products.

Films: Teenage Parenting Project of the Free Library of Philadelphia (Logan Square, Philadelphia, PA 19103). 1980.
An LSCA-funded project with professional previewing and selection based on the usefulness to the audience of this library system's Teenage Parenting project. Recommended filmstrips and pamphlets are also compiled, as well as rejects in each area, with full explanations and annotations.

Guide to Films on Reproductive Rights. Media Network and the Reproductive Rights National Network in Cooperation with the Film Fund (208 West 13th Street, New York, NY 10011). 1983.
An up-to-date guide to sixty recommended films, videotapes, and slide shows, plus program tips.

Media Catalog. Compiled by Pamela Wilson and Nancie Connolly. Sex Education Coalition (1309 L Street, NW, Washington, DC 20005). Annual.
This guide to family-life education audiovisual materials contains an annotated list of films and filmstrips available for loan in the Washington, D.C., area.

Selected Films for Young Adults. Young Adult Services Division, American Library Association (50 East Huron Street, Chicago, IL 60611). Annual.
Exhaustively previewed and selected by a hard-working and savvy committee. This well-annotated list varies in size and content from year to year.

Tactile Media for Sexuality Education. Compiled by George M.

Worthington for Planned Parenthood Federation of America (810 Seventh Avenue, New York, NY 10019). 1984.
An annotated alphabetical listing of catalogs from which three-dimensional models and teaching aids can be ordered.

Review Periodicals

Booklist. American Library Association (50 East Huron Street, Chicago, IL 60611). Semimonthly, monthly in July and August.
Lists twelve to fifteen critical and descriptive reviews of recommended films only. Gives suggested use in public libraries. Reviewing tends to be brief and level-headed.

Film and Video News (formerly *Film News*). Gorez Goz Publishing Co. (1058 Eighth Street, La Salle, IL 61301). Quarterly.
Community, religious, and feature films are evaluated regularly. Subject lists as well as articles on films and film programs at selected libraries, museums, and festivals.

Landers Film Reviews. Landers Associates (P.O. Box 69760, Los Angeles, CA 90069). Bimonthly.
Alphabetical descriptive listing of over fifty films per issue. Producers pay to have their films included in the looseleaf insert listing. Cumulated annual index.

Media and Methods. American Society of Educators (1511 Walnut Street, Philadelphia, PA 19102). Monthly.
Each issue has a few lengthy critical reviews of recommended feature-length and short films of interest to high-school humanities and social-studies teachers. Often has articles briefly noting recently released shorts of merit or comparing several films on one topic. Occasional issues are devoted solely to 16-mm film. Eccentric at times.

SIECUS Report. Sex Information and Education Council of the U.S. (80 Fifth Avenue, New York, NY 10011). Bimonthly.
Sexual-health topics with critical annotated reviews of print and nonprint materials. Leaders in the field of sex education and highly respected by the medical and social-work crowd.

Sight Lines (recently merged with *Film Library Quarterly*). Edu-

cational Film Library Association (45 John Street, Suite 301, New York, NY 10038). Quarterly.
Notes new films with a brief description. Rental prices as well as free-loan films are included. Includes articles on films and filmmaking plus thrice-a-year Film Review Index to reviews in film periodicals. (EFLA also puts out five of the best evaluation guides annually. Subscription with membership.)

Voice of Youth Advocates (3936 West Colonial Parkway, Virginia Beach, VA 23452). Bimonthly.
The "must-have" for all youth-service providers. This marvelous tool has pertinent reviews of print and nonprint materials in every issue as well as articles, trends, bibliographies, and program ideas.

Wilson Library Bulletin. H. W. Wilson Company (950 University Avenue, Bronx, NY 10452). Monthly except July and August.
Film reviewing tends to be very general and not particularly discriminating.

■ BIBLIOGRAPHY

Cabeceiras, James. *The Multimedia Library: Materials Selection and Use*. New York: Academic, 1978.

Crichton, Sarah. "Off the Beach Blanket and into the Bedroom: What on Earth Is Going On in Teenage Movies?" *Ms.*, June 1985, p. 90.

Monaco, James. *How to Read a Film: The Art, Technology, Language, History and Theory of Film and Media*. New York: Oxford University Press, 1977.

Pillon, Nancy Bach. *Reaching Young People Through Media*. Littleton, Colo.: Libraries Unlimited, 1983.

Rehrauer, George. *Film User's Handbook*. New York: Bowker, 1975.

Research on Adolescence for Youth Service: An Annotated Bibliography on Adolescent Development, Educational Needs and Media, 1978–1980, ed. Hodge and Bradburn. Chicago: Young Adult Services Division, Media and the Young Adult Committee, American Library Association, 1984.

Chapter 14

The Right Book at the Right Time

By now it should be apparent that there are plenty of good books about sex for teenagers. But by and large this body of literature is a national resource that is invisible and underutilized. The stigma of "what every young man should know" still clings to the popular perception of sex guides, and young adults searching for information in print are more likely to take their questions to parental copies of *Playboy* and *The Joy of Sex* than to look for something relevant to their own needs at the school or public library.

No serious modern study has ever been done on the relationship of private reading and adolescent sexual knowledge or behavior. Surveys that attempt to pin down the sources of sexual learning almost never include libraries as a choice and usually lump sex guides with "books and magazines" or even "media," categories that would encompass *Hustler* and *Porky's* as well as *Changing Bodies, Changing Lives*. Even more disturbing is the fact that government grants for community programs on sex education or adolescent pregnancy almost never perceive the library as an information center or even as an organization that might have an interest in being involved.

Why is it that this goldmine of information and guidance is not more widely used? Part of the blame lies in the lamentable history of the sex guide, as we have seen, and also in the policies of prudish librarians who kept "those books" locked in a back room. But even today many collections in public and school libraries and in youth agencies consist of a few titles chosen long ago almost at random and allowed to moulder away to laughable irrelevance. Even when teachers and librarians have a strong commitment to ongoing sexuality education, there is still a tendency to regard "a good book on sex" as "a good book on sex," without recognition of the many variables in reading level, sophistication, subject emphasis, literary quality, and liberal/conservative orientation.

A book that is exactly right for one adolescent may be exactly wrong for another. And an entirely different book may be right for both of them next year. Teenagers do not go to bookstores and buy sex guides. They are dependent on parents, teachers, librarians, and youth workers to put exactly the appropriate reading material into their hands at the moment when they need to read it. This is a job worth doing well.

▪ Background Reading for Adults

The first step in becoming an effective provider of sex information is to become comfortable with one's own sexuality. Parents as well as youth professionals may want to clear up confusions and bring their knowledge up to date with the very detailed and authoritative adult manual *Sex: The Facts, the Acts and Your Feelings*, by Michael Carrera.

Other preliminary background reading might be one of the many recent books based on surveys of adolescent sexual patterns in the U.S. Typically these involve formal data collected on a questionnaire from a large sampling of the teen population and a smaller number of personal interviews. The text is made up of general conclusions from the research and many juicy quotes from the interviews. There is very little scholarly apparatus—footnotes, charts, graphs—to give credibility. These are popular reading, and the treatment leans heavily toward the sensational and the explicit. Such books, while they are not to be taken too seriously as research, are eye-openers for those who are out of touch with the realities of adolescent life. An older book of this kind was *Sex and the American Teenager*, by Murray M. Kappelman, now out of date because the author attributes homosexuality to an imbalance in parental roles. Others are *Teenage Sexuality: A Survey of Teenage Sexual Behavior*, by Aaron Hass; *The Private Life of the American Teenager*, by Jane Norman and

Myron W. Harris; *Growing into Love: Teenagers Talk Candidly About Sex in the 1980s*, by Kathryn Watterson Burkhart; and *Sex and the American Teenager*, by Robert Coles and Geoffrey Stokes.

Parents, everyone agrees, should be the primary sex educators for their own children. Studies have consistently shown that teens who can talk with their parents about sex are much more likely to postpone intercourse and to use birth control when they do become sexually active. But the problem is that few parents are able to establish rapport with their offspring on such a touchy subject. In the last two years a bumper crop of excellent books have offered help with this problem.

Two of the best are *Sex Education Begins at Home: How to Raise Sexually Healthy Children* and *Parents' Guide to Teenage Sex and Pregnancy*, both by Howard and Martha Lewis. The authors speak intimately to parents, reassuring them as to their own competence ("It's more important to be approachable than to be a walking encyclopedia of sexual knowledge") and giving detailed suggestions on how to ease embarrassment, get used to talking about sex, and take advantage of the "teachable moment." At the same time they leave room for a variety of values. Like all other parent sex education books, they take great pains to demolish the myth so popular with the far right that sexual knowledge leads to sexual activity. *Sex Education Begins at Home* covers the basics, and *Parents' Guide to Teenage Sex and Pregnancy* deals with adolescent intercourse and its ramifications, including sexual dysfunctions, cohabitation, promiscuity, and the options for a problem pregnancy.

Some familiar and respected sex education names appear as authors of books for parents. Sol Gordon and his wife, Judith, tip their hats to the change in the American political climate with *Raising a Child Conservatively in a Sexually Permissive World*. Gordon defines his "conservatism" as a strong commitment to family values and a conviction that teenagers should not have sexual intercourse. But while he treads carefully around volatile issues like abortion, he is at pains to disassociate himself from those "who view the establishment of a 'Christian Republic' as the solution to the permissiveness around them." Dr. Mary Calderone, former head of the Sex Information and Education Council of the United States, and Eric Johnson, author of many sex guides for teens, have produced as a joint enterprise the thorough and dependable *Family Book About Sexuality.* Ruth Bell (an editor of *Changing Bodies, Changing Lives*) and Leni Zeiger Wildflower give practical and sympathetic advice on *Talking with Your Teenager*, and Elizabeth Winship draws on the letters she has received for her column "Ask Beth" (and her sex guide of the same title) to offer wise and friendly counsel on *Reaching Your Teenager.*

The impressive credentials of Katherine Oettinger give weight and credibility to the best book for the parents of a pregnant teenager—*Not My Daughter: Facing Up to Adolescent Pregnancy.* Dr. Oettinger has served as chief of the Children's Bureau for the Department of Health, Education, and Welfare; as Deputy Assistant Secretary for Population and Family Planning; as consultant and U.S. delegate to many international conferences on population and family health; and as coordinator for the Interhemispheric Conference on Adolescent Fertility. In all these positions and for many years she has worked hard to alleviate the complex social problems of too-early childbearing. *Not My Daughter* offers guidance on building healthy sexual communication in the home, educating boys as well as girls in the need for contraception, and making informed choices when teenage pregnancy happens. Although she has good words on personal decision-making and values, Dr. Oettinger is a politician, and her major emphasis is on working for community change. As examples she describes a number of national and local programs that have been effective.

For the one parent in ten whose child is homosexual, a comforting source of understanding and reassurance is *Now That You Know: What Every Parent Should Know About Homosexuality*, by Betty Fairchild and Nancy Hayward. Both authors have lived through the trauma of a teenage son or daughter's coming-out announcement and have learned to accept and take pride in their gay children. Fairchild and Hayward have been instrumental in founding the helping organization Parents of Gays. In their book they tell other parents going through the same emotional adjustment how to respond to their child, how to help (and not hurt), how to reconcile homosexuality with religion, and how to steer a young person toward a career where sexual preference will not be a handicap. With excerpts from the stories of dozens of gay men and women they show the range of homosexual life experiences and styles.

Librarians, teachers, and other youth professionals who have not had training in sexuality education may want to have on hand a copy of the basic college textbook on the subject: *The Sexual Adolescent*, by Sol Gordon, Peter Scales, and Kathleen Everly. Another dependable sourcebook for research and statistics is *Experiencing Adolescents*, edited by Richard Lerner and Nancy Galambos. This is a collection of well-documented scholarly articles on puberty and its psychological and social significance, adolescent sexuality and social relationships, drug and alcohol abuse, health issues in adolescence, and many other pertinent topics. A third resource for the professional shelf is *The Sexual Rights of Adolescents*, by Hyman Rodman and others, which summarizes for the educated lay reader the complex and changing legal ramifications of the teen years.

▪ Planning for Censorship

The librarian or teacher who takes an active role in promoting adolescent sexual literacy with a strong collection of books and films, staff training, and workshops and programs for parents and teens is sooner or later going to be confronted with individual parental protest or group censorship attack. This is a fact of life in our sex-negative society, but it is no excuse for backing away from this vital responsibility. Although parents and schools should be the basic providers of sound sex education, they seldom are. This leaves the library as the only source of sex information for young people, unless we want to abandon the job to sexploitation movies, rock lyrics, graffiti, and the dubious counsel of peers.

The best defense against censorship attempts is to be prepared. A written selection policy is essential. Librarians and teachers should be thoroughly familiar with the materials in the collection and should keep records of the reviews and recommendations that influenced the purchase decision. Even more important, a collection that is balanced is far less likely to draw attack. If protestors can be shown that while they may object to a particular book, there are other titles in the library that *do* reflect their views, they may be mollified. A well-handled complaint can be educational for both librarian and parent. A helpful source of techniques and strategies for heading off controversy is *The Front Lines of Sexuality Education: A Guide to Building and Maintaining Community Support*, by Peter Scales, who has forged his know-how in many a sex education battle. One of his more striking findings is that organized protest, although highly vocal, nearly always represents only a tiny minority of community opinion.

The American Library Association stands solidly behind intellectual freedom on all subjects (see Appendix III for the ALA Bill of Rights). The Young Adult Services Division of ALA went on record in January 1978 in support of sex education, adopting a policy statement that urges "all librarians and library educators to examine existing policies and practices, and to assume a leadership role in seeing that information is available for children and adolescents, their parents, and youth-serving professionals at the state and local level, to assure that comprehensive sex-related education materials, programs, referral and health services for youth are available and publicized." In practical terms the ALA Office for Intellectual Freedom offers advice and counsel on how to handle censorship cases. Director Judith Krug can be contacted at the American Library Association headquarters, 50 East Huron Street, Chicago, IL 60611.

▪ Review Sources

An invaluable resource for parents and professionals who are serious about their role as sex educators is the *SIECUS Report*. Published bimonthly by the Sex Information and Education Council of the United States, this slim but prestigious publication combines scholarly expertise with freshness and readability. Articles and reviews written by leading authorities evaluate the newest and most interesting and significant books and films on human sexuality and discuss trends, research, and discoveries in the field. In addition to the *Report* SIECUS publishes two frequently updated and highly selective lists of the best in sex education books: "Human Sexuality: Books for Everyone" and "Human Sexuality: A Selected Bibliography for Professionals." Other review journals in the following list cover a broad range of juvenile publishing including sex education and reflect the reviewers' background in library work with teenagers:

Booklist. Semimonthly, monthly in July and August. American Library Association, 50 East Huron Street, Chicago, IL 60611

School Library Journal. Monthly except June and July. R. R. Bowker Co., P.O. Box 1426, Riverton, NJ 08077

SIECUS Report. Bimonthly. 80 Fifth Avenue, New York, NY 10011

Voice of Youth Advocates. Bimonthly. 3936 West Colonial Parkway, Virginia Beach, VA 23452

Wilson Library Bulletin (column, "The Young Adult Perplex"). Monthly except July and August. 950 University Avenue, Bronx, NY 10452

▪ Evaluation Checklist

To focus the evaluation of new books, and to analyze and become familiar with the contents of older ones, the following checklist may be helpful. It is based on a list prepared by Dr. William S. Palmer, as quoted in the *Voice of Youth Advocates*, April 1982.

When evaluating new books, librarians should be alert for certain "instant disqualifiers": excessive description of sexual pathology, gross factual errors, (such as claiming that abortion is illegal or that homosexuals are child molesters), warnings of hellfire or other scare tactics, outdated "teen slang," or a heavily condescending tone. Critical attention should be given to areas in which research and attitudes are currently in flux, such as STD (especially AIDS), abortion, and homosexuality.

▪ Core Collections and Weeding Lists

We now come to the part of this book that sums up everything that has gone before. Appendix I is a set of core collection bibliographies for public and junior and senior high-school li-

A Checklist for Evaluating Sex Education Books

Physiological and related factors

Does the book contain information about the following:
- Sexual development?
- Sex organs and function?
- Menstruation?
- Masturbation?
- Intercourse?
- Homosexuality?
- Contraception?
- Pregnancy?
- Abortion?
- Childbirth?

Sociological aspects of intimate relationships

Does the book reflect an awareness of recent social changes in sexual attitudes and behavior?

Does the book stress the emotional as well as the physical aspects of lovemaking?

Does the book deal with the roles of men and women in sex equitably?

Moral aspects of intimate relationships

Does the book discuss the issue of sex before marriage?

Is support offered to those who wish to abstain from sexual activity?

For the sexually active, does the book stress the necessity of:
- Mutual consent?
- Caring and consideration for the partner?
- Responsible contraception?

Does the book recognize the validity of sexual moralities other than the one the author is advocating?

Problems with sex

Does the book discuss:

- Negative feelings about sex?
- Rape?
- Incest?
- Sexually transmitted diseases?

Amount and kind of information

Is the amount of basic sex information sufficient to make key concepts clear?

Does the book suggest further references and resources?

Reliability of information

Is the basic sex information accurate?

Does the book show an awareness of recent relevant changes in law and in scientific knowledge?

Is the author an expert in sex education?

Format and readability

Are the typeface and the composition of the page attractive and easy to read?

Are headings and subheadings used?

Is sentence structure simple and clear?

Does the book use illustrations that clarify basic sex information?

Are the young people shown in the illustrations easy for the reader to identify with?

Is there an index?

Is there a glossary?

Style

Does the writing style lend itself to the establishing of a rapport with the intended audience?

When possible, does the author use nonclinical nomenclature?

If humor or colloquialisms are used, is the inclusion effective?

braries both rich and poor. Appendix II is an even more important list—a guide to weeding existing collections.

Each title in these bibliographies has been discussed in the text and can be traced through the index. The core collections represent the best of the books that this author considers appropriate and valid in the field of adolescent sexuality. However, any such list must be a subjective choice and so should be considered only a tool, not Holy Scripture. Librarians may want to use these bibliographies as a general measure of the scope and validity of their holdings. Teachers and parents may also want to take them to the shelves of their school or public library to get a sense of how complete and current the collection is and, if necessary, to consult the lists as a basis for suggestions to the librarian. Youth professionals may want to use them for building office lending collections or for encouraging their local library to update and expand their sex education resources. They are meant for inspiration, not obligation.

It is important to note that only the edition cited is recommended. Note also that earnest effort has been made to include conservative as well as liberal titles. Only books published since 1977 (with a rare exception or two) have been included. In the case of fiction only a few particularly informative novels are listed, but the intention has not been to limit the collection to these titles. Some books are neither good enough to recommend for purchase nor bad enough to deserve weeding. While they have been discussed in previous chapters, such titles do not appear in the core collection or the weeding lists. If they are already in the library they can be left on the shelf for a year or two more, but they should not be replaced. Two lists are given for each type of library: one for those with restricted funds and an augmentation for those with more generous budgets. Some practical recognition has also been given to the more vulnerable censorship position of the school library.

For libraries or youth agencies in which the amount of money available for books on sexuality is really minuscule (not just hampered by a lack of commitment) pamphlets might be used to round out a small basic paperback collection. Although evaluation of such material is outside the scope of this volume, here is a list of some sources for excellent and inexpensive pamphlets:

Planned Parenthood Federation of America, 810 Seventh Avenue, New York, NY 10019

Rocky Mountain Planned Parenthood, RAJ Publications, Box 18599, Denver, CO 80218

Planned Parenthood of Syracuse, 1120 East Genesee Street, Syracuse, NY 13210

Public Affairs Pamphlets, 381 Park Avenue South, New York, NY 10016

Network Publications, 1700 Mission Street, Suite 203, Box 8506, Santa Cruz, CA 95061-8506

Life Skills Education, 280 Broad Street, Weymouth, MA 02188

American Social Health Association, 260 Sheridan Avenue, Palo Alto, CA 94306

Sundance Resource Center, 3207 Matthew NE, Albuquerque, NM 87107

Once collected, how should these books be displayed to attract the maximum number of young readers? The answer is "conspicuously—but not too conspicuously." In the public library they should be a matter-of-fact part of the young adult collection, not hidden away with the 600s in the adult section. Although occasional displays can be used to advertise the fact that the library has such materials, sex guides should not be routinely isolated in special bins or racks in a misguided attempt to get them noticed. The same rule applies to school libraries. In this situation they should be shelved in proper call-number order but with a modest sign to direct young searchers to the right place. A discreetly sheltered table nearby helps ease the embarrassment of teens who are not eager to let their friends see them reading a sex guide. That same discomfort will probably be responsible for a large number of copies leaving the library in a less-than-orthodox manner. This is the librarian's signal to buy multiple paperback copies of most-stolen titles and to rejoice that information needs are being met.

Good evaluation and selection are important, but energetic and informed weeding is even more vital in maintaining credibility with teenagers. It takes only one encounter with an antiquated sex guide to destroy any faith a young adult might have in the relevance of the library to his or her sex-information questions, regardless of how many other excellent books are shelved there. It may be tempting to keep an outdated book for just one more year until it wears out. It may be difficult to discard a book that seemed so au courant just a few years before or an expensive volume that has hardly been used at all. But it is essential to be ruthless. Throw it out—in the trash. Or give it to a research library to store as social history. But don't hand it over to the Friends of the Library for their annual book sale—it will do just as much harm there.

Once weeded, the collection must be periodically rechecked for creeping irrelevance. We have already discussed the subject areas that are changing rapidly: abortion, homosexuality, STD. But the future may bring other needs for reassessment. American sexual attitudes are as responsive as hemlines to changes in the social climate. If the pendulum should swing away from the present conservative mood (or swing even farther to the right), new books would be written and some old books would be out of phase. If the Supreme Court or a Constitutional amendment should reverse the legality of abortion, or if crucial new data are discovered on AIDS, or new contraceptive methods are perfected, the same would be true.

Sex guiding is a continuous and demanding responsibility, but in terms of human happiness and the future of the world, it is one of the very best services we can bring to youth.

■ BIBLIOGRAPHY

Bell, Ruth, and Leni Zeiger Wildflower. *Talking with Your Teenager: A Book for Parents.* New York: Random House, 1983.

Burkhart, Kathryn Watterson. *Growing into Love: Teenagers Talk Candidly About Sex in the 1980s.* New York: Putnam, 1981.

Calderone, Mary S., and Eric W. Johnson. *The Family Book About Sexuality.* New York: Harper and Row, 1981, 1983.

Carrera, Michael. *Sex: The Facts, the Acts and Your Feelings.* New York: Crown, 1981.

Coles, Robert, and Geoffrey Stokes. *Sex and the American Teenager.* New York: Harper and Row, Rolling Stone, 1985.

Fairchild, Betty, and Nancy Hayward. *Now That You Know: What Every Parent Should Know About Homosexuality.* New York: Harcourt, 1979.

Gordon, Sol, and Judith Gordon. *Raising a Child Conservatively in a Sexually Permissive World.* New York: Simon and Schuster, 1983.

Gordon, Sol, Peter Scales, and Kathleen Everly. *The Sexual Adolescent: Communicating with Teenagers About Sex*, 2nd ed. North Scituate, Mass.: Duxbury, 1979.

Hass, Aaron. *Teenage Sexuality: A Survey of Teenage Sexual Behavior*. New York: Macmillan, 1979.

Kappelman, Murray M. *Sex and the American Teenager: The Problems of Adolescent Sexuality—and How to Cope with Them in Today's Changing World*. New York: Crowell, 1977.

Lerner, Richard M., and Nancy L. Galambos, eds. *Experiencing Adolescents: A Sourcebook for Parents, Teachers, and Teens*. New York: Garland, 1984.

Lewis, Howard R., and Martha E. Lewis. *Parents' Guide to Teenage Sex and Pregnancy*. New York: St. Martin's, 1980.

——— . *Sex Education Begins at Home: How to Raise Sexually Healthy Children*. Norwalk, Conn.: Appleton-Century-Crofts, 1983.

Norman, Jane, and Myron W. Harris. *The Private Life of the American Teenager*. New York: Rawson, Wade, 1981.

Oettinger, Katherine B., and Elizabeth Mooney. *Not My Daughter: Facing Up to Adolescent Pregnancy*. New York: Prentice-Hall, 1979.

Rodman, Hyman, and others. *The Sexual Rights of Adolescents*. New York: Columbia University Press, 1984.

Scales, Peter. *The Front Lines of Sexuality Education: A Guide to Building and Maintaining Community Support*. Santa Cruz, Calif.: Network, 1984.

Winship, Elizabeth G. *Reaching Your Teenager*. Boston: Houghton Mifflin, 1983.

ADDENDA

The following books were published too late to be included in the body of the work:

Hyde, Margaret O., and Elizabeth H. Forsyth. *AIDS: What Does It Mean to You?* New York: Walker, 1986.
A well-researched and highly readable small book that carefully summarizes what is and is not known about this disease and makes a plea for national concern. First purchase for junior high, senior high, and public library core collections.

Landau, Elaine. *Sexually Transmitted Diseases*. Hillside, N.J.: Enslow, 1986.
A factually accurate but lifeless listing of symptoms and treatment. Stresses the worst possible outcome of each disease and lacks compassion and practicality. Not recommended for core collections.

Silverstein, Alvin, and Virginia B. Silverstein. *AIDS: Deadly Threat*. Hillside, N.J.: Enslow, 1986.
An excellent examination of the origins and progress of this disease with more biological detail than Hyde (see above). First purchase senior high and public library core collections. Second purchase junior high core collections.

Voss, Jacqueline, and Jay Gale. *A Young Woman's Guide to Sex*. New York: Holt, 1986.
A good, basic middle-of-the-road sex guide, somewhat overwritten and staid, but with sound, complete, and up-to-date information and advice. Outstanding discussions of contraceptive methods, acquaintance rape, and sexual decision-making. First purchase for junior high, senior high, and public library core collections.

Appendix I

Core-Collection Lists

▪ JUNIOR HIGH SCHOOL LIBRARY

(The following bibliography represents the basic minimum collection on sexuality for school libraries serving eleven- to fifteen-year-olds. Only the editions cited are recommended.)

Nonfiction

Bode, Janet. *Rape*. New York: Watts, 1979.
or
Booher, Dianna Daniels. *Rape*. New York: Messner, 1981.
Coleman, William L. *The Great Date Wait and Other Hazards*. Minneapolis: Bethany, 1982.
Comfort, Alex, and Jane Comfort. *The Facts of Love*. New York: Crown, 1979; New York: Ballantine, 1980.
Gardner-Loulan, JoAnn, Bonnie Lopez, and Marcia Quackenbush. *Period*, rev. ed. San Francisco: Volcano, 1981.
Gordon, Sol. *Facts About Sex for Today's Youth*, rev. ed. Fayetteville, N.Y.: Ed-U, 1985.
———. *Facts About STD*. Fayetteville, N.Y.: Ed-U, 1983.
Hettlinger, Richard F. *Growing Up with Sex*, new rev. ed. New York: Continuum, 1980.
Johnson, Eric W. *Love and Sex in Plain Language*, 4th rev. ed. New York: Harper and Row, 1985.
McCoy, Kathy. *The Teenage Body Book Guide to Sexuality*. New York: Simon and Schuster, 1983.
or

———. *The Teenage Body Book Guide to Dating*. New York: Simon and Schuster, 1983.

Madaras, Lynda, with Area Madaras. *What's Happening to My Body?* New York: Newmarket, 1983.

Madaras, Lynda, with Dane Saavedra. *The What's Happening to My Body? Book for Boys*. New York: Newmarket, 1984.

Miner, Jane Claypool. *Young Parents*. New York: Messner, 1985.

Pomeroy, Wardell B. *Boys and Sex*, rev. ed. New York: Delacorte, 1981.

———. *Girls and Sex*, rev. ed. New York: Delacorte, 1981.

Richards, Arlene Kramer, and Irene Willis. *Under 18 and Pregnant*. New York: Lothrop, Lee and Shepard, 1983.

or

Witt, Reni L., and Jeannine Masterson Michael. *Mom, I'm Pregnant*. New York: Stein and Day, 1982.

Fiction

Blume, Judy. *Forever*. Scarsdale, N.Y.: Bradbury, 1975; New York: Pocket Books, 1976.

Luger, Harriett. *Lauren*. New York: Viking, 1979; New York: Dell, 1981.

Miklowitz, Gloria D. *Did You Hear What Happened to Andrea?* New York: Delacorte, 1979; New York: Dell, 1981.

For special needs

Hopper, C. Edmund, and W. A. Allen. *Sex Education for Physically Handicapped Youth*. Springfield, Ill.: Thomas, 1980.

As funds become available, add titles given as alternates and also the following:

Nonfiction

Betancourt, Jeanne. *Am I Normal?* New York: Avon, 1983.

———. *Dear Diary*. New York: Avon, 1983.

Butler, John. *Christian Ways to Date, Go Steady, and Break Up*. Cincinnati: Standard, 1978.

Eagan, Andrea Boroff. *Why Am I So Miserable if These Are the Best Years of My Life?* rev. ed. New York: Avon, 1979.

Lindsay, Jeanne Warren. *Pregnant Too Soon: Adoption Is an Option.* Buena Park, Calif.: Morning Glory, 1980.
McCoy, Kathy. *The Teenage Survival Guide.* New York: Simon and Schuster, 1981.
———, and Charles Wibbelsman. *The Teenage Body Book.* New York: Simon and Schuster, 1978.
Roggow, Linda, and Carolyn Owens. *Handbook for Pregnant Teenagers.* Grand Rapids, Mich.: Zondervan, 1984.
Shedd, Charlie W. *The Stork Is Dead,* rev. ed. Waco, Texas: Word, 1982.
Simon, Nissa. *Don't Worry, You're Normal.* New York: Crowell, 1982.

Fiction

Blume, Judy. *Are You There God? It's Me, Margaret.* New York: Bradbury, 1970; New York: Dell, 1974.
———. *Then Again, Maybe I Won't.* New York: Bradbury, 1971; New York: Dell, 1974.
Hautzig, Deborah. *Hey Dollface!* New York: Greenwillow, 1978.
LeGuin, Ursula K. *Very Far Away from Anywhere Else.* New York: Atheneum, 1976; New York: Bantam, 1978.

▪ SENIOR HIGH SCHOOL LIBRARY

(The following bibliography represents the basic minimum collection on sexuality for school libraries serving fourteen- to eighteen-year-olds. Only the editions cited are recommended.)

Nonfiction

Balis, Andrea. *What Are You Using?* New York: Dial, 1981.
Bell, Ruth, et al. *Changing Bodies, Changing Lives.* New York: Random House, 1980.
Bode, Janet. *Rape.* New York: Watts, 1979.
or
Booher, Dianna Daniels. *Rape.* New York: Messner, 1981.
Cooney, Nancy Hennessy, with Anne Bingham. *Sex, Sexuality*

and You. Dubuque, Iowa: Brown, 1980 (*or* Reichert, *Sexuality and Dating*).
Gittelsohn, Roland B. *Love, Sex and Marriage: A Jewish View*, new ed. New York: Union of American Hebrew Congregations, 1980.
Gordon, Sol. *Facts About Sex for Today's Youth*, rev. ed. Fayetteville, N.Y.: Ed-U, 1978, 1985 (reluctant readers).
Hanckel, Frances, and John Cunningham. *A Way of Love, a Way of Life: A Young Person's Introduction to What It Means to Be Gay*. New York: Lothrop, Lee and Shepard, 1979.
Kelly, Gary F. *Learning About Sex*, rev. ed. Woodbury, N.Y.: Barron's Educational Series, 1977.
Lieberman, E. James, and Ellen Peck. *Sex and Birth Control*, rev. ed. New York: Harper and Row, 1981.
Lindsay, Jeanne Warren. *Pregnant Too Soon: Adoption Is an Option*. Buena Park, Calif.: Morning Glory, 1980.
———. *Teenage Marriage*. Buena Park, Calif.: Morning Glory, 1984.
———. *Teens Parenting*. Buena Park, Calif.: Morning Glory, 1981.
Lumiere, Richard, and Stephani Cook. *Healthy Sex and Keeping It That Way*. New York: Simon and Schuster, 1983 (*or* Neumann, *Dr. Neumann's Guide*).
McCoy, Kathy. *The Teenage Body Book Guide to Dating*. New York: Simon and Schuster, 1983.
or
———. *The Teenage Body Book Guide to Sexuality*. New York: Simon and Schuster, 1983.
Maddux, Hilary C. *Menstruation*. New York: Tobey, 1975 (*or* Voelckers, *Girls Guide to Menstruation*).
Neumann, Hans H., with Sylvia Simmons. *Dr. Neumann's Guide to the New Sexually Transmitted Diseases*. Washington, D.C.: Acropolis, 1983 (*or* Lumiere, *Healthy Sex*).
Reichert, Richard. *Sexuality and Dating: A Christian Perspective*. Winona, Minn.: St. Mary's Press, Christian Bros., 1981 (*or* Cooney, *Sex, Sexuality and You*).
Richards, Arlene Kramer, and Irene Willis. *Under 18 and Pregnant*. New York: Lothrop. Lee and Shepard, 1983 (*or* Witt, *Mom, I'm Pregnant*).
Short, Ray E. *Sex, Dating and Love*. Minneapolis: Augsburg, 1984

or

———. *Sex, Love, or Infatuation.* Minneapolis: Augsburg, 1978.

Voelckers, Ellen. *Girls Guide to Menstruation.* New York: Rosen, 1975 (*or* Maddux, *Menstruation*).

Witt, Reni L., and Jeannine Masterson Michael. *Mom, I'm Pregnant.* New York: Stein and Day, 1982 (*or* Richards, *Under 18 and Pregnant*).

Fiction

Blume, Judy. *Forever.* Scarsdale, N.Y.: Bradbury, 1975; New York: Pocket Books, 1976.

LeGuin, Ursula. *Very Far Away from Anywhere Else.* New York: Atheneum, 1976; New York: Bantam, 1978.

Luger, Harriett. *Lauren.* New York: Viking, 1979; New York: Dell, 1981.

Mazer, Norma. *Up in Seth's Room.* New York: Delacorte, 1979; New York: Dell, 1981.

Miklowitz, Gloria D. *Did You Hear What Happened to Andrea?* New York: Delacorte, 1979; New York: Dell, 1981.

Peck, Richard. *Are You in the House Alone?* New York: Viking, 1976; New York: Dell, 1977.

Stephensen, A. M. *Unbirthday.* New York: Avon, 1982.

For special needs

Doughten, Susan, Marlyn B. Minkin, and Laurie E. Rosen. *Signs for Sexuality.* Seattle: Planned Parenthood of Seattle/King County, 1978.

As funds become available, add titles given as alternates and also the following:

Nonfiction

Booher, Dianna Daniels. *Love.* New York: Messner, 1985.

Butler, John. *Christian Ways to Date, Go Steady, and Break Up.* Cincinnati: Standard, 1978.

Corsaro, Maria, and Carole Korzeniowsky. *STD.* New York: Holt, 1982.

Eagan, Andrea Boroff. *Why Am I So Miserable if These Are the Best Years of My Life?*, rev. ed. New York: Avon, 1979.

Ewy, Donna, and Rodger Ewy. *Teen Pregnancy: The Challenges We Faced, the Choices We Made.* New York: New American Library, 1985.

Hamilton, Eleanor. *Sex, with Love.* Boston: Beacon, 1978.

Hettlinger, Richard F. *Growing Up with Sex*, new rev. ed. New York: Continuum, 1980.

McCoy, Kathy. *The Teenage Survival Guide.* New York: Simon and Schuster, 1981.

———, and Charles Wibbelsman. *The Teenage Body Book.* New York: Simon and Schuster, 1978.

McGuire, Paula. *It Won't Happen to Me.* New York: Delacorte, 1983; New York: Delta, 1983.

Miner, Jane Claypool. *Young Parents.* New York: Messner, 1985.

Rice, Max, and Vivian Rice. *When Can I Say, "I Love You"?* Chicago: Moody, 1977.

Roggow, Linda, and Carolyn Owens. *Handbook for Pregnant Teenagers.* Grand Rapids, Mich.: Zondervan, 1984.

Stafford, Tim. *A Love Story.* Grand Rapids, Mich.: Zondervan, 1977.

Fiction

Mazer, Harry. *Hey, Kid! Does She Love Me?* New York: Crowell, 1985.

Mazer, Norma Fox. *Someone to Love.* New York: Delacorte, 1983; New York: Dell, 1985.

▪ Public Library Young Adult Section

(The following bibliography represents the basic minimum collection on adolescent sexuality for a public library. Only the editions cited are recommended.)

Nonfiction

Balis, Andrea. *What Are You Using?* New York: Dial, 1981.

Bell, Ruth, et al. *Changing Bodies, Changing Lives.* New York: Random House, 1980.

Bode, Janet. *Rape.* New York: Watts, 1979.

or

Booher, Dianna Daniels. *Rape*. New York: Messner, 1981.

Coleman, William L. *The Great Date Wait*. Minneapolis: Bethany, 1982.

Comfort, Alex, and Jane Comfort. *The Facts of Love*. New York: Crown, 1979; New York: Ballantine, 1980.

Gordon, Sol. *Facts About Sex for Today's Youth*, rev. ed. Fayetteville, N.Y.: Ed-U, 1978.

———. *Facts About STD*. Fayetteville, N.Y.: Ed-U, 1983.

Hanckel, Frances, and John Cunningham. *A Way of Love, a Way of Life*. New York: Lothrop, Lee and Shepard, 1979.

Hettlinger, Richard F. *Growing Up with Sex*, new rev. ed. New York: Continuum, 1980.

Hopper, C. Edmund, and William A. Allen. *Sex Education for Physically Handicapped Youth*. Springfield, Ill.: Thomas, 1980.

Johnson, Eric W. *Love and Sex in Plain Language*, 4th rev. ed. New York: Harper and Row, 1985.

Kelly, Gary F. *Learning About Sex*, rev. ed. Woodbury, N.Y.: Barron's Educational Series, 1977.

Lieberman, E. James, and Ellen Peck. *Sex and Birth Control*, rev. ed. New York: Harper and Row, 1981.

Lindsay, Jeanne Warren. *Pregnant Too Soon: Adoption Is an Option*. Buena Park, Calif.: Morning Glory, 1980.

———. *Teenage Marriage*. Buena Park, Calif.: Morning Glory, 1984.

———. *Teens Parenting*. Buena Park, Calif.: Morning Glory, 1981.

McCoy, Kathy. *The Teenage Body Book Guide to Dating*. New York: Simon and Schuster, 1983.

or

———. *The Teenage Body Book Guide to Sexuality*. New York: Simon and Schuster, 1983.

Madaras, Lynda, with Area Madaras. *What's Happening to My Body?* New York: Newmarket, 1983.

Madaras, Lynda, with Dane Saavedra. *The What's Happening to My Body? Book for Boys*. New York: Newmarket, 1984.

Miner, Jane Claypool. *Young Parents*. New York: Messner, 1985.

Pomeroy, Wardell B. *Boys and Sex*, rev. ed. New York: Delacorte, 1981.

———. *Girls and Sex*, rev. ed. New York: Delacorte, 1981.

Richards, Arlene Kramer, and Irene Willis. *Under 18 and Pregnant*. New York: Lothrop, Lee and Shepard, 1983 (*or* Witt, *Mom, I'm Pregnant*).

Short, Ray E. *Sex, Dating and Love*. Minneapolis: Augsburg, 1984.

or

———. *Sex, Love, or Infatuation*. Minneapolis: Augsburg, 1978.

Westheimer, Ruth, and Nathan Kravetz. *First Love: A Young People's Guide to Sexual Information*. New York: Warner, 1985 (red cover, ISBN 0-446-34294-7).

Witt, Reni L., and Jeannine Masterson Michael. *Mom, I'm Pregnant*. New York: Stein and Day, 1982 (*or* Richards, *Under 18 and Pregnant*).

Fiction

Blume, Judy. *Forever*. Scarsdale, N.Y.: Bradbury, 1975; New York: Pocket Books, 1976.

Davis, Gary Lee. *What Now, McBride?* Orem, Utah: Raymont, 1982.

Filichia, Peter. *A Matter of Finding the Right Girl*. New York: Fawcett Juniper, 1985.

Garden, Nancy. *Annie on My Mind*. New York: Farrar, Straus, 1982.

Hautzig, Deborah. *Hey Dollface!* New York: Greenwillow, 1978.

Hermes, Patricia. *A Solitary Secret*. New York: Harcourt, 1985.

Klein, Norma. *Beginner's Love*. New York: Dutton, 1983; New York: Fawcett Juniper, 1984.

LeGuin, Ursula K. *Very Far Away from Anywhere Else*. New York: Atheneum, 1976; New York: Bantam, 1978.

Luger, Harriett. *Lauren*. New York: Viking, 1979; New York: Dell, 1981.

Mazer, Harry. *Hey, Kid! Does She Love Me?* New York: Crowell, 1985.

Mazer, Norma Fox. *Someone to Love*. New York: Delacorte, 1983; New York: Dell, 1985.

———. *Up in Seth's Room*. New York: Delacorte, 1979; New York: Dell, 1981.

Miklowitz, Gloria D. *Did You Hear What Happened to Andrea?* New York: Delacorte, 1979; New York: Dell, 1981.

Peck, Richard. *Are You in the House Alone?* New York: Viking, 1976; New York: Dell, 1977.
Stephensen, A. M. *Unbirthday*. New York: Avon, 1982.
Strasser, Todd. *A Very Touchy Subject*. New York: Delacorte, 1985.
Sweeney, Joyce. *Center Line*. New York: Delacorte, 1984; New York: Dell, 1985.

As funds become available, add titles given as alternates and also the following:

Booher, Dianna Daniels. *Love*. New York: Messner, 1985.
Butler, John. *Christian Ways to Date, Go Steady, and Break Up*. Cincinnati: Standard, 1978.
Cooney, Nancy Hennessy, with Anne Bingham. *Sex, Sexuality and You*. Dubuque, Iowa: Brown, 1980.
Eagan, Andrea Boroff. *Why Am I So Miserable if These Are the Best Years of My Life?*, rev. ed. New York: Avon, 1979.
Ewy, Donna, and Rodger Ewy. *Teen Pregnancy: The Challenges We Faced, the Choices We Made*. New York: New American Library, 1985.
Foster, Sallie. *The One Girl in Ten*. Claremont, Calif.: Arbor, 1981.
Frank, Daniel B. *Deep Blue Funk and Other Stories*. Chicago: University of Chicago Press, 1983.
Fricke, Aaron. *Reflections of a Rock Lobster*. Boston: Alyson, 1981.
Gittelsohn, Roland B. *Love, Sex and Marriage*. New York: Union of American Hebrew Congregations, 1980.
Hamilton, Eleanor. *Sex, with Love*. Boston: Beacon, 1978.
Heron, Ann, ed. *One Teenager in Ten*. Boston: Alyson, 1983.
McCoy, Kathy. *The Teenage Survival Guide*. New York: Simon and Schuster, 1981.
———, and Charles Wibbelsman. *The Teenage Body Book*. New York: Simon and Schuster, 1978.
McGuire, Paula. *It Won't Happen to Me*. New York: Delacorte, 1983; New York: Delta, 1983.
Reichert, Richard. *Sexuality and Dating: A Christian Perspective*. Winona, Minn.: St. Mary's Press, Christian Bros., 1981.

Rice, Max, and Vivian Rice. *When Can I Say, "I Love You"?* Chicago: Moody, 1977.
Roggow, Linda, and Carolyn Owens. *Handbook for Pregnant Teenagers*. Grand Rapids, Mich.: Zondervan, 1984.
Shedd, Charlie W. *The Stork Is Dead*, rev. ed. Waco, Texas: Word, 1982.
Simon, Nissa. *Don't Worry, You're Normal.* New York: Crowell, 1982.
Stafford, Tim. *A Love Story*. Grand Rapids, Mich.: Zondervan, 1977.
Young, Gay and Proud!, 2nd. ed. Boston: Alyson, 1985.

Children's Room

(In addition to other books on sexuality appropriate for younger readers, the following should be shelved with the children's collection.)

Betancourt, Jeanne. *Am I Normal?* New York: Avon, 1983.
———. *Dear Diary*. New York: Avon, 1983.
Blume, Judy. *Are You There God? It's Me, Margaret*. Scarsdale, N.Y.: Bradbury, 1970; New York: Dell, 1974.
———. *Then Again, Maybe I Won't*. Scarsdale, N.Y.: Bradbury, 1971; New York: Dell, 1974.
Gardner-Loulan, JoAnn, Bonnie Lopez, and Marcia Quackenbush. *Period*, rev. ed. San Francisco: Volcano, 1981.
Rosenberg, Ellen. *Growing Up Feeling Good*. New York: Beaufort, 1983.

Adult Section

(In addition to other books on sexuality appropriate for adults and those mentioned in the bibliography for Chapter 14, the following should be shelved with the adult collection.)

Corsaro, Maria, and Carole Korzeniowsky. *STD*. New York: Holt, 1982.
———. *A Woman's Guide to Safe Abortion*. New York: St. Martin's, 1980; New York: Holt, 1983.
Doughten, Susan, Marlyn B. Minkin, and Laurie E. Rosen. *Signs for Sexuality*. Seattle: Planned Parenthood of Seattle/King County, 1978.

Francke, Linda Bird. *The Ambivalence of Abortion.* New York: Random House, 1978; New York: Dell, 1978.
Hansen, Caryl. *Your Choice.* New York: Avon, 1980.
Luker, Kristin. *Abortion and the Politics of Motherhood.* Berkeley: University of California Press, 1984.
Lumiere, Richard, and Stephani Cook. *Healthy Sex and Keeping It That Way.* New York: Simon and Schuster, 1983.
Maddux, Hilary C. *Menstruation.* New York: Tobey, 1975.
Neumann, Hans H., with Sylvia Simmons. *Dr. Neumann's Guide to the New Sexually Transmitted Diseases.* Washington, D.C.: Acropolis, 1983.
Reagan, Ronald. *Abortion and the Conscience of the Nation.* Nashville, Tenn.: Nelson, 1984.
Voelckers, Ellen. *Girls Guide to Menstruation.* New York: Rosen, 1975.

Appendix II

Weeding Guide

Discard all nonfiction books on sexuality published in 1977 or earlier, with these exceptions:

Eagan, *Why Am I So Miserable. . . .* 1976.

Kelly, *Learning About Sex.* 1977.

Maddux, *Menstruation.* 1975.

Rice and Rice, *When Can I Say, "I Love You"?* 1977.

Stafford, *A Love Story.* 1977.

Voelckers, *Girls Guide to Menstruation.* 1975.

Remove the editions cited of the following books:

Nonfiction

Aseltine, Gwen Pamenter. *Honest Answers About Dating and Sex.* Old Tappan, N.J.: Revell, 1982.

Burgess-Kohn, Jane. *Straight Talk About Love and Sex for Teenagers.* Boston: Beacon, 1979.

Carlson, Dale. *Loving Sex for Both Sexes.* New York: Watts, 1979.

Coleman, William L. *The Great Date Wait and Other Hazards.* Minneapolis: Bethany, 1982.

Cooper, Darien B. *How to Be Happy Though Young.* Old Tappan, N.J.: Revell, 1979.

Dobson, James. *Preparing for Adolescence.* Ventura, Calif.: Vision House, 1978.

Gale, Jay. *A Young Man's Guide to Sex.* New York: Holt, 1984.

Gordon, Sol. *Facts About VD for Today's Youth,* new ed. Fayetteville, N.Y.: Ed-U, 1979.

———. *The Teenage Survival Book.* New York: Times, 1981.

———. *You Would if You Loved Me.* New York: Bantam, 1978.

Hartley, Fred. *Update.* Old Tappan, N.J.: Revell, 1977, 1982.

Johnson, Eric W. *VD*, rev. ed. Philadelphia: Lippincott, 1978.

Kaplan, Helen Singer. *Making Sense of Sex.* New York: Simon and Schuster, 1979.

Landau, Elaine. *The Teen Guide to Dating.* New York: Messner, 1980.

Langone, John. *Like, Love, Lust.* Boston: Little, Brown, 1980.

Mayle, Peter, and Arthur Robins. *Congratulations! You're Not Pregnant.* New York: Macmillan, 1981.

Tippit, Sammy, as told to Jerry Jenkins. *You Me He.* Wheaton, Ill.: Victor, 1978.

Westheimer, Ruth, and Nathan Kravetz. *First Love: A Young People's Guide to Sexual Information.* New York: Warner, 1985 (white cover, ISBN 0-446-34092-8).

White, Joe. *Looking for Love in All the Wrong Places.* Wheaton, Ill.: Tyndale, 1982.

Wood, Barry. *Questions Teenagers Ask About Dating and Sex.* Old Tappan, N.J.: Revell, 1981.

Fiction

Benton, John. *Carmen.* Old Tappan, N.J.: Revell, 1970 (and all others in the "New Hope Books" series).

Eyerly, Jeannette. *Bonnie Jo, Go Home.* Philadelphia: Lippincott, 1972.

Head, Ann. *Mr. and Mrs. Bo Jo Jones.* New York: Putnam, 1967: New York: New American Library, 1973.

Johnson, Lissa Halls. *Just Like Ice Cream.* Palm Springs, Calif.: Haynes, 1982.

Zindel, Paul. *My Darling, My Hamburger.* New York: Harper and Row, 1969; New York: Bantam, 1978.

Appendix III

Library Bill of Rights

The American Library Association affirms that all libraries are forums for information and ideas, and that the following basic policies should guide their services.

1. Books and other library resources should be provided for the interest, information, and enlightenment of all people of the community the library serves. Materials should not be excluded because of the origin, background, or views of those contributing to their creation.
2. Libraries should provide materials and information presenting all points of view on current and historical issues. Materials should not be proscribed or removed because of partisan or doctrinal disapproval.
3. Libraries should challenge censorship in the fulfillment of their responsibility to provide information and enlightenment.
4. Libraries should cooperate with all persons and groups concerned with resisting abridgment of free expression and free access to ideas.
5. A person's right to use a library should not be denied or abridged because of origin, age, background, or views.
6. Libraries which make exhibit spaces and meeting rooms available to the public they serve should make such facilities available on an equitable basis, regardless of the beliefs or affiliations of individuals or groups requesting their use.

Adopted June 18, 1948. Amended February 2, 1961, June 27, 1967, and January 23, 1980, by the ALA Council.

Index